PATTERNS & PRACTICE
in Chinese Medicine

PATTERNS & PRACTICE

in Chinese Medicine

Zhao Jingyi & Li Xuemei

EASTLAND PRESS ❖ SEATTLE

Published by Eastland Press, Inc.
P.O. Box 99749
Seattle, WA 98139, USA
www.eastlandpress.com

Library of Congress Catalog Card Number: 92-85309
ISBN: 978-0-939616-75-6

2   4   6   8   10   9   7   5

Book design by Gary Niemeier

Contents

Acknowledgements

We would like to thank and express our appreciation for all the help we received from our teachers, professors, and colleagues at the Beijing College of Chinese Medicine, the National Academy of Chinese Medicine, Dongzhimen Hospital, Guanganmen Hospital, and our friends both in China and abroad.

We are greatly indebted to Charles Gannon, who gave a great deal of his time and energy in editing the English language version in a most thorough manner. Especially in view of the time devoted to explaining Chinese medical terminology, we are particulary aware of the importance of his work.

We are also grateful to Dr. Josephine Freeney, who did so much work for us on the companion volume, *Acupuncture Patterns & Practice,* and who continued to provide great support to us in the writing of this book.

We greatly appreciate the expert advice and excellent editing of Dr. Dan Bensky and John O'Connor at Eastland Press, who worked hard to bring this book to press.

Finally, we would like to acknowledge the support of our friends Dr. Primoz Rozman of Slovenia; Dr. Max Hilfiker-Wissmann, Dr. Charlotte Wissmann Hilfiker, and Dr. Marian Caflisch of Switzerland; Dr. Eleonora Lalli of Canada; Marianne Rasmussen of Denmark; and Melanie King of the United States.

Preface

This book follows the same principle as its companion, *Acupuncture Patterns & Practice*, in outlining a method for applying the basic theories of Chinese medicine in clinical practice to readers who already have a certain amount of basic theory and training in Chinese medicine and acupuncture. In order to improve diagnostic and treatment skills, and to facilitate the transition from the classroom to the clinic, the same format has been retained as in the first volume.

There are, however, two major changes in this book. First, the explanations of the treatment principles have been extended. Not only must practitioners know the details of the treatment methods in each case, they must also understand why a particular treatment should be applied. Practitioners will benefit from this knowledge when tackling more complicated cases in the future.

Second, many cases have been chosen in which Chinese herbs and other materia medica, or a combination of acupuncture and herbs, were prescribed. Acupuncture is but one of the treatment modalities used in Chinese medicine, and treatment with herbs is of equal importance. However, the theory underlying the use of each modality is considerably different. Often, the classical formulas on which the herbal prescriptions are based were modified to some extent to fit the particular circumstances of the case. We have therefore explained not only the basic theory for the use of a particular herbal remedy, but each of the modifications as well. Furthermore, because there are no fixed principles governing the combined use of acupuncture and herbal therapy, it is hoped that the student can learn various approaches through the practical case studies described in this volume.

Asthma

CASE 1: **Male, age 44**

Main complaint

Wheezing and cough

History

In the past after a bad cold this patient would regularly develop a cough without any wheezing. The recovery would be rapid, and did not require medication. Twelve years ago the coughing began to last longer, often up to a month or two, and was accompanied by wheezing, a stifling sensation in the chest and copious sputum. The symptoms gradually worsened, and wheezing became the main problem. A change in the weather would bring on an attack, especially during winter. When the symptoms became very severe the patient resorted to a sitting position in order to breathe more easily (orthopnea); at night, he was unable to lie flat. During such attacks he used conventional medication, including aminophylline and ephedrine. At the beginning this gave some relief, but later had little effect.

The present attack occurred during winter. The patient has wheezing, a stifling sensation in the chest, shortness of breath, and a copious amount of white, sticky sputum which is easy to expectorate. During these recent two nights, the patient has slept very little as he finds it difficult to lie flat. He is therefore suffering from fatigue, lacks energy, and has no appetite. Urine and bowel movements are normal, and his complexion is pale.

Tongue

Pale, with a white, moist coating

Pulse

Slippery

Analysis of symptoms

1. History of recurrent cough—injury to Lung qi.
2. Attack associated with change in weather or during winter—
   dysfunction or weakness of protective qi.
3. Wheezing, coughing, and stifling sensation in the chest—stagnation of Lung qi.
4. Copious, sticky sputum—retention of phlegm.
5. Fatigue, lack of energy, and poor appetite—qi deficiency.
6. Pale face, pale tongue with white coating—qi deficiency and cold.
7. Slippery pulse—retention of phlegm.

Basic theory of case

Cough and wheezing are both common symptoms of Lung disorders. In the clinic they often occur together, and there is a similarity in their pathological mechanisms. (The reader is referred to the chapter on cough in our companion volume *Acupuncture Patterns & Practice*.) In the cases presented here the main complaint is wheezing; there may also be mild or severe cough, but it is certainly not the main complaint.

Physiologically, the Lung has the functions of dispersing and descending, which means that the qi of this Organ moves upward and downward, in two different directions. The movement of Lung qi in turn controls the movement of qi throughout the entire body *(Fig. 1-1)*.

The Lung's dispersing function encompasses the following three aspects:

- transporting the food essence, which is produced by the Spleen, to the upper burner, and from there to the whole body
- spreading the protective qi to the body surface
- exhaling and removing the turbid or waste qi from the body.

The Lung's descending function likewise has three aspects:

- inhaling the clear qi from the environment into the Lung
- transporting the clear qi to the Organs
- causing the fluids from the upper burner to descend to other parts of the body, especially to the lower burner.

Fig. 1-1

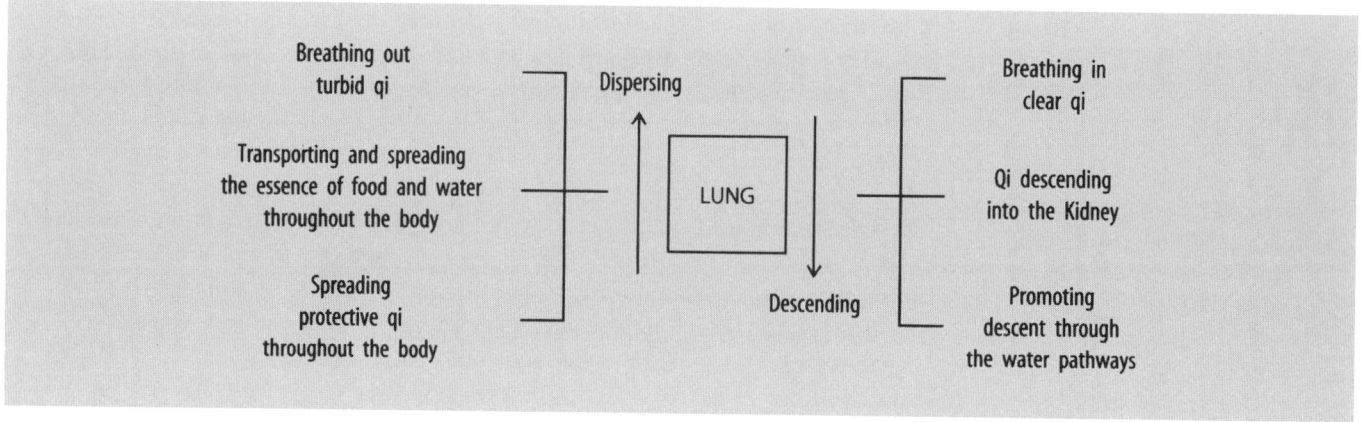

Cause of disease

Phlegm

In this case there are symptoms of wheezing, a stifling sensation in the chest, and copious, sticky sputum. All of these symptoms suggest retention of phlegm in the chest. The cause of disease is therefore phlegm.

Site of disease

Lung

The long history of wheezing and cough, stifling sensation in the chest, and copious sputum are evidence of a Lung disorder.

Pathological change

Dispersing and descending of Lung qi is a synchronized, harmonious function. If there is a dysfunction in either aspect, the movement of Lung qi will become disharmonious and give rise to various symptoms.

The long-term illness and the recurrent cough has weakened the functioning of the Lung, that is, its dispersing and descending aspects. This has caused the reversal or rebellion of Lung qi—manifested as wheezing—which can further aggravate the injury to the Lung qi and lead to a worsening of the symptoms.

Protective qi wards off pathogenic factors and protects the surface of the body.

When the dispersal of Lung qi is impaired, the protective qi cannot be transported to the skin. The patient then becomes vulnerable to attack by pathogenic factors, and has little tolerance to changes in the weather or to wintry conditions.

The stifling sensation in the chest, wheezing, and inability to lie flat are caused by the stagnation of qi in the chest and retention of phlegm. The stagnant qi affects water metabolism, such that the transportation of fluids in the upper burner is impaired. Fluids accumulate in the upper burner and become phlegm. The retention of phlegm also affects the qi function in the chest and causes it to stagnate.

The control of qi by the Lung also means that the Lung regulates the production and activity of qi throughout the body. In this case, the already weakened state of the Lung qi has diminished the body's qi in general, and this deficiency of qi has led to fatigue and lack of energy. The moist tongue coating and slippery pulse are signs of retention of phlegm.

Fig. 1-2

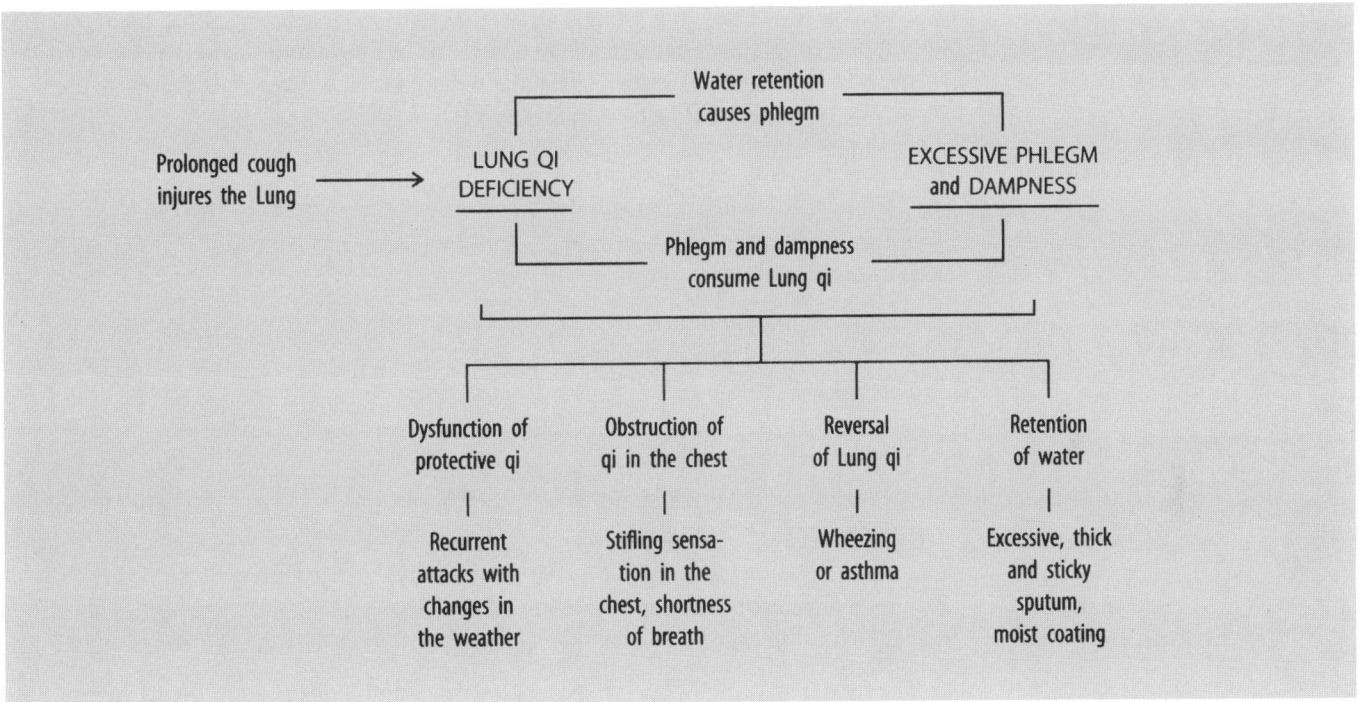

| Pattern of disease | The pattern in this case is of the interior, because the site of disease is in the Lung and there are no exterior symptoms at all (e.g., no aversion to cold). |

The pattern in this case is of the interior, because the site of disease is in the Lung and there are no exterior symptoms at all (e.g., no aversion to cold).

There is no fever, the sputum is white, the tongue is pale, and the coating is white and moist. This is therefore a cold pattern.

Because the patient has suffered from this Lung disorder for a long period of time, the Lung qi is weakened. Yet there is also retention of phlegm. Thus the pattern is one of both deficiency and excess.

Additional notes

1. Is there Spleen qi deficiency in this case?

In Chinese medicine the Lung controls the qi, and the Spleen is the source of qi and blood production. According to five-phase theory, the Spleen and Lung have a mother-child relationship, and Lung deficiency causes Spleen qi deficiency. It would therefore be natural for the practitioner to raise the question of Spleen dysfunction with respect to this patient's lack of appetite and general qi deficiency. Does this include Spleen qi deficiency? In terms of Spleen symptoms, there is only his poor appetite; his bowel movements are normal and there are otherwise no Spleen-related symptoms. At this time the diagnosis is therefore mainly Lung qi deficiency.

2. What causes the pale complexion and pale tongue?

The normal complexion and tongue are both slightly red. Very often, pallor indicates poor circulation of qi and blood resulting from cold or malnourishment related to blood deficiency. Because there is no evidence here of blood deficiency or severe cold, the main problem is that qi deficiency causes poor circulation in the body, leading to a pale complexion and a pale tongue. This pathological change is different from a simple pattern of blood deficiency or cold.

3. What is the relationship between the patterns of excess and deficiency in this case?

The weakness of Lung and general qi here pertains to deficiency, while the retention of phlegm pertains to excess. The wheezing, stifling sensation in the chest and inability to lie flat are all associated with phlegm; the main pattern is therefore one of excess, while deficiency is secondary.

Conclusion

1. According to the eight principles:
   Interior, cold, both excess and deficiency (deficiency within excess)

2. According to etiology:
   Retention of phlegm

3. According to Organ theory:
   Retention of phlegm in the Lung,
   Lung qi deficiency

Treatment principle

1. Disseminate the Lung qi.

2. Remove the phlegm and calm the wheezing.

3. Tonify the qi.

Explanation of treatment principle

The main difference between the treatment principle (*zhì zé*) and treatment method (*zhì fǎ*) is as follows:

- The treatment principle is the foundation or essential direction of the treatment, and is determined in accordance with the diagnosis. It serves as a guide for selecting among various methods.
- The treatment method includes such elements as the selection of acupuncture points or herbal formula, and the manner of needle manipulation (reinforcing or reducing).

Determination of the treatment principle in the clinic is thus very important, as it provides a basis for assuring the accuracy and underlying purpose of a particular treatment.

This patient suffers from Lung qi stagnation and Lung qi deficiency, as well as retention of phlegm, which is characteristic of excess. It is important to remove the phlegm and disseminate the Lung qi in order to calm the wheezing; the qi cannot circulate well if the stagnation is not relieved.

With this patient it is necessary to find a balance between reducing and tonifying. Since the patient's qi was previously deficient, a strong reducing method will weaken the Lung qi. The best solution is to use a combination of tonifying and reducing, as long as the tonifying method is not so strong that it impedes the removal of the pathogenic factor.

Selection of points

Prescription one:	Prescription two:
GV-14 *(da zhui)*	PC-6 *(nei guan)*
CV-22 *(tian tu)*	CV-12 *(zhong wan)*
ding chuan (M-BW-1)	S-40 *(feng long)*
	CV-22 *(tian tu)*
	BL-13 *(fei shu)*

Explanation of points

GV-14 *(da zhui)*. *Dà* means big and *zhuī* means vertebra. The location of this point is below the posterior process of the seventh cervical vertebra, which is big and obvious. In addition to expelling pathogenic factors, this point serves an important function in strengthening the yang in the channels and regulating the qi. The tonifying method is utilized at this point in order to draw upon the yang qi in the governing vessel to tonify the antipathogenic factors in the body. This point can also help clear and calm the spirit, as the patient has been feeling very groggy for lack of sleep.

CV-22 *(tian tu)*. *Tiān* generally means heaven, but here it means high up; *tū* means projecting, or, in this context, pronounced. This point is located in the depression immediately above the sternum (suprasternal notch), which is like the opening of a chimney. In Chinese medicine it is regarded as the passageway of the Lung qi.

In the treatment of wheezing this is an important point that can be directly used for removing stagnant qi. The qi obstruction in this case is very severe because the Lung qi is blocked by phlegm. This point has a local function and also serves to promote the dispersion and regulation of Lung qi. The reducing method should be used at this point.

ding chuan (M-BW-1) is an extra or miscellaneous point that is located 0.5 unit lateral to the process of the seventh cervical vertebra. *Dìng* in Chinese means settle and *chuǎn* means wheezing; the name is thus derived from the function of the point. This is an empirical point that is very effective in calming wheezing.

There are only three points in the first prescription, all of which are located very close to the neck. The purpose of this prescription is to regulate the qi and remove the obstruction from the upper part of the Lung. This is a typical example of promoting the dispersing function of the Lung. The needling technique for this prescription is a combination of reinforcing at GV-14 *(da zhui)*, and reducing at CV-22 *(tian tu)* and *ding chuan* (M-BW-1).

PC-6 *(nei guan)* is the connecting point of the Pericardium channel. The meaning of *nèi* is internal or medial, and *guān* means pass. The point is found behind the *guān mài* or middle pulse position. It can be used for regulating the qi in the upper burner to relieve the stifling sensation in the chest. It also serves to calm the spirit and thereby remove stress, and assists S-40 *(feng long)* in removing phlegm.

S-40 *(feng long)*. *Fēng* means big and *lóng* means abundant. This name is derived from the abundance of muscles at the site of this point. This is the connecting point of the Stomach channel. It is important for removing phlegm and dampness. Here the retention of phlegm, which causes stagnation of qi, is the major problem. The patient has copious white phlegm, which he finds easy to bring up. S-40 *(feng long)* is a good point for this condition.

CV-12 *(zhong wan)* is the alarm point of the Stomach. *Zhōng* means middle and *wǎn*, which can mean empty vessel, here signifies the inside of the Stomach. This point tonifies and regulates the qi of the middle burner. It also strengthens the water metabolism functions of the Spleen and Stomach, and promotes the function of the middle burner in transporting the turbid yin of the body downward. The middle burner is where phlegm is produced; hence, regulating the middle burner and removing dampness is intended to resolve the root of the phlegm problem and help the function of Lung qi.

BL-13 *(fei shu)*. *Fèi* means Lung and *shū* means point. This refers to the Lung qi which accumulates on the back. This point is mainly used to treat Lung disorders, hence its name. As the associated point of the Lung on the back it serves to tonify and regulate the Lung qi and calm the wheezing. It is the only point on the back in the second prescription. In this prescription it is punctured first, and then withdrawn. The patient is then asked to lie on his back, and the other four points are punctured.

Combination of points

GV-14 *(da zhui)* and CV-22 *(tian tu)* are both very close to the neck. CV-22 *(tian tu)* is on the front, GV-14 *(da zhui)* on the back; one is on the conception vessel, the other on the governing vessel. These points form a combination of yin and yang, and, in terms of needling technique, of reinforcing and reducing. The purpose of this combination is to fortify the yang qi of the body, promote the dissemination of the Lung qi, and calm the wheezing.

The combination of PC-6 *(nei guan)*, CV-12 *(zhong wan)*, and S-40 *(feng long)* regulates the qi in the upper and middle burners. These three points as a group help regulate the qi, adjust the middle burner, and remove the phlegm. PC-6 *(nei guan)* is a connecting point on the arm; S-40 *(feng long)* a connecting point on the leg. CV-12 *(zhong wan)* is located in the middle burner, and is an alarm point of the Stomach. Hence the combination is composed of two connecting points, which are used to regulate the qi, and one alarm point, which is used to remove the obstruction. S-40 *(feng long)* is a special point for removing phlegm. This is a typical combination that can be used for removing phlegm by regulating qi.

GV-14 *(da zhui)* and *ding chuan* (M-BW-1) are two points, but utilize three needles (M-BW-1 is punctured bilaterally). These points are separated by only 0.5 unit. While it may appear illogical to select points so close to each other, in fact different needling methods are used at the two points: GV-14 *(da zhui)* is reinforced and *ding chuan* (M-BW-1) is reduced. This combination is used to calm the wheezing.

Which prescription should be used?

Prescription one strives to remove the stagnation of qi in the Lung, especially by promoting the dispersing function of the Lung. When the patient has very severe wheezing and a stifling sensation in the chest, prescription one is the best. When the wheezing begins to improve and the removal of phlegm becomes more important, prescription two is used.

Follow-up

During the first week the patient was treated once every day. Prescription one was used for the first two days. The symptoms then improved: the patient was able to lie flat, and he stopped taking conventional medication. Prescription two was then utilized for another two days. After the fourth visit there was a substantial reduction in phlegm. As there was less phlegm but still significant wheezing during the fifth and sixth visits, the first prescription was again used. An obvious improvement in most of the symptoms ensued.

In the second week treatment was given every other day for another two weeks. After this period the wheezing disappeared and treatment was stopped. The patient remained well for the following six months and only occasionally suffered some shortness of breath and a stifling sensation after catching a cold. He was treated, and the symptoms completely disappeared. The patient was advised to begin exercising outdoors as soon as the weather became warm, and to continue exercising during the winter and thereafter.

The patient was followed for three more years. During this time he had only a few colds. When these occurred he was given further treatment and only experienced slight wheezing or shortness of breath.

There is no fixed principle for terminating conventional medication once treatment with Chinese medicine begins. In this case conventional medications were stopped early in the treatment for two reasons. First, after two days the results of treatment were very good and the wheezing was already markedly relieved. Second, this particular patient had been taking conventional medications for twelve years before the wheezing began. At first the medications brought good results, but later they did not. The patient himself had stopped taking his medications several times during this period. Thus, because this was not the first time medication had been terminated, we were more confident about this decision.

CASE 2: **Male, age 34**

Main complaint

Asthma

History

The asthma began four years ago after the patient had used pesticide at a farm. An asthmatic attack could be brought on by simply smelling a similar chemical from an empty pesticide bottle, or out in a field. He complained that from then on he suffered three or four asthma attacks a year. Recently, during the present year, the symptoms worsened: catching a cold can now bring on an attack. During a severe attack he resorts to taking anti-asthmatic and cortisone tablets. When he came to the clinic his asthmatic attack had lasted for ten hours. He presented with a severe stifling sensation in the chest, rapid, strong, heavy and loud breathing, orthopnea, and gurgling in the throat. The patient can barely speak and sweats excessively. Between attacks he is intolerant of wind and cold, and is afraid to take off his clothes. He usually suffers from shortness of breath, but sleeps well, and his appetite, bowel movements, and urine are all normal. His lips are purple in color.

Tongue

Dark purple with a white coating

Pulse

Slippery, rapid, and forceless

Analysis of symptoms

1. History of recurrent asthma attacks—
   retention of the pathogenic factor in the body injuring the Lung qi.
2. Stifling sensation in the chest, asthma, and strong, heavy breathing—
   stagnation of Lung qi.
3. Gurgling in the throat—obstruction of the airway by phlegm.
4. Excessive sweating and intolerance of wind and cold—
   lowered resistance on the surface of the body.
5. Purple lips and tongue—poor circulation of blood.
6. Slippery pulse—retention of phlegm.

Basic theory of case

In Chinese medicine the word for the disease known as asthma is *xiāo chuǎn*. These are words for two traditional symptoms that involve a problem in breathing. When the problem is severe, the patient is unable to lie flat on their back (known as orthopnea), and must move their chest and shoulders, as well as open their mouth, to relieve the difficulty in breathing.

The symptoms referred to by *xiāo* and *chuǎn* have certain different characteristics. We translate *chuǎn* as wheezing (others translate it as panting or dyspnea). This term includes various types of difficulty in breathing that often results from colds or influenza without any allergic factor. It can also refer to the wheezing or panting that accompanies physical overexertion. It is not a problem that is necessarily associated with regular attacks (*Fig. 1-3a*).

We translate the traditional term *xiāo* as asthma. It is characterized by an attack of dyspnea with gurgling (literally "with a phlegm-like sound in the throat"). Most patients with asthma have a definite history of some type of allergy with regular

Fig. 1-3a

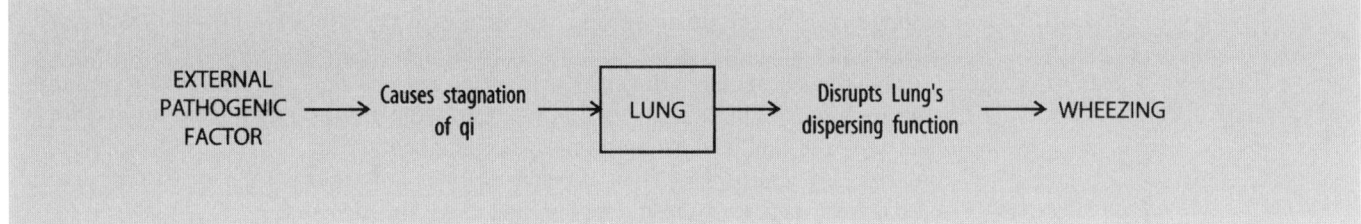

attacks. The disorder usually begins in childhood, and the asthma is often caused by the same precipitating factors.

A characteristic of asthma in Chinese medicine is retention of phlegm deep in the Lung. This is called dormant phlegm *(sù tán)*. Because dormant phlegm remains deep in a fixed location, the patient usually does not show any obvious symptoms. It can, however, become activated by a variety of pathogenic factors including the six exogenous pathogenic factors, improper foods, certain kinds of smells from food, animals, chemicals, or a strong emotional episode. It then moves into the airway, causing sudden and severe dyspnea. The obstruction of the airway and breathing difficulty caused by the movement of phlegm leads to gurgling in the throat. When the pathogenic factor eases, the obstruction of the airway caused by retention of phlegm gradually diminishes or disappears, and the symptoms are relieved. Yet because the dormant phlegm has not been completely removed, it may

Fig. 1-3b   cause recurrent attacks and thus a prolonged history of the disease *(Fig. 1-3b)*.

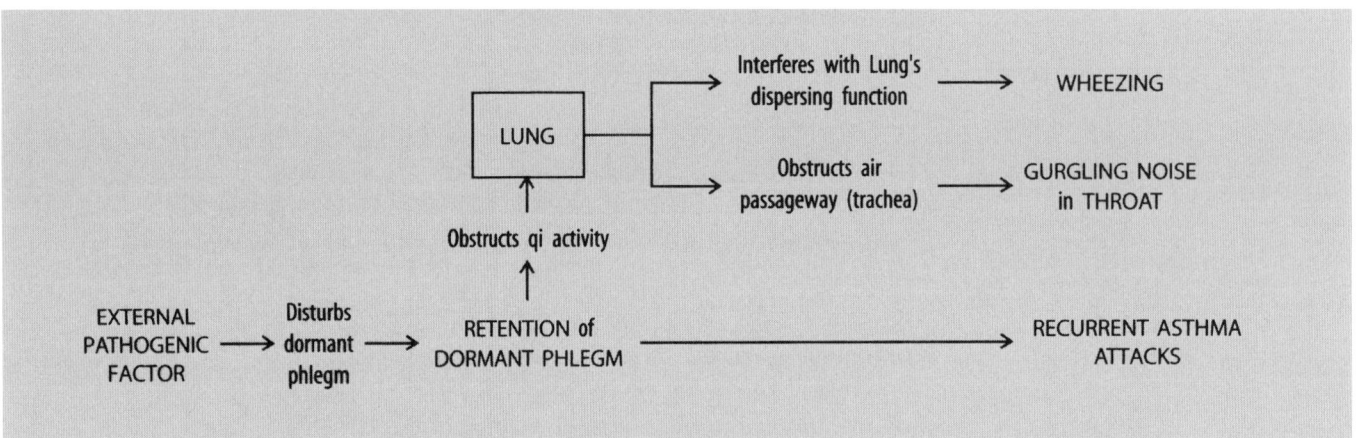

Cause of disease	Phlegm
	The patient has a stifling sensation in the chest and gurgling in the throat, indicating stagnation of Lung qi and obstruction caused by phlegm.
Site of disease	Lung
	Asthma and strong, heavy breathing are the main symptoms, suggesting a disorder of the Lung.
Pathological change	There is asthma in this case because of the clear precipitating factor and characteristic presentation. The recurrent asthma was caused by the retention of the phlegm deep in the Lung (dormant phlegm). In the early stages the precipitating factor was relatively simple. Later, as the Lung qi became injured, the symptoms gradually became more severe. Lung qi deficiency led to a lowering of the body's resistance in this case, such that asthma is triggered even when the patient catches

Fig. 1-4

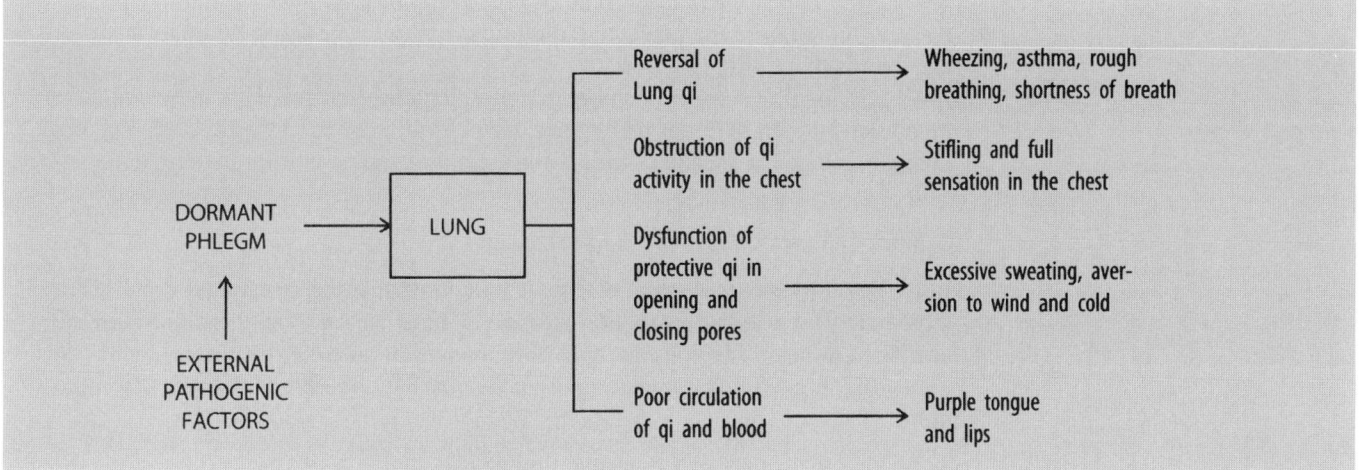

a common cold (*Fig. 1-4*).

Because the phlegm blocks the airway, leading to poor circulation of qi in the chest, the patient experiences a stifling sensation in the chest and gurgling in the throat. Meanwhile, the Lung qi that has been obstructed by the pathogenic factor loses its normal ability to disperse, which means that the pathogenic factor and the stagnation have together become too strong, causing rapid and strong, loud breathing.

Although the patient has been perspiring excessively, he has not had a fever or any other symptom associated with a heat pattern. The sweating does not, therefore, indicate heat. The stagnation of Lung qi can lead to the failure of the protective qi in spreading to the body surface, interfering with the opening and closing of the pores; the body fluids thereupon flow out through the pores, which results in sweating. Similarly, because the protective qi cannot maintain its normal function of keeping the body surface warm, the patient has become intolerant of cold. This explains why he is reluctant to remove any clothing.

In Chinese medicine the general function of circulating the qi, which is the responsibility of the Lung, also contributes to the circulation of blood. Stagnation of Lung qi leads to poor blood circulation, thus the patient has purple lips and tongue.

The white coating on the tongue indicates cold. The slippery pulse suggests the presence of phlegm, and its forceless quality indicates deficiency.

This patient usually suffers from shortness of breath, pointing to injury to the Lung qi. His appetite, sleep, bowel movements and urine are all normal, which means that there are no significant problems with his other Organs.

Pattern of disease

This patient has a long history of Lung disorder; the pattern can thus be traced to the interior.

In this case there is no evidence of heat, such as fever, thirst, or constipation. The patient has a dark complexion, and there is a white coating on the tongue, both of which suggest a cold pattern.

Fullness, the stifling sensation in the chest, and the strong, loud breathing all indicate a pattern of excess. The patient often has shortness of breath, which is caused by Lung qi deficiency. This case, therefore, represents a combination of excess and deficiency.

Additional notes

1. Is there any evidence of an exterior pattern in this case?

The patient is intolerant of cold, which in clinical practice is similar to the symptom of aversion to cold. There are two disorders associated with this feeling of being cold: one is the exterior pattern caused by an invasion of a pathogenic factor, and the other is the protective qi deficiency pattern caused by impairment of the Lung's dispersing function.

While the first scenario is more common than the second, there is no evidence of invasion by an external pathogenic factor in this case. Thus the cold problem here pertains to the second type of disorder, indicating an interior pattern, not exterior.

2. What causes the rapid pulse in this case?

In the section on pathological change it was noted that the sweating did not result from heat, because there was no evidence of heat. Neither can the rapid pulse be attributed to heat. The pulse is rapid *but forceless*, indicating that the deficiency of qi is providing too little strength to drive the circulation of blood, leading to a rapid pulse.

3. What is the source of the dormant phlegm?

Dormant phlegm in the Lung is one of the characteristic pathological changes in asthma sufferers.

The cause of dormant phlegm in Chinese medicine is rather complicated. There are, generally speaking, two major causes. One is a congenital imbalance of yin and yang, which leads to the accumulation of phlegm inside the body. The other is recurrent invasion by pathogenic factors, or chronic illness which is not thoroughly treated, resulting in first the production and then the retention of phlegm within the body.

In clinical practice it is often the case that the initial cause of dormant phlegm cannot be ascertained with certainty. And because the dormant phlegm can remain deep in the Lung, the patient may not present with excessive sputum, either during asthma attacks or in between. This is what happened in this case. While the use of a farm chemical four years earlier may have caused the patient's first asthma attack, it does not explain the existence of the dormant phlegm. Exposure to the chemical was merely the triggering event: an allergic substance which provoked the pathogenic factor in the Lung (the dormant phlegm) to cause the symptoms.

Conclusion

1. According to the eight principles:
   Interior, cold, and both excess and deficiency. Excess is the main problem.

2. According to etiology:
   Dormant phlegm

3. According to Organ theory:
   Stagnation of Lung qi with Lung qi deficiency

Treatment principle

1. Disseminate the Lung qi.

2. Calm the asthma.

Explanation of treatment principle

There are acute and chronic stages in asthma, and the governing treatment principle differentiates between them. During the acute stage, treatment aims at relieving the stifling or suffocating sensation in the chest, and in calming the wheezing. Treatment is therefore similar to that of a wheezing pattern. The principle here is to regulate the Lung's functions of dispersing and descending in order to relieve the asthma.

This particular patient has mainly suffered from stagnation of Lung qi, in other words, impairment of the Lung's dispersing function. The emphasis here is on promoting the proper functioning of the Lung.

During the second stage of the asthma pattern, acute symptoms such as wheezing and the stifling sensation in the chest have been relieved. However, the dormant pathogenic factor has not been removed, and thus treatment must be continued. The treatment principle at this stage mainly aims at augmenting the antipathogenic factor. Strengthening body resistance is essential for expelling pathogenic factors. Because the pathogenic factor in this type of case is retained deep in the body, treatment should last for three to six months in ordinary cases, and as long as one to two years in severe cases.

Selection of points

BL-12 *(feng men)*
BL-13 *(fei shu)*
BL-14 *(jue yin shu)*

Explanation of points

The name *fēng mén* means "gate of wind." This point is used to remove wind, especially pathogenic wind, from the exterior of the body, and is thus an important point for removing exterior patterns. This patient perspires and is intolerant of wind and cold, but has no exterior pattern. This indicates that the protective qi on the surface of the body is not strong enough. The patient therefore catches cold very easily, which in turn triggers the asthma. This is why BL-12 *(feng men)* is used to help strengthen the protective qi on the surface of the body.

BL-13 *(fei shu)* is used to disseminate Lung qi, calm the asthma, and regulate the qi. This is the associated point of the Lung on the back.

BL-14 *(jue yin shu)*. The words *jué yīn* means "terminal yin" and *shū* means "associated point." This point settles the Heart and calms the spirit, and is used for disorders in the chest, Heart, and diaphragm. It regulates the qi, stops the cough, and is a very good point for removing the stifling sensation in the chest. This point is the associated point on the back for the terminal yin channel. It also helps the blood system.

Needling

The threading method is used with this prescription. Two 2.5 unit needles are used: one is threaded from BL-12 *(feng men)* to BL-14 *(jue yin shu)*, passing BL-13 *(fei shu)*, while the other needle is threaded from BL-14 *(jue yin shu)* to BL-12 *(feng men)*, also passing BL-13 *(fei shu)*. It does not matter which side is threaded. Simultaneously, moxibustion is used with smokeless moxa sticks. The smokeless stick is less irritating to an asthma patient, and also produces very strong heat.

Combination of points

In this case only two points are punctured, BL-12 *(feng men)* on one side and BL-14 *(jue yin shu)* on the other, but in fact three pairs of three points are stimulated: BL-12 *(feng men)*, BL-13 *(fei shu)*, and BL-14 *(jue yin shu)*. The combination comprises associated points on the back for the Lung and terminal yin (Pericardium) channels, plus BL-12 *(feng men)*. This is an important combination for removing a pathogenic factor from the upper burner through the "gate of wind."

BL-13 *(fei shu)* is identified more with qi, while BL-14 *(jue yin shu)*, an associated point for the Pericardium channel on the back, is identified more with blood. The combination of these two points thus regulates the qi and blood. Regulating the blood helps to regulate the qi, and also helps calm the spirit and alleviate the patient's feeling of stress. The combination of these two back associated points with BL-12 *(feng men)* helps remove the external pathogenic factor from the upper burner.

Basic herbal formula

Minor Bluegreen Dragon Decoction *(xiao qing long tang)* is the name of a formula found in the classic *Discussion of Cold-induced Disorders (Shang han lun)*. This formula was originally used to treat cough and asthma caused by an invasion of pathogenic wind and cold, plus retention of congested fluids in the Lung.

The primary indications are aversion to cold, fever, absence of sweating, cough, wheezing, difficulty in lying flat, copious, watery and white sputum, a white and moist tongue coating, and a superficial pulse. The pathological change for this pattern is an invasion by pathogenic wind and cold on the surface of the body; it is thus an exterior pattern. Because the Lung qi is obstructed by external pathogenic factors, and there is accumulation of dormant phlegm in the Lung (an internal pathogenic factor), a relatively severe Lung qi disorder has been caused, which leads to a reversal or rebellion of Lung qi. This is manifested in such symptoms as severe cough and wheezing or asthma with copious sputum.

The basic formula consists of the following ingredients:

Herba Ephedrae *(ma huang)* 9g
Ramulus Cinnamomi Cassiae *(gui zhi)* 6g
Radix Paeoniae Lactiflorae *(bai shao)* 9g
Rhizoma Zingiberis Officinalis *(gan jiang)* 9g
Herba cum Radice Asari *(xi xin)* 3g
Rhizoma Pinelliae Ternatae *(ban xia)* 9g
Fructus Schisandrae Chinensis *(wu wei zi)* 3g
Radix Glycyrrhizae Uralensis *(gan cao)* 6g

Explanation of basic herbal formula

In this formula, Herba Ephedrae *(ma huang)* and Ramulus Cinnamomi Cassiae *(gui zhi)* are the chief ingredients. Both are acrid in flavor and warm in nature. They are very effective in promoting sweating, releasing exterior patterns, and expelling the external pathogenic factors of wind and cold. These two herbs can remove the obstruction to the Lung qi.

Herba cum Radice Asari *(xi xin)* and Rhizoma Zingiberis Officinalis *(gan jiang)* are deputy herbs; the former is acrid and warm, the latter acrid and hot. Both are associated with the Lung and are ideal for warming it and removing pathogenic cold. They also serve to warm and resolve cold phlegm and congested fluids in the Lung.

There are three assistant herbs: Rhizoma Pinelliae Ternatae *(ban xia)*, Fructus Schisandrae Chinensis *(wu wei zi)*, and Radix Paeoniae Lactiflorae *(bai shao)*. Rhizoma Pinelliae Ternatae *(ban xia)* is warm and dry and is used to dry and resolve phlegm and dampness, helping Rhizoma Zingiberis Officinalis *(gan jiang)* and Herba cum Radice Asari *(xi xin)*. Fructus Schisandrae Chinensis *(wu wei zi)* is sour and warm and is able to restrain the Lung qi; it is used for a pattern of chronic cough or asthma caused by Lung qi deficiency, or the failure of the Kidney to grasp the qi. Radix Paeoniae Lactiflorae *(bai shao)* is sour and slightly cold and is often used for nourishing the yin and blood. Fructus Schisandrae Chinensis *(wu wei zi)* and Radix Paeoniae Lactiflorae *(bai shao)* are used to buffer the acrid, warm, and dry herbs so as to prevent injury to the Lung qi, yin, and blood.

Radix Glycyrrhizae Uralensis *(gan cao)* is an envoy herb that strengthens the Stomach and protects the antipathogenic factors, while harmonizing the dispersing and astringent characteristics of the other herbs.

Modified herbal formula

Herba Ephedrae *(ma huang)* 6g
Ramulus Cinnamomi Cassiae *(gui zhi)* 10g
Semen Pruni Armeniacae *(xing ren)* 10g
Cortex Magnoliae Officinalis *(hou po)* 8g
Radix Paeoniae Lactiflorae *(bai shao)* 10g
Rhizoma Zingiberis Officinalis *(gan jiang)* 10g
Herba cum Radice Asari *(xi xin)* 3g
Rhizoma Pinelliae Ternatae *(ban xia)* 10g
Fructus Schisandrae Chinensis *(wu wei zi)* 10g
Fructus Zizyphi Jujubae *(da zao)* . . . . 4 pieces
Radix Glycyrrhizae Uralensis *(gan cao)* 10g

Explanation of modified herbal formula

This is Minor Bluegreen Dragon Decoction *(xiao qing long tang)* with the addition of Semen Pruni Armeniacae *(xing ren)*, Cortex Magnoliae Officinalis *(hou po)*, and Fructus Zizyphi Jujubae *(da zao)*.

In this case there is no invasion of external pathogenic factors, but the stagnation of qi in the Lung and retention of phlegm are very severe. Because it is necessary to disseminate the Lung qi, Minor Bluegreen Dragon Decoction *(xiao qing long tang)* was selected as the basic formula in view of its role in promoting the dispersing function of the Lung, removing the cold pathogenic factor, warming and transforming cold-phlegm, and improving the ascending and decending functions of the Lung qi.

The prescription in this case still retains most of the characteristics of the original Minor Bluegreen Dragon Decoction *(xiao qing long tang)*, but with a few modifications. The original formula's action in promoting sweating and removing the exterior pattern is diminished, as Herba Ephedrae *(ma huang)* is reduced from 9g to 6g. Cortex Magnoliae Officinalis *(hou po)* and Semen Pruni Armeniacae *(xing ren)* have been added to assist in disseminating the Lung qi and calming the asthma. Increasing the dosage of Fructus Schisandrae Chinensis *(wu wei zi)* and adding Fructus Zizyphi Jujubae *(da zao)* helps strengthen the antipathogenic factors.

Follow-up

To relieve the acute symptoms, the patient was treated twice a day with acupuncture. After the first day's treatment the symptoms were much improved, and after three days of treatment the asthma was brought under control. The modified herbal formula was then prescribed to remove the phlegm and disseminate the Lung qi. The formula was taken for a week: one half dose taken twice daily. After the first week the formula was replaced by a prepared medicine, Two-Cured Pills *(er chen wan)*. One pill was taken twice daily for a period of three months, during which the symptoms gradually abated. The patient experienced only one, very slight attack, which lasted just a few hours. After three months, treatment was terminated and all the symptoms disappeared. The patient was advised to avoid exposure to allergic agents.

During the winter of the following year the patient twice caught cold and experienced some asthma, but the attacks were not as severe as before. He was given the same acupuncture treatment, which controlled the symptoms. During the remainder of the two year follow-up he reported no significant breathing problems.

CASE 3: **Female, age 60**

Main complaint

Wheezing and cough

History

The patient has suffered from recurrent wheezing and cough for over ten years. Three days ago, for no apparent reason, she began coughing and wheezing and experienced a stifling sensation in the chest, accompanied by shortness of breath, which was aggravated by any sort of physical exertion. She also had copious yellow and sticky sputum. She did not experience any chest pain.

The patient also complained of a hot sensation in the upper part of the body with heavy sweating, aversion to wind, poor appetite, and intolerance of cold food and drink. She had little desire to drink much water. She also had loose stools three times a day, without abdominal pain.

Tongue

Swollen, slightly dark and purple, with tooth marks on the border and a thick, yellow and white, greasy coating

Pulse

Sunken, thin, and slippery

Analysis of symptoms

1. Cough, wheezing, and stifling sensation in the chest—stagnation of Lung qi
2. Shortness of breath becoming worse with physical exertion—qi deficiency
3. Copious yellow and sticky sputum—excessive accumulation of phlegm-heat inside the Lungs
4. Hot sensation in the upper part of the body and excessive sweating—heat in the upper burner
5. Aversion to wind—protective qi fails in its external function
6. Lack of thirst, poor appetite, intolerance of cold food, and loose stools—Spleen yang deficiency
7. Purple, dark tongue—poor circulation of qi and blood
8. Thick, greasy tongue coating—phlegm
9. Swollen, tooth-marked tongue and thin, sunken pulse—yang deficiency

Basic theory of case

In traditional Chinese medicine, phlegm is of two types: visible (formed) and invisible (unformed). (For a fuller discussion of this topic, see page 42 of *Acupuncture Patterns & Practice*.) The phlegm associated with wheezing, asthma, and cough is of the visible type. It is caused by dysfunction of the Lung qi leading to a Lung disorder in controlling the water metabolism; fluids thereupon accumulate in the Lung and transform into phlegm. In addition to phlegm, there is a similar type of pathogenic factor, congested fluids *(yǐn)*, which is watery and clear in quality, and is often seen in clinical practice.

Phlegm and congested fluids are both yin pathogenic factors. They often cause symptoms associated with obstruction of yang qi and accumulation of internal dampness: a feeling of being cold, cold limbs or extremities, pale complexion, watery and clear sputum, lack of thirst or unwillingness to drink, pale tongue with white and greasy coating, and a slippery (but not rapid) pulse.

Phlegm and congested fluids may also become mixed with heat, resulting in a rather complicated pathogenic factor: phlegm-heat. The heat may derive from a variety of sources, e.g., when phlegm blocks the circulation of qi, causing qi stagnation which leads to heat from constraint *(yù rè)*; or when a patient has a yang constitution, which means that the internal heat is pre-existing.

Phlegm-heat is formed when heat, which is of a yang nature, combines with phlegm or congested fluids, which is yin and cold. The nature of the pathogenic factor changes from yin to yang, and the manifestations likewise reflect the presence of heat: generalized sensation of heat, sweating, red complexion, and yellow, sticky sputum. Some patients have difficulty expectorating. There may also be yellow urine, dry or normal stools, red tongue, yellow, thick and greasy coating on the tongue, and a slippery and rapid pulse. Patients may complain of a lack of thirst, or may feel thirsty but not want to drink much. The reason for this apparent contradiction is that there is *both* phlegm and heat (yin and yang) coexisting in the body at the same time *(Fig. 1-5)*.

Cause of disease

Phlegm-heat

The patient presents with wheezing and coughing, excessive yellow and sticky sputum, a feeling of heat in the upper part of the body, and excessive sweating. These symptoms are characteristic of phlegm in the Lung and heat from constraint. The cause of the illness is accordingly phlegm-heat.

Site of disease

Lung and Spleen

Evidence of a Lung disorder is reflected in the chronic, recurrent attacks of coughing and wheezing, which are aggravated by physical exertion.

Evidence of a Spleen disorder can be found in the poor appetite and loose stools.

Fig. 1-5

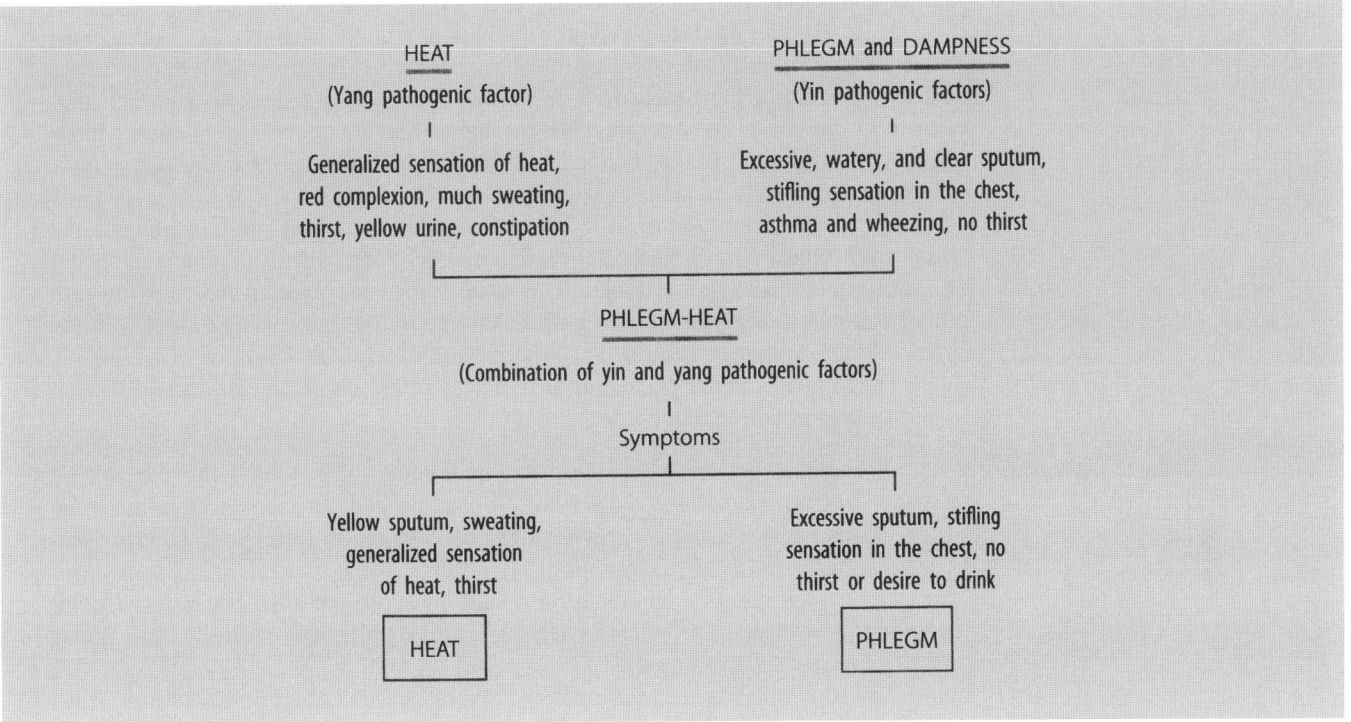

Pathological change

Fig. 1-6

The symptoms in this case can be divided into two groups. The first indicates heat in the Lung, the second, cold in the Spleen. The patient has a ten-year history of cough and wheezing, which has severely injured the Lung qi. The most recent attack, with shortness of breath, stifling sensation in the chest, and abundance of phlegm, indicates retention of phlegm (phlegm-heat in this case) and stagnation of qi in the chest. Physical exertion depletes the qi and aggravates the Lung qi deficiency; the symptoms therefore worsen upon physical exertion. The patient is intolerant of wind because the protective qi is not circulating as it should on the body surface; this leads to a failure in controlling the opening and closing of the pores, one of the functions of the protective qi.

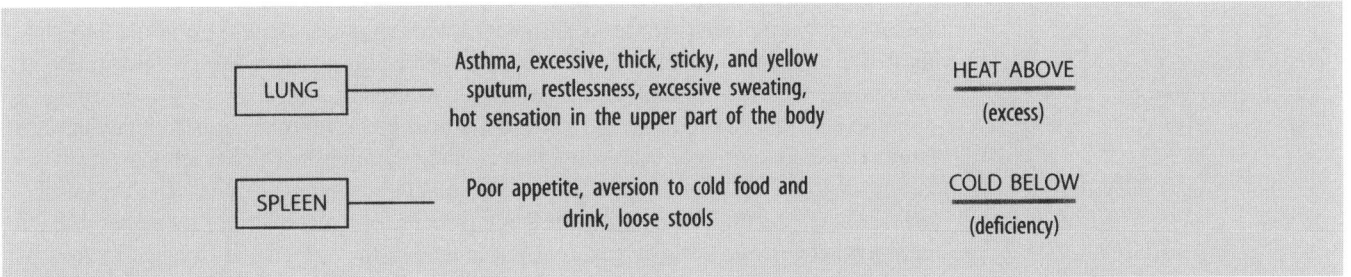

As in the previous case, this patient exhibits excessive sweating, but the difference here is that the sweating is accompanied by a sensation of heat in the upper part of the body. This indicates a different pathological mechanism: retention of phlegm-heat in the Lung. Excessive heat in the upper burner pushes the body fluids outward, which explains why the patient sweats and feels hot in the upper part of the body.

There is also internal cold from Spleen deficiency here. The impaired ability of the Spleen to transform and transport food means that food cannot be digested properly, which results in a poor appetite. The long history of deficiency has injured the yang, and yang deficiency causes internal cold, which can be aggravated by eating cold food; this explains the patient's intolerance of cold food. Spleen deficiency can lead to the failure of food essence to ascend. Instead, it drains downward to the Large Intestine where, combined with water and dampness (which arises from the failure of water metabolism due to Spleen deficiency), it causes loose stools. This patient is not inclined to drink, which indicates that the body fluids have not been injured.

The swollen, tooth-marked tongue is characteristic of retention of phlegm and dampness caused by Spleen yang deficiency. Its dark, purplish color is a sign of poor circulation of qi and blood. The thick and greasy coating indicates phlegm and dampness. The presence of both heat and cold in this case is reflected in the color of the tongue coating, which is a mixture of white and yellow.

The slippery nature of the pulse indicates retention of phlegm, while its thin and sunken qualities suggest deficiency.

Pattern of disease

In this case the disorder, which has lasted over ten years, is in the Lung and Spleen. Although the patient complains of a hot sensation with an aversion to wind, these conditions are not caused by an invasion of exogenous pathogenic factors. This pattern, therefore, is of the interior.

The case presents a combination of hot and cold patterns, because there are symptoms of heat (hot feeling, sweating, yellow phlegm) as well as cold (loose stools, aversion to cold food).

Retention of phlegm is a symptom of excess, but insufficiency of an antipathogenic factor is a sign of deficiency. This case, therefore, involves patterns of both excess and deficiency.

Additional notes

1. How should we characterize the Lung disorder in this case, as deficiency or excess?

The Lung disorder here involves both deficiency and excess, with retention of phlegm-heat in the Lung (excess) and injury to the Lung following the long history of the disease (deficiency). Initially, however, the stifling sensation in the chest and the wheezing caused by retention of phlegm-heat is the main complaint, thus the diagnosis of Lung deficiency is not considered. The present diagnosis for the Lung is one of excess.

2. Is there any relationship between the disorders of the Lung and Spleen?

In this case the Spleen disorder is associated with yang deficiency; Lung disorders involve qi deficiency and retention of a pathogenic factor. Discussion of this question should therefore consider each of these two aspects.

With regard to deficiency, in Chinese medical theory chronic qi deficiency can eventually lead to injury of the yang, that is, yang deficiency. The Spleen yang deficiency in this case was caused by a chronic illness which preceded the present attack of wheezing. The Lung qi deficiency here also resulted from chronic and recurrent wheezing. According to five-phase theory, the Spleen and Lung influence each other in a mother and child relationship, that is, a Spleen disorder can disrupt the function of the Lung and vice versa.

With regard to excess, retention of phlegm-heat in the Lung is the primary cause of the present wheezing attack. This pathological change is independent; it has no relationship to the Spleen yang deficiency.

3. Is there blood stasis in this case?

Purple lips and a dark tongue are characteristic of a severe attack of wheezing or asthma. These symptoms were found in both this and the previous case. In pathological terms, this is because qi stagnation leads to poor circulation of blood. The poor circulation here is not limited to any particular part of the body, hence the absence of localized, sharp pain. And because this generalized stagnation of blood is a result of long-term qi stagnation, and is not severe, a diagnosis of blood stasis would be inappropriate.

Conclusion

1. According to the eight principles:
   Interior, both heat and cold (heat above, cold below),
   both excess and deficiency.

2. According to etiology:
   Retention of phlegm-heat.

3. According to Organ theory:
   Retention of phlegm-heat in the Lung,
   Spleen yang deficiency.

Treatment principle

1. Clear the heat and remove the phlegm.

2. Disseminate the Lung qi and calm the wheezing.

3. Concurrently tonify the qi.

Explanation of treatment principle

This case is a difficult one to treat because heat and cold are both present. Clearing heat may consume the body's yang, while tonifying yang may strengthen the pathogenic heat. When this dilemma occurs, the basic principle is to avoid using a strong treatment method of tonifying yang or clearing heat; instead, try using a gentle and neutral method in order to regulate the balance of yin and yang. Strengthening the qi can be useful in these circumstances.

In this case, because the cold and heat are located in different parts of the body, treatment should focus on those channels and herbs that are associated with the affected Organs to avoid unecessary complications. Extremes of hot and cold should be avoided. Strengthening the qi serves to support the function of the Spleen, and can also assist in the removal of phlegm-heat from the Lung. After the phlegm-heat has been removed, the yang can then be tonified.

Selection of points

ding chuan (M-BW-1)
S-40 *(feng long)*
LU-5 *(chi ze)*
SP-3 *(tai bai)*

Explanation of points

ding chuan (M-BW-1) is an effective and commonly-used point in clinical practice. It is used to calm wheezing because it disseminates the Lung qi. The reducing method is used in this case, the purpose being to disperse the pathogenic heat and remove the obstruction and stagnation of qi in order to regulate the Lung qi and calm the wheezing.

S-40 *(feng long)* is the connecting point of the Stomach and is therefore associated with both the Spleen and Stomach channels. It removes phlegm and calms wheezing. It also calms the spirit and regulates the function of the Intestines. This point is useful in promoting the qi function of descending. It helps drain the phlegm, following the tendency of the turbid yin (phlegm in this case) to drain from the body. The reducing method is also used at this point.

LU-5 *(chi ze)*. A *chǐ* is a Chinese unit of measurement, three of which constitute one meter. According to *Records of the State (Ling shu gu du)*, the distance from the wrist to the elbow is one *chǐ*. As this point is located in the area of the elbow, the word *chǐ* is used in its name. *Zé* means moisture. According to the theory of the five transporting points, this is a sea point of the Lung channel, which is associated with water, hence the use of this word in its name. This point clears heat from the Lung, promotes the descending of Lung qi, and harmonizes the Stomach and

Intestines. It also removes heat through the blood and helps relieve toxicity. The reducing method is used. As the needle is withdrawn, it should be rotated in order to enlarge the punctured point. The needle is then fully withdrawn, a three-edged needle is inserted, and the bleeding method is used to extract about one milliliter of blood. The purpose of this is to remove the strong heat from the Lung.

SP-3 *(tai bai). Tài bái* literally means "very white," and refers to the Chinese name for the planet Venus. This point is located on the medial aspect of the big toe, at the juncture of the pale skin of the sole and the darker skin of the upper part of the foot. As this area of pale skin is very large, the word "very" is used in the name. This is also a stream point associated with earth, which promotes metal *(jin)*. It is the source point of the Spleen channel, which tonifies the Spleen and harmonizes the middle burner. It can also regulate the qi, remove dampness, and improve digestion. In this instance, an even movement is used in manipulating the needle at this point; although phlegm-heat has accumulated in the Lung, the patient presents with some Spleen yang deficiency, for which a strong reinforcing method would be inappropriate. An even movement is used first to regulate the qi, and when the wheezing improves, gentle reinforcing can be used in order to tonify the Spleen yang. Moxibustion is inappropriate at this stage because it may increase the heat in the upper burner.

Combination of points:

ding chuan (M-BW-1) and S-40 *(feng long)* function to disperse and cause to descend. The point *ding chuan* (M-BW-1) disseminates the Lung qi; S-40 *(feng long)* promotes the descending function of the Lung qi. Both points calm wheezing and are therefore helpful in regulating qi activity to remove the phlegm. The reducing method is used at both points, the purpose being to remove the qi obstruction.

S-40 *(feng long)* and LU-5 *(chi ze)* combine to draw on the qi from the greater yin channels. LU-5 *(chi ze)* is an arm greater yin channel point, while S-40 *(feng long)* is the connecting point on the leg yang brightness channel with the leg greater yin channel. These points thus help both the related yin Organs (Lung and Spleen) which are the site of the disease in this patient. In addition, S-40 *(feng long)* and LU-5 *(chi ze)* regulate the function of the Intestines and Stomach; they help the digestive system and reduce heat.

Basic herbal formulas

Two classic formulas were the basis for the prescription in this case: Ephedra, Apricot Kernal, Gypsum, and Licorice Decoction *(ma xing shi gan tang)* and Two-Cured Decoction *(er chen tang)*.

First formula

Ephedra, Apricot Kernel, Gypsum, and Licorice Decoction *(ma xing shi gan tang)* was first described in the Han dynasty medical book *Discussion of Cold-induced Disorders (Shang han lun)*, and contains the following ingredients:

Herba Ephedrae *(ma huang)* 5g
Semen Pruni Armeniacae *(xing ren)* 9g
Radix Glycyrrhizae Uralensis *(gan cao)* 6g
Gypsum *(shi gao)* 18g

This formula has an acrid, cool nature that is suitable for promoting the Lung's functions of dispersing and descending. It clears heat from the Lungs and calms wheezing. The formula was originally used to treat a disorder of the greater yang caused by an invasion of wind and cold. Upon invading the body, these pathogenic factors were transformed into a heat pattern after the sweating method had failed to remove the exterior pattern. The symptoms of this disorder are sweating, wheezing, and asthma. In the original source this formula is said to be useful in the treatment of wheezing and sweating.

Subsequently, the formula has been used not only for interior heat resulting from an invasion of wind-cold, but also for other patterns of heat accumulated in the Lung from various causes. The principal pattern is described as retention of severe heat in the Lung with symptoms such as a hot sensation or fever, wheezing, asthma, shortness of breath, thirst, and rapid pulse. The formula can be used whether or not there is sweating. It is considered suitable for all these conditions, and has brought consistently good results.

Explanation of herbs in first formula

Herba Ephedrae *(ma huang)* is the chief herb in this formula. It is acrid in flavor, warm in nature, and facilitates the expulsion of pathogenic heat from the body surface by promoting dispersal of the Lung qi.

Gypsum *(shi gao)* is acrid, cold, and sweet and is used as a deputy herb to control the warmth of Herba Ephedrae *(ma huang)*. The dosage of Gypsum *(shi gao)* is much greater than that of Herba Ephedrae *(ma huang)*. In addition to buffering the warmth of Herbal Ephedrae *(ma huang)*, Gypsum *(shi gao)* also clears heat from the Lung.

Semen Pruni Armeniacae *(xing ren)* is an assistant herb and is combined with Herba Ephedrae *(ma huang)* to promote the descent of Lung qi and calm the wheezing.

Radix Glycyrrhizae Uralensis *(gan cao)* is an envoy herb that helps tonify the qi in order to strengthen the antipathogenic factors.

In clinical practice, the ratio of Herba Ephedrae *(ma huang)* to Gypsum *(shi gao)* must be adjusted in accordance with the condition of the patient, the primary considerations being the severity of heat in the Lung and the stagnation of Lung qi.

Second formula

Two-Cured Decoction *(er chen tang)* is the second formula on which the prescription in this case is based. It is used for treating patterns associated with phlegm and retention of congested fluids, and contains the following ingredients:

Rhizoma Pinelliae Ternatae *(ban xia)* 15g
Pericarpium Citri Reticulatae *(chen pi)* 15g
Sclerotium Poriae Cocos *(fu ling)* 9g
Radix Glycyrrhizae Uralensis *(gan cao)* 5g

Patterns associated with retention of phlegm or dampness can give rise to such symptoms as cough, asthma, wheezing, stifling sensation in the chest, abdominal distention, nausea, vomiting, dizziness, and palpitations.

Explanation of herbs in second formula

Rhizoma Pinelliae Ternatae *(ban xia)* is the chief herb. It is acrid and warm, dries dampness, and resolves phlegm.

Pericarpium Citri Reticulatae *(chen pi)* is a deputy herb. It is acrid, warm, regulates qi, and resolves phlegm. Together with the previous herb, it removes formed phlegm and dampness while promoting qi activity.

Sclerotium Poriae Cocos *(fu ling)* is an assistant herb. It benefits the Spleen and resolves dampness. In clinical practice, the source of phlegm is said to be a disorder of the Spleen. This is an ideal herb for treating the source of phlegm.

Radix Glycyrrhizae Uralensis *(gan cao)* is an envoy herb which strengthens the qi of the middle burner. Combined with Sclerotium Poriae Cocos *(fu ling)*, it can reduce phlegm.

Modified herbal formula

Herba Ephedrae *(ma huang)* 6g
Semen Pruni Armeniacae *(xing ren)* 10g
Cortex Magnoliae Officinalis *(hou po)* 10g
Cortex Mori Albae Radicis *(sang bai pi)* 10g
Fructus Trichosanthis *(gua lou)* 10g
Pericarpium Citri Reticulatae *(chen pi)* 10g

Rhizoma Pinelliae Ternatae *(ban xia)* 8g
Radix Scutellariae Baicalensis *(huang qin)* 10g
Sclerotium Poriae Cocos *(fu ling)* 15g
Rhizoma Atractylodis Macrocephalae *(bai zhu)* 10g
Radix Glycyrrhizae Uralensis *(gan cao)* 6g

Explanation of modified herbal formula

The two basic formulas above were combined, with some modifications. Although Ephedra, Apricot Kernel, Gypsum, and Licorice Decoction *(ma xing shi gan tang)* is used to treat heat in the Lung, because the phlegm-heat was very strong in this case, Two-Cured Decoction *(er chen tang)* and a few other herbs that clear heat from the Lung were used to clear the heat, resolve the phlegm, and remove the damp-heat from the Lung. Furthermore, because the patient also has symptoms associated with Spleen yang deficiency, Gypsum *(shi gao)* was omitted because of the risk that it would aggravate the injury to the yang of the middle burner.

The absence from this prescription of a very cold herb to clear the heat, and a very hot herb to tonify the yang; is noteworthy, since the treatment principle included the removal of phlegm-heat from the Lung and the promotion of Spleen qi in the middle burner. In contrast to Gypsum *(shi gao)*, which is associated with the Lung and Stomach, herbs associated with the Lung channel, including Radix Scutellariae Baicalensis *(huang qin)*, Fructus Trichosanthis *(gua lou)*, and Cortex Mori Albae Radicis *(sang bai pi)*, were prescribed in order to avoid injuring the Spleen yang. Likewise, Rhizoma Atractylodis Macrocephalae *(bai zhu)* helps Sclerotium Poriae Cocos *(fu ling)* promote the Spleen qi while gently strengthening the antipathogenic factors. Hence the demands of this case in clearing the heat while avoiding injury to the yang qi were met.

Follow-up

At first, acupuncture was administered once a day. After four treatments the wheezing, shortness of breath, and stifling sensation in the chest were substantially relieved, but there was still a fair amount of yellow sputum. The loose stools also continued once or twice a day. The treatment principle was therefore changed to tonification of the Spleen and Lung, and removal of the phlegm. The acupuncture prescription was changed accordingly: LU-5 *(chi ze)* was replaced by LU-7 *(lie que)*, using even manipulation of the needle, and CV-12 *(zhong wan)* was added, using a reinforcing method. At this stage the herbal remedy was introduced: one dosage, divided into two, taken each day.

After one-and-a-half weeks during which acupuncture was administered once a day, the wheezing had almost disappeared, the appetite had improved a little, and the phlegm had diminished in volume and become white and thin. Acupuncture was then stopped, but the herbs were continued for another three weeks, with slight adjustments as the condition changed, until the symptoms had almost subsided. The herbs were then stopped, and acupuncture resumed with the revised prescription described above for about three more weeks. Treatments were administered three times a week, every other day, in order to tonify the Spleen and Lung and remove the last of the phlegm.

Thereafter, the patient returned only once a month for a check-up. A very mild herbal remedy for regulating the body was also prescribed:

Radix Astragali Membranacei *(huang qi)* 15g
Sclerotium Poriae Cocos *(fu ling)* 10g
Rhizoma Atractylodis Macrocephalae *(bai zhu)* 10g
Radix Dioscoreae Oppositae *(shan yao)* 30g
Pericarpium Citri Reticulatae *(chen pi)* 10g
Semen Pruni Armeniacae *(xing ren)* 8g
Radix Platycodi Grandiflori *(jie geng)* 6g
Fructus Perillae Frutescentis *(su zi)* 6g

Radix Glycyrrhizae Uralensis *(gan cao)* 10g

The patient took this remedy over four months. It was taken for one week each month: one dose a day for six days, and then none until the following month. The symptoms subsided, and the patient had much more energy.

The following year the patient experienced no further attacks of wheezing. He was advised to engage in more physical exercise in order to strengthen the body's resistance, which would prevent further attacks. He was followed for another four years, during which time he had only two mild attacks. On those occasions he was treated with acupuncture and herbal medicine, based on very similar treatment principles.

CASE 4: **Female, age 70**

Main complaint

Wheezing and shortness of breath

History

The patient has suffered from this condition for several decades. She has a very weak constitution, is prone to a variety of illnesses, has a long history of chronic wheezing and difficulty in recovering. Severe wheezing attacks may occur either in summer or winter. During attacks she may experience severe shortness of breath and a stifling sensation in the chest. She has a copious amount of watery, clear, or frothy sputum, sweats easily, and experiences coldness in her limbs. She finds it very difficult to lie flat. She has been hospitalized many times for treatment.

During the intervals between her wheezing attacks the patient still suffers from shortness of breath and a stifling sensation in the chest. Physical activity proves to be difficult and leads to wheezing. She either sits up or stays in bed. To ease the symptoms, she uses various conventional medications (including steroid inhalers) as well as some Chinese prepared medicines, such as Reduce Cough and Wheezing *(xiao ke chuan)* and Citrus and Tangerine Pills *(zhi ke ju hong wan)*.

At the moment, the patient breathes weakly and has severe shortness of breath. Her sputum is clear and watery, and her voice is very weak. She has a very poor appetite, but does not feel thirsty. Her limbs are cold. When she moves, she sweats spontaneously; any physical activity increases the sweating, and leads to fatigue. She does not sleep soundly. She has little urine and it is clear. Her stools are watery and loose. She has one or two bowel movements every day. The patient is very frail and emaciated. Her complexion is gray, dark, and lusterless. Her lips are purplish.

Tongue

Dark, pale, and swollen with a white, thick, and moist coating

Pulse

Sunken, thin, and forceless; both proximal positions are very weak

Analysis of symptoms

1. Long history of illness, weak constitution, inability to engage in physical activity—severe injury to the antipathogenic factors.

2. Wheezing, stifling sensation in the chest, severe shortness of breath—problems with grasping the qi.

3. Weakness and shortness of breath, very weak voice, spontaneous sweating which is aggravated by physical activity—Lung qi deficiency.

4. Coldness and cold extremities—yang deficiency.

5. General lassitude, fatigue, watery and loose stools—dysfunction of the Spleen in its transportive and transformative functions.

6. Gray and dark complexion, purple tongue and lips—poor circulation of blood.

7. White, thick, and moist tongue coating, sunken, thin, and forceless pulse—yang deficiency.

8. Very weak and forceless pulse, especially in both proximal positions—Kidney deficiency.

Basic theory of case

In Chinese medicine the Lung and Kidney nourish each other through their yin aspects. This refers to the mutual generation relationship between water and metal: metal (Lung) is the mother of water (Kidney). The Kidney yin also supports the Lung yin. In addition, the Lung governs breathing and the Kidney is responsible for the grasping and storing of qi *(Fig. 1-7)*. Breathing in Chinese medicine means inhaling clear or pure yang, which not only enters the Lung, but is also transported downward to be stored in the Kidney. The Kidney yang thereby continuously receives yang qi from the external environment.

Other Organs are also dependent upon the nourishment from the clear qi. Thus, the ability of the Kidney to grasp the qi is very important for producing and supplementing the yang qi of the entire body. This is why the Kidney is referred to as "the root of qi."

The grasping of qi by the Kidney is not due entirely to the Kidney itself; it is brought about by the coordinated, balanced effort of the Lung and Kidney. That is to say, the Lung is responsible for the qi descending, and the Kidney for storing it. Thus, when the Lung is severely ill, the Kidney may appear to be dysfunctional in grasping and storing the qi. In practice, this is a very severe type of wheezing.

Fig. 1-7

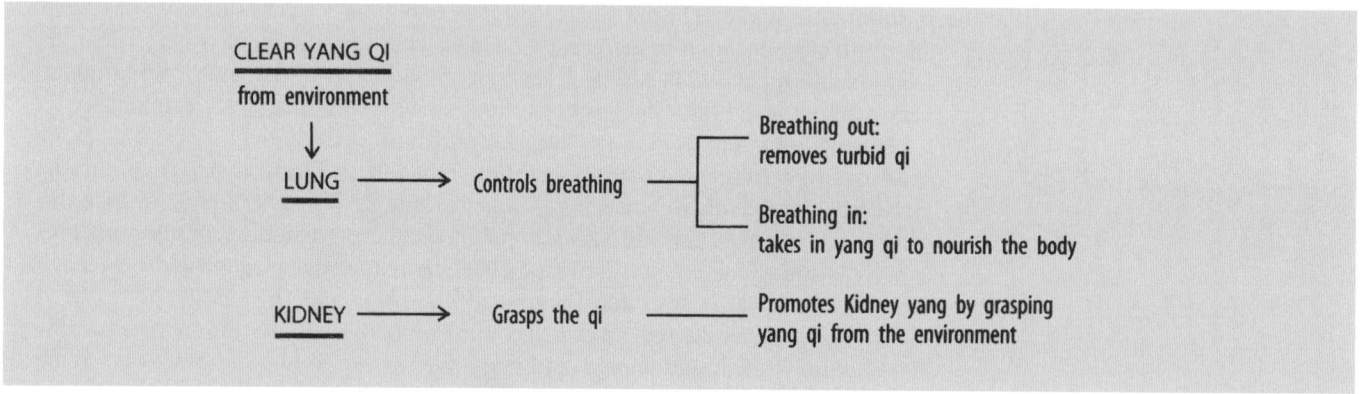

CLEAR YANG QI

from environment

LUNG → Controls breathing —
- Breathing out: removes turbid qi
- Breathing in: takes in yang qi to nourish the body

KIDNEY → Grasps the qi — Promotes Kidney yang by grasping yang qi from the environment

Cause of disease

Phlegm

The patient has white, clear, watery, and copious sputum, which indicates the retention of phlegm in the Lung as the cause of disease.

Site of disease

Lung, Kidney, Spleen

The patient has a long history of shortness and weakness of breath and recurrent attacks of wheezing. During the attacks, she experiences severe and continuous shortness of breath; this is the main evidence suggesting that the site of the disease is the Lung and Kidney. Her poor appetite and loose stools implicate the Spleen as well.

Pathological change

In clinical practice, chronic cough and wheezing injure the Lung at an early stage, interfering with its ability to control breathing. If this condition persists, the Kidney's functions of grasping and storing the qi may also be affected. This can lead to deficiency of both the Lung and Kidney. That is what happened in this case.

The patient's Lung qi was injured by persistent illness, which interfered with the dispersal of the protective qi to the superficial layers of the body where it is needed to fend off pathogenic factors. As a result, external pathogenic factors invaded the body with little resistance. This accounts for her recurrent attacks of asthma, and her propensity to become ill.

The persistence of this condition further injures the antipathogenic factors, and leads to a vicious circle of chronic illness. Although the patient is not presently suffering from an acute attack, the Lung's ability to control breathing and the Kidney's ability to grasp the qi are both seriously impaired. The qi activity in the chest is also affected, causing poor circulation and stagnation of qi, which accounts for the stifling sensation in her chest. Because the qi is not received into the body in the normal manner, the patient suffers from irregular bouts of weakness and shortness of breath.

The Lung controls both the ascending and descending of qi. The ascending aspects include removal of turbid qi, spreading the body fluids and the essence of food from the Spleen to the entire body, including the surface (skin and hair), and dispersing the protective qi to regulate the opening and closing of the interstices and pores, and to control sweating. The descending aspects include inhaling the qi from the external environment, and transporting clear qi and fluids to the lower part of the body. Where (as here) there is deficiency of Lung qi and yang qi, the ascending and descending functions will be disrupted. The body fluids will not be disseminated throughout the body, but will accumulate instead in the Lungs. This results in excessive, watery, clear, and frothy sputum. The severe injury to the Lung qi impairs its ability to support speech, hence the weak voice. The weakness of protective qi limits its ability to properly open and close the pores on the surface of the body, causing spontaneous sweating. And because of the yang deficiency, the body cannot maintain its proper temperature; the patient feels cold and has cold extremities. There is no injury to the body fluids, hence the absence of thirst, and the clarity of her urine.

The poor appetite, general lassitude, loose, watery stools, and emaciation are all evidence of Spleen deficiency. This can be traced to the yang qi deficiency in both the Lung and Kidney, which deprives the Spleen yang qi of its normal support; the Spleen's transportive and transformative functions are accordingly weakened.

The patient has a gray, lusterless complexion, purple tongue and lips, which indicate that—again due to qi and yang deficiency—internal cold constricts the vessels and causes poor circulation of blood. The pale, swollen tongue with its thick, white, and moist coating, and the sunken, thin, and forceless pulse all indicate yang deficiency and a preponderance of internal cold. The forceless pulse at both proximal positions indicates Kidney deficiency *(Fig. 1-8)*.

Pattern of disease

The patient has a history of a chronic disorder which has severely injured the Lung, Spleen, and Kidney; there is an absence of such symptoms as fever or aversion to cold. We may therefore conclude that hers is an interior pattern.

The cold extremities and feeling of coldness, clear urine, loose, watery stools, and dark, pale tongue with a white, moist coating indicate a cold pattern.

This condition has persisted for many years and consequently has left the patient with a very weak constitution. She has suffered a variety of disorders—among them general fatigue, lassitude, weak breathing and voice—all of which are evidence of deficiency.

Fig. 1-8

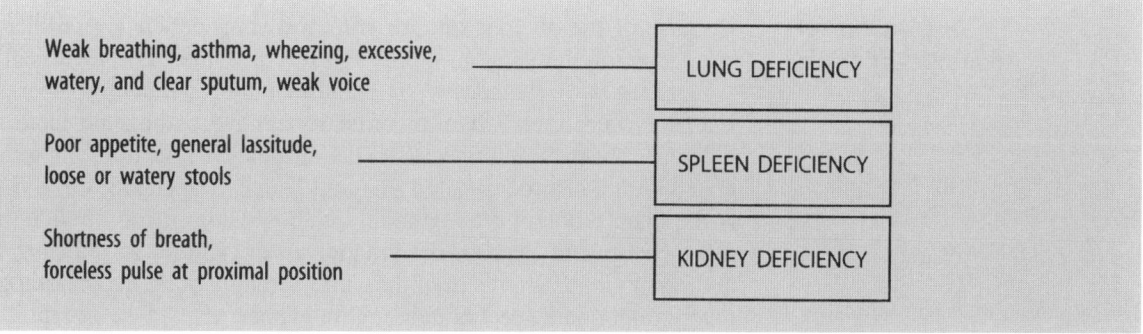

Weak breathing, asthma, wheezing, excessive, watery, and clear sputum, weak voice	LUNG DEFICIENCY
Poor appetite, general lassitude, loose or watery stools	SPLEEN DEFICIENCY
Shortness of breath, forceless pulse at proximal position	KIDNEY DEFICIENCY

Additional notes

1. Is there a pattern of excess in this case?

As noted in the previous cases, the presence of wheezing, asthma, stifling sensation in the chest, and copious sputum may support a diagnosis of both deficiency and excess, in which the pattern of excess is predominant. Why, then, does the diagnosis in this case suggest only deficiency?

Examine the symptoms once again. When the patient came to the clinic, her main complaint was shortness and weakness of breath. This indicates a deficient pattern. Her breathing was not rough or loud, and the nature of her wheezing provided little evidence of excess.

2. Is there yang deficiency in the Spleen and Kidney?

A Kidney disorder mainly involves symptoms of the Kidney's inability to grasp the qi, which may implicate either Kidney yang deficiency or Kidney qi deficiency. In this case, in addition to the Kidney's inability to grasp the qi, there is a feeling of cold as well as cold extremities. These are general symptoms of internal cold, which point to Kidney yang deficiency. There is also loose, watery stools and a swollen tongue with a moist coating, indicating Spleen yang deficiency. We accordingly diagnose Kidney and Spleen yang deficiency.

3. How does one distinguish between wheezing caused by Lung qi deficiency from that associated with the Kidney's inability to grasp the qi?

A weak cough and wheezing can be associated with either Lung qi deficiency or with the Kidney's inability to grasp the qi. What distinguishes them are the characteristics of the wheezing and the degree of severity of the disorder. The Kidney's inability to grasp the qi is characterized by weak, short, but very rapid breathing. Another telling sign is that there is more difficulty with inhalation than with exhalation.

This particular patient has a desire to breathe deeply, but finds it difficult to do so; clinically, her breathing is quite shallow. Although a patient with Lung qi deficiency suffers from shortness of breath and wheezes weakly, the difficulty in inhaling is not as pronounced as in a patient with a Kidney disorder. Kidney dysfunction is a much more severe disorder than Lung qi deficiency.

Conclusion

1. According to the eight principles:
   Interior, cold, deficiency

2. According to etiology:
   Retention of phlegm

3. According to Organ theory:
   Deficiency of Lung qi, failure of Kidney to grasp the qi,
   phlegm and retention of dampness in the Lung,
   Spleen and Kidney yang deficiency

Treatment principle

1. Warm the yang of the body and strengthen the qi.

2. Resolve the phlegm and calm the wheezing.

Explanation of treatment principle

Because of the obvious interior cold and yang deficiency problems in this case, strengthening the yang and tonifying the qi is the basic treatment principle. The yang of the body provides warmth and maintains the body temperature; it can also improve water metabolism in order to remove pathogenic factors (in this case, phlegm). The patient wheezes and has shortness of breath, symptoms that are associated with a disorder of the Lung and Kidney, especially the Kidney, which here is the main problem. Strengthening Kidney yang qi can provide the Kidney with more energy and improve the function of the Kidney in grasping the qi. Thus, in addition to tonifying the qi of the Lung, strengthening the yang qi of the Kidney is a very important aspect of calming the wheezing.

In this case, the wheezing is part of a deficiency pattern. It is important to distinguish between the treatment of deficient and excessive wheezing. Strengthening the dispersing function of the Lung cannot be used in cases of deficient wheezing; it is only appropriate for expelling pathogenic factors (including external pathogenic factors that obstruct the Lung qi, as well as the stagnation of qi in the chest, which is generally caused by qi obstruction resulting from an accumulation of excessive qi).

Patients with deficient wheezing may have either Lung qi deficiency or Lung and Kidney qi deficiency. If the patient has a dysfunction of the Kidney in grasping the qi, it means that the qi of the body floats in the upper burner and cannot be received ("grasped") into the lower part of the body. This is the primary pathological change for patients with deficiency of Lung and Kidney qi.

If, when dealing with this type of patient, the Lung is strengthened by using the dispersing method, the antipathogenic factor may be pushed further upward and outward. The floating of qi in the upper part of the body and the patient's shortness of breath can cause the wheezing to worsen, and may even lead to a very dangerous pattern of floating of deficient yang. This approach must therefore be avoided.

The correct method for treating this type of condition in the acute stage is to apply the basic treatment principle of strengthening the Kidney's function of grasping the qi, either through acupuncture or herbs, and also to promote the descent of the qi. Meanwhile it is also necessary to use some herbs or acupoints to promote the ascent of the Lung qi in order to regulate the qi activity in the Lung. However, in doing so one must ensure that promoting the dispersing function of the Lung is pursued less vigorously than promoting the descending function of the Lung. During the interval (that is, after an acute attack), the Lung and Spleen qi must be strengthened so that the Kidney yang can be tonified. This is the main method.

Selection of points

Because this patient was particularly weak and could not visit the clinic for regular acupuncture and moxibustion treatments, the ear acupuncture method was recommended. Instead of subcutaneous needling, a seed named Semen Vaccariae Segetalis *(wang bu liu xing)* was used with pressure on the acupoints of the ear *(Fig. 1-9)*.

FRONT OF EAR:

Calm Wheezing, Trachea, Lung, Triple Burner, Liver, Spleen, Kidney, Lower Tragus, Shenmen, Subcortex

BACK OF EAR:

Superior Root of Ear, Upper Root of Ear

Explanation of points

One group of points was chosen to promote the dispersing and descending functions of the Lung, and for calming the wheezing. These include Calm Wheezing, Lung, Trachea, Lower Tragus, and Superior Root of Ear *(shang er gen)*. A second group was chosen to strengthen the functions of the Organs. Shenmen and Subcortex calm the mind and regulate the blood circulation. The Spleen and Triple Burner points promote water metabolism, tonify the Spleen, and resolve the phlegm. The Liver point regulates the body's general qi activity, and the Kidney point tonifies the Kidney and promotes the Kidney's function of grasping the qi to assist in calming the wheezing.

According to modern research, ear acupuncture points have five separate functions that are relevant to this case. These are noted below along with the points used in this case that serve that particular function.

- Provide relief from allergies—
  Lung, Trachea, Upper Tragus, Superior Root of Ear
- Regulate the endocrine system—Liver, Kidney

Fig. 1-9

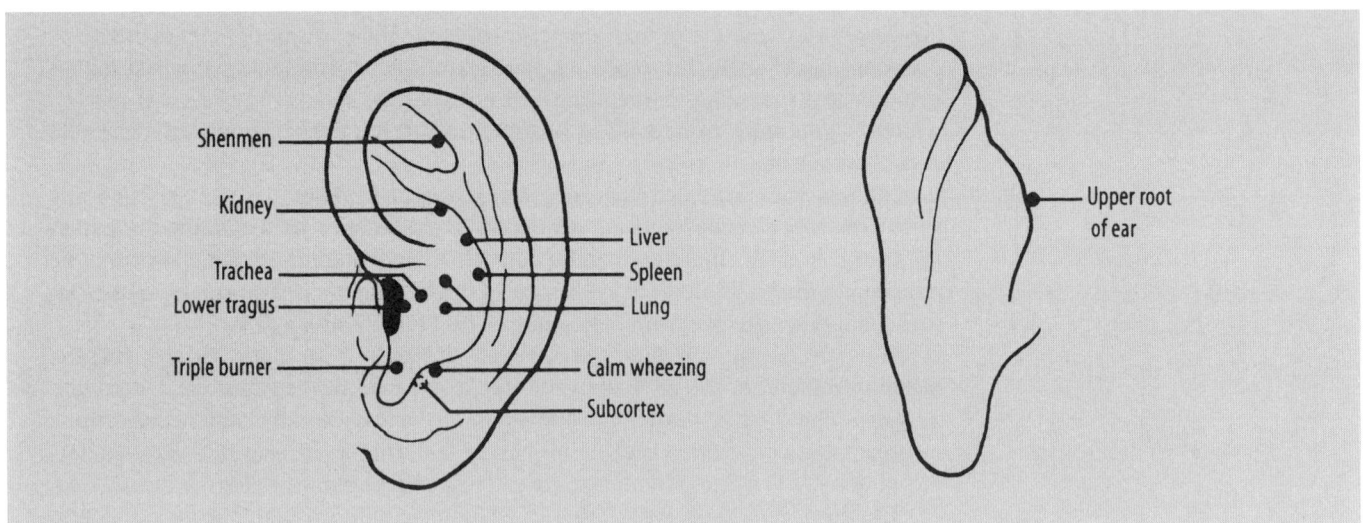

- Anti-infectious effect—Shenmen
- Regulate the autonomic nervous system—Subcortex
- Resolve mucus—Spleen, Triple Burner

Basic herbal formula

Perilla Fruit Decoction for Directing Qi Downward *(su zi jiang qi tang)* is used for reversal of Lung qi, along with Kidney yang deficiency and the failure of the Kidney to grasp the qi. This type of pathological change results in symptoms such as cough, asthma, shortness of breath, wheezing, copious sputum, and a stifling sensation in the chest, along with soreness, weakness, and a sensation of cold in the lower back or edema of the limbs. The tongue coating is moist and white. The original formula contains the following ingredients:

Fructus Perillae Frutescentis *(su zi)* 9g

Rhizoma Pinelliae Ternatae *(ban xia)* 9g

Pericarpium Citri Reticulatae *(chen pi)* 9g

Radix Peucedani *(qian hu)* 6g

Cortex Magnoliae Officinalis *(hou po)* 6g

Cortex Cinnamomi Cassiae *(rou gui)* 3g

Radix Angelicae Sinensis *(dang gui)* 6g

Radix Glycyrrhizae Uralensis *(gan cao)* 6g

Explanation of basic herbal formula

In this formula, Fructus Perillae Frutescentis *(su zi)* is the chief herb and is used for promoting the Lung qi in descending, eliminating phlegm, and calming wheezing.

Rhizoma Pinelliae Ternatae *(ban xia)*, Pericarpium Citri Reticulatae *(chen pi)*, Cortex Magnoliae Officinalis *(hou po)*, and Radix Peucedani *(qian hu)* comprise a group of deputy herbs that resolve and expel phlegm, stop coughing, and calm wheezing. The chief herb and the four deputies are all associated with the Lung; they promote the descent of qi in the body, and are therfore used when a reversal of Lung qi leads to a pattern involving cough, wheezing, and copious sputum. With the exception of Radix Peucedani *(qian hu)*, which is cold, the other four herbs are acrid and warm, and thus the combination is particularly good for a pattern of cold-phlegm retention in the Lung.

Cortex Cinnamomi Cassiae *(rou gui)* is acrid, sweet, and hot. It is associated with the Heart, Spleen, and Kidney and strongly promotes the yang of the body, and removes internal cold. It can be used for such problems as a constant feeling of being cold, coldness in the limbs, cold pain in the abdominal and epigastric regions, soreness and weakness in the lower back and knees, urinary frequency, and loose stools when caused by Kidney and Spleen yang deficiency. It is especially useful for Kidney yang deficiency with an accumulation of internal cold in the lower burner. In this formula the herb is used to warm the body and strengthen the Kidney yang in order to expel cold from the body, and to promote the Kidney's ability to grasp the qi, so as to calm the wheezing. The herb is used here in the role of assistant.

Radix Angelicae Sinensis *(dang gui)* is acrid and warm and is always used to nourish the blood and dispel blood stasis. In this formula it is used to prevent the other dry and warm herbs from injuring the yin and blood of the body. It therefore functions as an assistant.

Radix Glycyrrhizae Uralensis *(gan cao)* regulates the function of the middle burner, and harmonizes the other herbs in the formula. It is used here as an envoy herb.

Modified herbal formula	Radix Ginseng *(ren shen)* 10g
	Radix Astragali Membranacei *(huang qi)* 15g
	Cortex Cinnamomi Cassiae *(rou gui)* 5g
	Rhizoma Zingiberis Officinalis *(gan jiang)* 5g
	Radix Rehmanniae Glutinosae Conquitae *(shu di huang)* 10g
	Fructus Perillae Frutescentis *(su zi)* 10g
	Rhizoma Pinelliae Ternatae *(ban xia)* 10g
	Pericarpium Citri Reticulatae *(chen pi)* 6g

Explanation of modifed herbal formula

The patient in this case presented with Lung and Kidney deficiency, together with dysfunction of the Kidney in grasping the qi. Thus, the wheezing pertains to a pattern of deficiency. There was also yang deficiency of the Spleen and Kidney, giving rise to symptoms associated with an accumulation of internal cold. Perilla Fruit Decoction for Directing Qi Downward *(su zi jiang qi tang)* was prescribed as the basic formula to promote the descent of qi, and thereby calm the wheezing. However, because the patient was not suffering an acute attack, the wheezing and reversal of qi in this case were not very severe. Rather, shortness of breath and symptoms of general deficiency were the main problems. Because the original formula emphasizes the expulsion of pathogenic factors but has relatively little effect in reinforcing the antipathogenic factor, additional herbs which tonify the yang and qi were added to compensate.

This formula differs from the original primarily in its change of emphasis to that of strengthening the antipathogenic factors. This is accomplished by warming and tonifying the Spleen and Kidney yang qi.

Because the pathogenic factors are not very strong in this case, only three of the five herbs that were included in the original formula to expel them were retained in the modified formula. The dosage of Cortex Cinnamomi Cassiae *(rou gui),* used in the original prescription for strengthening the antipathogenic factors, was increased. Other herbs were added to tonify the Lung qi and warm the Spleen yang. Radix Angelicae Sinensis *(dang gui)* was replaced by Radix Rehmanniae Glutinosae Conquitae *(shu di huang)*. Although the function of these herbs is similar, the emphasis of the first is on nourishing the blood, while that of the latter herb is on strengthening the Kidney, hence the substitution.

Follow-up

Because the condition of this patient was very poor, and she was physically quite weak, she came to the clinic only once every two weeks for a refill of her herbs and placement of seeds in the ear. After one month, the symptoms were alleviated. They were not as erratic or changeable, and the patient noticed that the stifling sensation in her chest, wheezing, and shortness of breath were all slightly improved, as was her physical energy. During the first month of treatment, she had no acute attacks of wheezing and she was able to rest for short periods of time lying down.

Treatment was continued for another two months, maintaining the same principle of strengthening the antipathogenic factors. Minor changes were made to the herbal formula to accommodate the patient's condition. She experienced only two acute wheezing attacks, for which she used an inhaler and some conventional medications, but did not require hospitalization. Also during this period, she occasionally found that she was able to walk around without suffering from as much physical exhaustion as before.

The ear seed treatment was continued, but the herbal remedy was stopped for a month as the weather was becoming warmer. Prepared herbal remedies were prescribed, alternating Stabilize the Root of Coughing and Wheezing Pills *(gu ben ke chuan pian)* and Six-Gentlemen Pills with Aucklandia and Amomum *(xiang sha liu jun zi wan)* with Six-Ingredient Pill with Rehmannia *(liu wei di huang wan)*. The frequency and intensity of the acute wheezing attacks were greatly diminished, and she was able to engage in some very light physical activities.

Maintaining this principle, each year the patient was given a modified version of Perilla Fruit Decoction for Directing Qi Downward *(su zi jiang qi tang)* for three to four months during the winter, followed by a one month break. As preparing decoctions every day at home proved to be too much during the summer, she took prepared herbal formulas when her condition stabilized. She continued to use seeds in her ear when her condition was relatively unstable, primarily in the winter.

Conventional medicine was used for three years to treat heart failure. She suffered acute heart failure twice during this time, for which she was hospitalized. Her condition did not worsen and the treatment was satisfactory. However, following a third episode of heart failure, she suffered severe decompensation and damage to the heart and lungs, and passed away.

This is an example of a chronic case that involves severe heart failure. Most patients of this type suffer a great deal and have a miserable life when the illness develops to this stage. Nevertheless, it can be seen here that the ear seed treatment and herbal remedies reduced this patient's suffering and improved her general condition and quality of life during her last few years.

Diagnostic Principles for Asthma

In Chinese medicine there are two different types of asthma and wheezing. One is called *chuǎn*, the other *xiāo*. The word *chuǎn* means difficulty in breathing and shortness of breath. The patient must open his mouth to breathe, and the shoulders move up and down as the accessory muscles of respiration are used. Lying flat becomes difficult. When there is wheezing along with a gurgling noise in the throat, this condition is known as *xiāo*. These two conditions cover most types of what is diagnosed as asthma in modern biomedicine.

Cause of disease and pathological changes

Causes of asthma include invasion of external pathogenic factors and disorders of the internal Organs *(Fig. 1-10)*. Of the six external pathogenic factors, asthma most often results from an invasion of wind-cold or wind-heat. The pathological change is the entrance of external pathogenic factors through the skin, nose, and mouth into the Lung, causing Lung qi stagnation and a dysfunction of the Lung in dispersing the qi. This type of asthma is associated with excess.

Asthma related to an internal disorder can be either excessive or deficient. That which is associated with excess is often caused by retention of phlegm and dampness, resulting in obstruction of the Lung qi's functions of dispersing and descending. Common examples of asthma associated with deficiency are Lung qi

Fig. 1-10

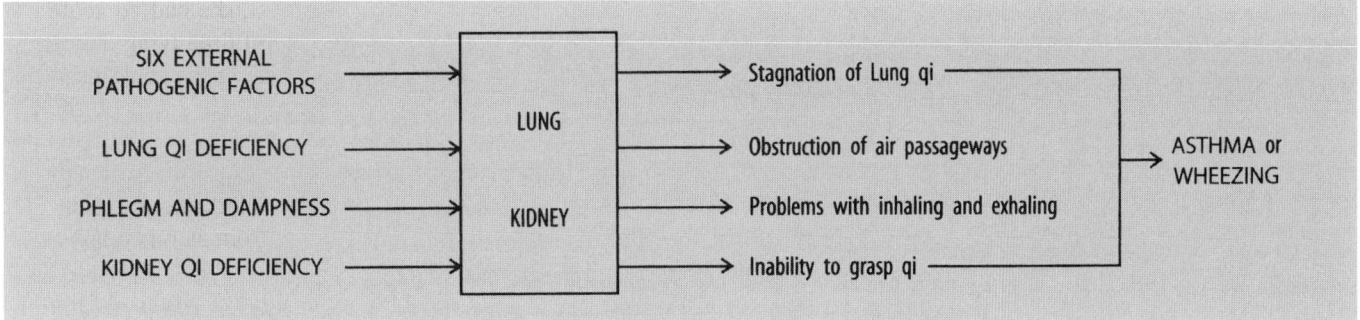

deficiency and Kidney qi deficiency. Both can lead to an inability of the body's qi to properly ascend and descend, resulting in asthma.

For additional information, see "Diagnostic principles for cough" on pages 33-35 of *Acupuncture Patterns & Practice.*

Differentiation of asthma

The focus of diagnosis in asthma is to determine whether it is of a deficient or excessive nature.

The excessive type is characterized by acute onset, and does not last long. Breathing is usually rough and is accompanied by wheezing and restlessness; in severe cases there is orthopnea. Lying flat cannot be tolerated and there is a full and stifling sensation in the chest. Exhaling is difficult and requires much effort. If the asthma or wheezing is caused by an invasion of pathogenic wind-cold, the patient will usually present with an aversion to cold, fever, cough, clear, white, and watery phlegm, slightly red tongue with a thin white coating, and a floating, tight pulse.

If the pattern is caused by an invasion of wind-heat, or if the heat pattern is caused by cold leading to constraint, the patient will feel hot around the body and will have a red complexion, sweating, thirst, and a stifling sensation or pain in the chest. The phlegm is usually yellow, sticky, and thick. The urine is yellow and the stools are dry. The tongue is red with a yellow coating, and the pulse is rapid.

If the patient has retention of phlegm-dampness or damp-heat, there will be severe or paroxysmal coughing, profuse sputum, stifling sensation in the chest, and a feeling of being generally cold or hot.

The deficient type of asthma is chronic, long-lasting, and is characterized by a slow onset. There is weak wheezing with considerable shortness of breath. Patients usually have a weak voice, experience difficulty inhaling, and have insufficient energy to do so. They often feel so short of breath that they can hardly continue breathing. The asthma may be aggravated by any kind of physical exertion. Other symptoms include fatigue, general lassitude, spontaneous sweating, pale tongue with a moist, white coating, and a forceless (deficient) pulse.

Asthma associated with a pattern of Lung qi deficiency usually presents with forceless or very weak wheezing as the primary symptom. In this pattern the Kidney's ability to grasp or receive the qi is impaired, and there is shallow breathing; exhalation is more pronounced than inhalation. There is severe shortness of breath, and some patients have urinary incontinence *(Fig. 1-11).*

Fig. 1-11

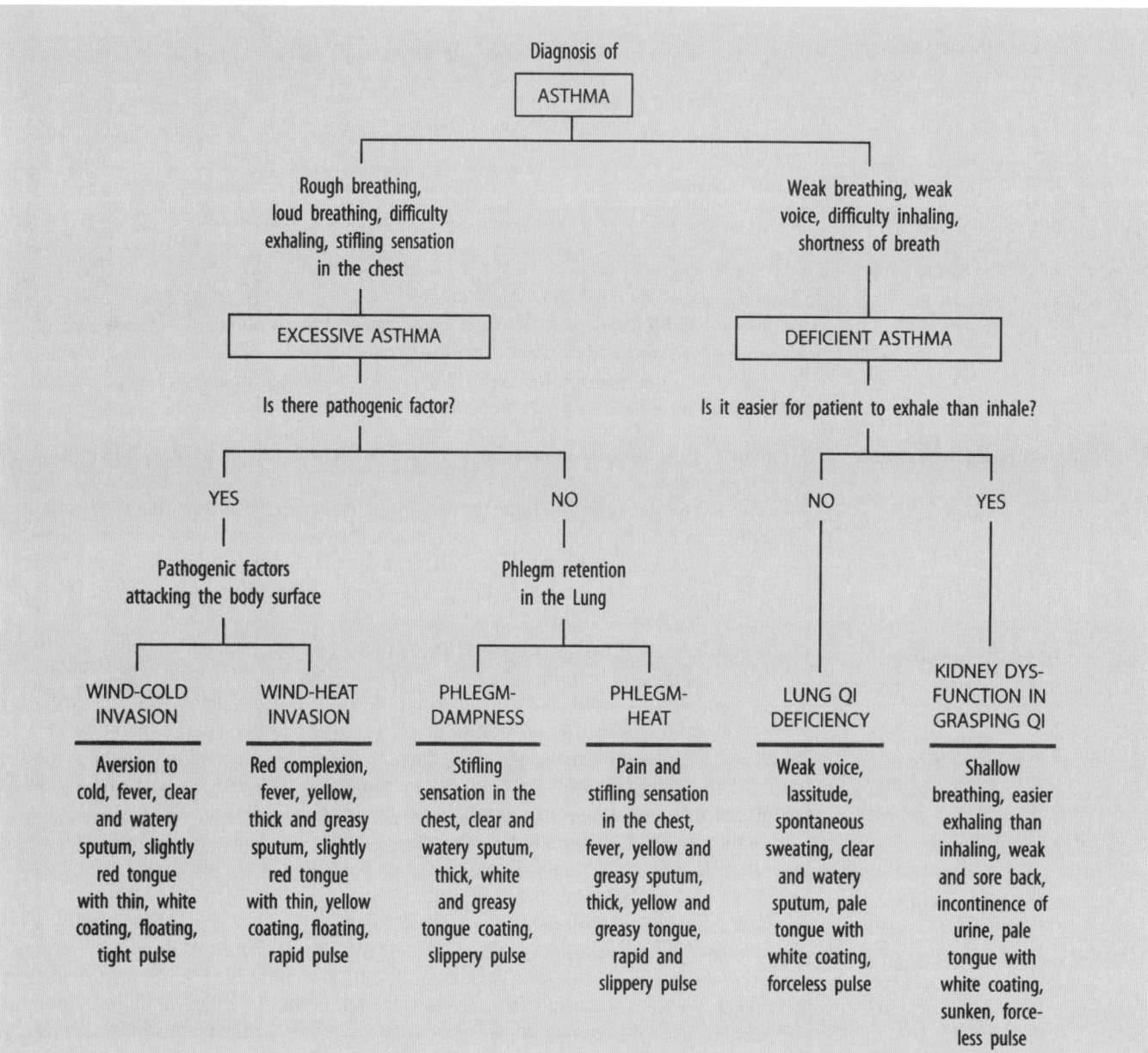

Facial Disorders

CASE 5: **Female, age 60**

Abnormal sensations on the right side of the face

The patient came to the clinic in mid-winter when it was extremely cold. Because of long periods of time spent outdoors, she felt cold, numbness, and pain on her face, ears, and nose, which had become slightly red. Whenever she came back indoors it took a while to get over these sensations, and she noticed that, over time, it took longer and longer to do so.

About three weeks ago the symptoms gradually worsened, especially on the right side of the face. Not only did it feel numb, but the skin felt thicker. It also began to lack sensitivity, and developed a tingling sensation. All of these complaints were aggravated by exposure to cold. The skin in this area had now become pale, and even when she returned to a warm room, the symptoms would no longer be completely relieved. The patient feels that the muscles on the right side of her face are stiff and tense, but there is no deviation of the mouth and eyes, that is, no motor impairment. One week ago she discovered that her sense of taste had diminished on the right side of the tongue; the rest of her mouth was normal.

The patient remembered that when she was a teenager she suffered from low blood pressure. She used to experience episodic dizziness, but she seldom had syncope. She received no particular treatment for this condition. At the moment, apart from the facial symptoms, her appetite is normal. She can become slightly fatigued and her sleep is not very sound. She often wakes early in the morning and finds it difficult to fall asleep again.

Examination revealed diminished superficial sensitivity on the right side of the face, normal muscle strength, and no motor impairment. The skin color was normal, as was sensitivity in the rest of the body, and the strength and movement of the limbs. The patient's cholesterol level, which had been checked three months previously, was within normal limits. There is no history of heart or cerebrovascular disease.

Slightly pale, with a thin, white coating

Sunken, slightly slow

1. Appearance of symptoms after exposure to cold—invasion of pathogenic cold.
2. Pain, cold, and numbness of the face—obstruction of channels and collaterals by invasion of pathogenic cold.

3. Abnormal numbness and sensation of thickness, together with diminished sensitivity in the face—obstruction in the channels and collaterals due to blood deficiency and malnourishment of the channels and collaterals.

4. Tension and stiffness in the facial muscles—malnourishment of the vessels and sinews.

5. Unsound sleep, waking early, and difficulty in falling back to sleep—malnourishment of Heart spirit.

6. History of dizziness—blood deficiency.

7. Pale tongue, white coating, slow pulse—cold pattern.

Basic theory of case

There are two types of pathogenic cold: internal and external. External cold comes from the environment and invades the body, after which symptoms develop. Internal cold implies a deficiency of yang qi and hypofunction of the body resulting in internal cold as a pathological change, with attendant symptoms.

The common cold is the most frequently encountered disorder in the clinic, and is caused by an external invasion of pathogenic cold. Pathogenic cold invades the superficial aspect of the body, blocks the normal circulation of protective qi, and gives rise to an exterior pattern.

Because the channel and collateral system exists both on the surface as well as inside the body, pathogenic cold can invade the body through this system. Although this condition is an exterior pattern in the general sense, it differs from the typical exterior pattern, which affects the whole surface of the body. In patterns relating to disorders of the channels and collaterals, the site of disease is slightly deeper than an exterior pattern, and the symptoms frequently manifest on the limbs, head, face, etc. Pathologically, cold, a yin pathogenic factor, injures the yang qi of the body. When it invades the channels and collaterals, the yang qi—which is the force that drives the circulation of qi and blood in the system—is injured, and the circulation of qi and blood is consequently reduced. In addition, a characteristic of cold is constriction, thus cold can directly cause stagnation of blood. Both of these causes can lead to poor circulation of qi and blood, which results in an obstruction, such that the affected area loses the normal warmth and nourishment provided by the yang qi and blood. This is why there may be localized pallor, cold, numbness, pain, and purplish discoloration. In severe cases there may also be ulcers and even necrosis of the tissues.

Although the characteristics of external and internal cold and their related disorders are very different, both types of cold are also closely related and can influence each other. Patients with internal cold caused by yang deficiency can very easily contract cold from the environment. On the other hand, if external cold invades the body and remains too long, it can injure the body's yang qi. In this way internal cold can develop from external cold.

Fig. 2-1

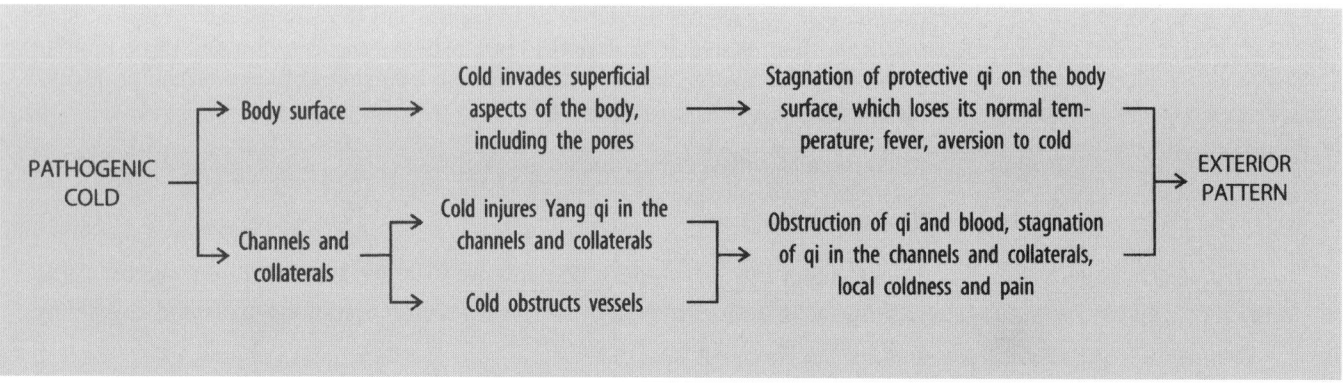

Cause of disease	External cold pathogenic factor

The occurrence of the disorder in this case is clearly related to the invasion of pathogenic cold. Local symptoms include pallor of the skin, cold, numbness, and pain, all of which are aggravated by cold temperatures and alleviated by warmth. This is evidence of external pathogenic cold injuring the yang qi of the body and obstructing the qi and blood. External pathogenic cold is accordingly the cause of disease.

Site of disease — Channels and collaterals

Because the symptoms are confined to just one side of the face, mainly on the skin where there is an abnormal sensation, the disorder is associated with the channels and collaterals.

Pathological change

The onset of this disorder occurred in winter. From the very beginning, the patient's discomfort was associated with going out into a cold environment. The skin on the face, ears, and nose felt cold, painful, and numb. This means that the channels and collaterals were invaded by pathogenic cold from the external environment. Because the yang qi of the channels and collaterals was unable to circulate normally to the face, symptoms developed. At first the symptoms were not very severe; thus, when the patient came indoors (warmth), the yang qi of the body could still repel the coldness from the channels and collaterals, the qi and blood circulation could recover, and the symptoms would therefore disappear. However, the repeated exposure to severe cold, during which the pathogenic and antipathogenic factors fought each other, eventually depleted the yang qi of the channels and collaterals. The symptoms lasted longer, and eventually could not be relieved by warmth. The skin on one side of the face became numb, felt thicker than usual and developed a tingling sensation, and its sensitivity diminished.

In Chinese medicine this is called paresthesia and numbness *(má mù)*. These two words refer to two different, but somewhat related, disorders of the senses. Paresthesia refers to a subjective alteration of sensation caused by a dysfunction of qi; numbness is an objective sensory disturbance associated with a deficiency of blood. (For a more detailed discussion, see case 20 in *Acupuncture Patterns & Practice*.) In this case, the abnormal sensations involve both paresthesia and numbness, which has evolved to the point that warmth cannot relieve the symptoms. This indicates that, in addition to the pathogenic cold that remains in the channels and collaterals causing an obstruction of qi, there is also blood deficiency causing malnourishment of the skin, channels, and collaterals of the face.

The muscular tension and stiffness on the right side of the patient's face indicates that qi has stagnated in the channels and collaterals, and that the sinews and vessels are malnourished due to local blood and qi deficiency. There is no deviation of the mouth and eyes, or any other motor impairment, indicating that the condition is not severe. The diminished sensation of taste on one side of the tongue can be attributed to a dysfunction of the qi and blood circulation in the channels and collaterals.

The patient reported a history of episodic dizziness, which began when she was a teenager. At that time there was deficiency of qi and blood causing malnourishment of the head, and the inability of clear yang to properly rise. Considering her history in conjunction with the present complaints of insomnia, tendency to wake early and difficulty in falling back to sleep, and bearing in mind that there are no heat symptoms like restlessness or anxiety, we may conclude that the patient suffers from blood deficiency, which has led to malnourishment of Heart spirit *(Fig. 2-2)*.

Further evidence of blood deficiency is the slightly pale color of the tongue. The presence of cold is suggested by the white coating and slightly slow pulse.

Fig. 2-2

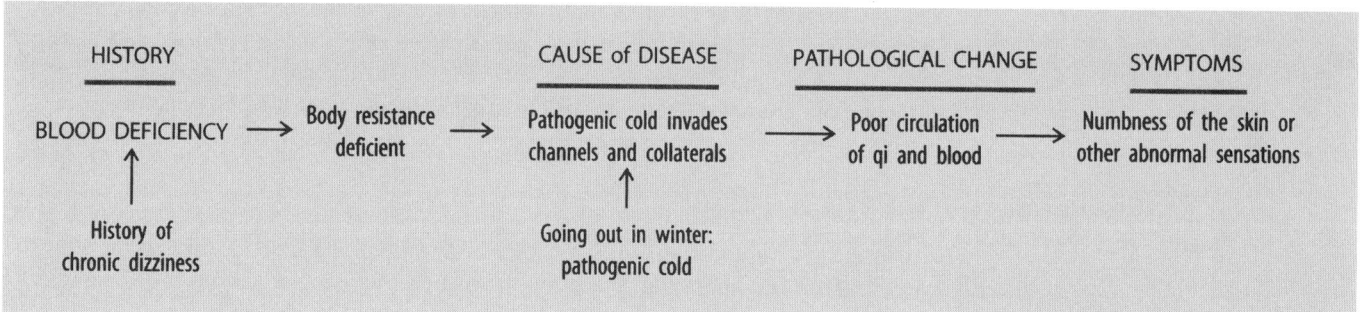

HISTORY		CAUSE of DISEASE	PATHOLOGICAL CHANGE	SYMPTOMS
BLOOD DEFICIENCY →	Body resistance deficient →	Pathogenic cold invades channels and collaterals →	Poor circulation of qi and blood →	Numbness of the skin or other abnormal sensations
↑		↑		
History of chronic dizziness		Going out in winter: pathogenic cold		

Pattern of disease

There is an obvious history of invasion by external pathogenic factors. Because the symptoms are localized on the skin of the face, and there are no general symptoms involving fever or an aversion to cold, we may conclude that the disorder is located in the channels and collaterals. A disorder of the channels and collaterals is classified as an exterior pattern, but not as a typical exterior pattern.

A pattern of cold is evidenced by the facial pain, cold, and pallor, which symptoms are aggravated by cold and alleviated by warmth.

In the early stage of the disorder, pathogenic cold, which was strong, invaded the channels and collaterals. This suggests that the pattern is one of excess. However, as there was already a deficiency of blood in the channels when the patient came to the clinic, these symptoms, in addition to reflecting a pattern of excess, also reveal a pattern of deficiency. The pattern here is thus a combination of excess and deficiency.

Additional notes

1. What is the evidence supporting a diagnosis of blood deficiency?

From the patient's history we know that as a teenager she suffered from episodic dizziness, which suggests that she had blood deficiency at the time, although it was not severe and did not require treatment. This blood deficiency could have remained latent in the channels and collaterals, and, at a later stage of the patient's life, made her vulnerable to invasion by pathogenic cold.

At first the abnormal sensation in her face occurred when she went out into the cold, and a return to warmth alleviated the symptoms. But by the time she came to the clinic the symptoms were continuous and could not be relieved by warmth. This indicates that what had begun as a simple invasion by an external pathogenic factor had transformed into a combination of blood deficiency plus retention of the excessive pathogenic factor. Nevertheless, the blood deficiency is not very severe, and it is mainly localized in the channels and collaterals.

2. How does one explain the thin, white tongue coating and the slow, sunken pulse?

The thin tongue coating suggests an exterior pattern, the sunken pulse an interior pattern. In this case the disorder of the channels and collaterals pertains to an exterior pattern, hence the appearance of the tongue. The sunken pulse exists because the cold pathogenic factor retained in the channels and collaterals has blocked the circulation of yang qi, causing it to stagnate. This explains why the pulse has become slow and sunken, reflecting a cold pattern, but not an interior cold pattern in this instance.

Conclusion

1. According to the eight principles:
   Channel-collateral pattern, cold, combination of deficiency and excess (deficiency within excess).

2. According to etiology:
   Invasion of cold pathogenic factor.

3. According to theory of channels and collaterals:
   Cold pathogenic factor invades the yang brightness channels and collaterals.

4. According to theory of qi, blood, and body fluids:
   Blood deficiency of the channels and collaterals.

Treatment principle

1. Disperse the pathogenic cold, warm the channels, and remove the obstruction from the channels and collaterals.

2. Nourish the blood of the channels and collaterals.

Explanation of treatment principle

In Chinese medicine there are two ways of treating pathogenic cold: disperse the cold *(sàn hán)* and warm the yang *(wēn yáng)*. The former is used in treating exterior cold patterns, the latter in treating interior cold patterns. Both methods use warmth and heat.

In order to disperse external cold, it must be removed through the body surface. This method is appropriate for patterns associated with an external invasion of cold (that is, from the environment) which accumulates on the surface of the body or remains in certain channels and collaterals. On the other hand, to warm the yang one must tonify and warm the yang qi inside the body. This method is appropriate for treating internal cold that has accumulated in the body, for example, in the Organs.

Under certain conditions internal cold may become very severe. For example, if there is a collapse of yang qi, or if external cold directly enters the body, the yang qi of the Organs will be injured. In these circumstances, warming the yang and dispersing the cold must be combined, but warming the yang always takes precedence.

In this case, dispersing the cold, and warming and removing obstruction from the channels and collaterals, are the principle methods. Because there is also blood deficiency in the channels and collaterals, it is necessary to nourish the blood to help disperse the pathogenic factors and remove the pathogenic cold.

Basic herbal formula

Tangkuei Decoction for Frigid Extremities *(dang gui si ni tang)* is one of the classic formulas from *Discussion of Cold-induced Disorders (Shang han lun)*. The formula contains the following ingredients:

Radix Angelicae Sinensis *(dang gui)* 12g
Herba cum Radice Asari *(xi xin)* 1.5g
Ramulus Cinnamomi Cassiae *(gui zhi)* 9g
Medulla Tetrapanacis Papyriferi *(tong cao)* 3g
Radix Paeoniae Lactiflorae *(bai shao)* 9g
Fructus Zizyphi Jujubae *(da zao)* . . . . 8 pieces
Radix Glycyrrhizae Uralensis *(gan cao)* 5g

Explanation of basic herbal formula

The indications for this formula are a pale complexion and cold in the limbs, or pain in the lower back and legs, especially when the symptoms are aggravated by cold and relieved by warmth; pale tongue with a white coating; and a thin, sunken pulse. The pathogenesis associated with this pattern is that cold invades a patient with constitutional blood deficiency, which affects the channels and collaterals such that the normal circulation of qi and blood is obstructed, and then stagnates.

The chief herb in this formula is Radix Angelicae Sinensis *(dang gui)*. It is sweet, acrid, and warm. It is associated with the Liver channel, dispels blood stasis, and nourishes and tonifies the blood.

There are three deputy herbs. Radix Paeoniae Lactiflorae *(bai shao)*, sour and cold, is associated with the Liver channel, and assists Radix Angelicae Sinensis *(dang gui)* in nourishing the blood. Ramulus Cinnamomi Cassiae *(gui zhi)*, acrid, sweet, and warm, is associated with the Heart, Lung, and Bladder channels. Herba cum Radice Asari *(xi xin)*, acrid and warm, is associated with the Lung and Kidney channels. The latter two herbs, when combined, are used to warm the channels and collaterals, and to remove cold from this system, as well as from the blood vessels. They strengthen the effect of the yang qi in propelling the circulation of blood in the channels and collaterals, in order to treat the invasion of pathogenic cold in the channels and collaterals.

Three herbs serve as both assistant and envoy: Medulla Tetrapanacis Papyriferi *(tong cao)* is sweet, bland, and cold, and is associated with the Lung and Stomach channels. This herb was originally used for clearing heat and promoting the metabolism of water, but here is used to remove obstruction from the channels and collaterals. Fructus Zizyphi Jujubae *(da zao)* is sweet and warm; Radix Glycyrrhizae Uralensis *(gan cao)* is sweet and neutral; both herbs are associated with the Spleen and Stomach channels. They promote the qi and antipathogenic factors, strengthen the Spleen, and harmonize the twin functions of the herbs in the formula: tonifying the antipathogenic factors and removing the pathogenic factors.

Modified herbal formula

Radix Angelicae Sinensis *(dang gui)* 10g
Radix et Caulis Jixueteng *(ji xue teng)* 15g
Ramulus Cinnamomi Cassiae *(gui zhi)* 6g
Ramulus Sangjisheng *(sang ji sheng)* 8g
Radix Paeoniae Lactiflorae *(bai shao)* 10g
Fructus Zizyphi Jujubae *(da zao)* . . . . 6 pieces
Rhizoma et Radix Ligustici *(gao ben)* 6g
Radix Glycyrrhizae Uralensis *(gan cao)* 5g

Explanation of modified herbal formula

Because the diagnosis in this case is very similar to the indications for Tangkuei Decoction for Frigid Extremities *(dang gui si ni tang)*, that formula was chosen as the basis for our prescription here, with the following modifications. Because the pathogenic cold was not very severe when the patient came to the clinic for treatment, Rhizoma et Radix Ligustici *(gao ben)* was substituted for Herba cum Radice Asari *(xi xin)* in the original formula, as the latter is very acrid and warm and might therefore aggravate the injury to the yin and blood. Also, Radix et Caulis Jixueteng *(ji xue teng)* and Ramulus Sangjisheng *(sang ji sheng)* were added to strengthen the formula's effect in nourishing the blood, and to remove the obstruction from the channels and collaterals, which is essential in this case.

Follow-up

The patient was given one packet of herbs daily, divided into two doses. After one week, the tension and numbness on the face had disappeared, and the skin was no longer pale. In addition, the abnormal sensation in the tongue was gone, the patient's sense of taste had returned to normal, and she only complained of cold and pain in the face when she went outdoors. This would suggest that the pathogenic cold had been removed by this stage, but the blood deficiency had not fully recovered. The treatment principle was therefore changed to nourishing the blood and tonifying the qi. A prepared medicine, *Renshen guipi wan*, which is based on Restore the Spleen Decoction *(gui pi wan,*.was then prescribed. The patient took one pill twice a day for a period of two months.

As the weather became warmer and the symptoms disappeared, it was unnecessary to continue taking this remedy. The following winter the patient returned for a check-up. There had been no recurrence of symptoms, and therefore no further treatment was indicated.

CASE 6: **Female, age 69**

Main complaint

Pain on the right side of the face

History

Six months ago, while vacationing with her family, the patient visited a place where there was a large waterfall. The wind was very strong, and she felt it blowing over the right side of her face. When she returned to the hotel, this side of her face, as well as the forehead, nose, and lips, were painful — especially the forehead. She noticed that the skin had become very red, swollen, and covered with papulae around the affected areas. Since then she has suffered constant, severe pain, which at times becomes aggravated. The occurrence and duration of these aggravated episodes varies; between attacks she experiences slight pain, discomfort, and stiffness. During the attacks, the pain affects her sleep; it also radiates to her teeth, causing discomfort when she eats.

After returning from vacation, the patient went to a hospital for a check-up and was diagnosed with trigeminal neuralgia. She was given conventional medication, mainly in the form of pain killers. Because the results have been far from satisfactory, she decided to try acupuncture.

At the present time her facial pain is much the same as before, although the papulae have subsided. There are no red and swollen areas on the right side of the face. The patient is obese and suffers from shortness of breath after physical activity. She has no fever or aversion to cold, and her appetite, bowel movements, and urination are all normal.

Tongue

Pale, soft, and swollen, with a white, moist coating

Pulse

Sunken and moderate

Analysis of symptoms

1. Disorder occurring after exposure to wind and cold—invasion of external pathogenic factor.
2. Pain on the right side of the face—obstruction of channels and collaterals.
3. Pain in the forehead, nose, lips, and teeth, but primarily in the forehead—obstruction by pathogenic factors of the yang brightness channels.
4. Obesity and shortness of breath after physical activity—qi deficiency.
5. Absence of fever or aversion to cold—no invasion of pathogenic factors on the surface of the body.
6. Pale, soft, and swollen tongue, with white, moist coating—insufficiency of yang qi.
7. Moderate pulse—insufficiency of antipathogenic factors.

Basic theory of case

In clinical practice a patient's inherent constitution can often be determined on the basis of their somatotype *(Fig. 2-3)*. Different somatotypes are associated with a tendency towards certain types of illness. For example, strong, muscular people do not easily fall ill, but when they do, it generally involves patterns of heat and excess. Slim, weak people on the other hand often suffer from deficiency, from which a pattern of either cold or heat may develop.

Among the defining aspects of somatotype are the following:

- Bone structure: strong or weak, thick or thin.
- Muscle quality: muscular people have well-defined muscles, whereas weak and slim people do not.
- Skin: moist, lustrous, soft, dry, or wrinkled.
- Thorax: wide or narrow.

In Chinese medicine, obese people often have yang deficiency, Spleen qi deficiency, or retention of dampness. Because the Spleen governs the muscles and limbs,

Fig. 2-3

	BASIC CONSTITUTIONAL CHARACTERISTICS	CHARACTERISTICS of ILLNESS	TREATMENT PRINCIPLE
NORMAL STRONG CONSTITUTION	Strong resistance	Acute disease, excess pattern, heat pattern	Expel pathogenic factors
OBESE PATIENTS	Deficiency of yang qi, easily accumulates dampness and produces phlegm	Damp-phlegm or damp-heat, Spleen qi deficiency	Strengthen the Spleen and expel dampness
EMACIATED PATIENTS	Deficiency of antipathogenic factors, easily catches illness	Chronic disease, deficiency pattern, and either cold or heat pattern	Strengthen the antipathogenic factors

obese people tend to require much more food essence and body fluids, which are supplied by the Spleen and Stomach, to nourish and support the muscles and limbs. They also need more yang qi to maintain proper circulation of qi and blood in the channels and collaterals, and to provide the energy required to support other physiological functions. Hence the Spleen and Stomach qi, and the yang qi of the body, may, in comparison with normal people, appear to be relatively deficient among those who are obese, with corresponding symptoms. When there is deficiency or insufficiency of Spleen and Stomach qi, the transportive aspect of water metabolism can diminish, resulting in retention of dampness or phlegm.

This does not imply, however, that all obese people will have this condition. Rather, it is only a tendency, and each case must be judged individually on the basis of whether the patient presents with the relevant symptoms.

Cause of disease

Pathogenic wind and cold

The patient's problem arose from exposure to wind. The disorder developed very quickly, and is aggravated at irregular intervals. This is evidence that it was caused by pathogenic wind, which can give rise to symptoms that vary in intensity and location, and that appear suddenly.

The main symptom is pain. Cold causes constriction of the tissues, vessels, and channels, leading to obstruction of the channels and collaterals, and thus pain. We may therefore conclude that this disorder was caused by pathogenic wind and cold.

Site of disease

Channels and collaterals

The symptoms are localized on one side of the face, and there are no apparent accompanying symptoms of a general nature. Thus the site of disease is the channels and collaterals.

Pathological change

As described above, obese people have a tendency towards Spleen qi deficiency, insufficiency of yang qi, or retention of dampness. In this case the patient is obese and suffers from shortness of breath after physical activity. This indicates that she already suffers from general qi deficiency, which means that her body resistance is weak and unable to ward off invasion by pathogenic factors. She is therefore easily affected by changes in the external environment. We may therefore conclude that pathogenic wind and cold invaded the channels and collaterals of the face, where they caused an obstruction of qi and blood. This resulted in pain, which is the main symptom here.

The leg yang brightness Stomach channel begins at the side of the nose. It proceeds upward, meeting the leg greater yang channel at the inner canthus, continues downward, and encircles the mouth and lips, where it connects with the teeth. It then passes through the lower edge of the mandible, turns upward, travels past the front of the ear to the hairline, and then reaches the forehead. The area of pain in this case is mainly on the right side of the forehead, as well as the nose, lips, and teeth. This clearly indicates that pathogenic wind and cold has invaded the leg yang brightness Stomach channel. Yet the invasion has affected only a portion of the channel, not the entire channel or the whole body surface: the patient exhibits no exterior symptoms of a general nature, such as fever or an aversion to cold.

Other signs in this case—including the pale, swollen, and soft tongue with a white, moist coating—do suggest qi and yang deficiency. However, the patient's appetite and bowel movements are both normal, demonstrating that the deficiency in the Spleen and Stomach is not significant, and there is no evidence of phlegm retention.

The sunken, moderate pulse reflects the inability of the deficient qi to properly circulate the blood.

Pattern of disease

This patient has a history of invasion by external pathogenic factors. As the symptoms are localized on the skin of the face, and there are no general symptoms such as fever or aversion to cold, the disorder is limited to the channels and collaterals, and thus pertains to a channel-collateral pattern.

When this patient came to the clinic she did not complain of thirst, nor did she have dry stools; her tongue was pale with a white, moist coating, and her pulse was moderate. This suggests a cold pattern.

Retention of wind and cold in the channels and collaterals indicates that the pathogenic factor is strong, hence a pattern of excess. And because the patient has a constitutional deficiency of yang qi, and suffers from shortness of breath after any physical exertion, there is deficiency. There are, accordingly, patterns of both deficiency and excess.

Additional notes

1. During the first stage of this disorder the skin on a portion of the patient's face was red, swollen, and covered by papulae. How is this explained in Chinese medicine?

When the patient's channels and collaterals were initially invaded by pathogenic wind and cold, the body's antipathogenic factors, that is, the qi and blood (especially the protective qi), were dispersed outward to the locality of the face to fend off the pathogenic factors. The struggle between the pathogenic and antipathogenic factors caused the face to become red and swollen. The appearance of the papulae was due to increased blood circulation, which enlarged the vessels on the surface of the skin.

If the symptoms were to disappear after the skin becomes red and swollen and the papulae appear, it would signify that the antipathogenic factors were strong, and were able to completely expel the pathogenic factors. In this case, however, the pain has continued, indicating that the antipathogenic factors are not strong enough to completely expel the pathogenic factors.

2. Is there any evidence of pathogenic dampness in this case?

This particular patient's disorder began while standing before a waterfall. The presence of the waterfall may lead one to conclude that there may have been an invasion of pathogenic dampness and water. There are three possibilities: an invasion of external dampness, wind-dampness, or cold-dampness.

As we know, diagnosis in Chinese medicine relies heavily on the evidence at hand. Dampness is a substantial pathogenic factor; it causes the yang qi of the body to stagnate, and has a heavy, turbid quality. When a patient is exposed to pathogenic dampness (including wind-dampness or cold-dampness) the main symptoms will involve local heaviness and pain, sometimes with the addition of a distending sensation. In this case there was a very rapid onset, indicating that wind is one of the pathogenic factors. Pain suggests the presence of cold, which can cause the qi and blood to stagnate, and in turn obstruct the channels and collaterals. However, there is no evidence of dampness in this case.

3. What distinguishes this case from the previous one?

There are many similarities between this case and the previous one, especially in the eight-principle diagnosis: both cases involve a disorder of the channels and collaterals, and a pattern of cold. The etiology of the previous case involved cold, while in this case there is both wind and cold.

The main difference is that in the previous case there was blood deficiency, while here there is qi and yang deficiency. Because qi and yang are both yang aspects of the body, while blood and yin pertain to yin, the treatment principles in these two cases are obviously different. No matter if one chooses acupuncture or herbs, a warming and heating method must be used for qi and yang deficiency in order to tonify the qi and yang of the body, expel the pathogenic factors, and strengthen the antipathogenic factors. The warming method would also be appropriate in the previous case, but one must be cautious to avoid using too much heat, as this can easily aggravate the blood disorder there.

Fig. 2-4

	CAUSE of DISEASE	SITE of DISEASE	SYMPTOMS	TREATMENT PRINCIPLE
CASE 5	Pathogenic cold	Channels and collaterals, blood deficiency	Continuous numbness	Nourish the blood, remove obstruction from channels and collaterals
CASE 6	Pathogenic wind and cold	Channels and collaterals, yang qi deficiency	Severe paroxysmal pain	Warm and tonify the yang qi, remove obstruction from channels and collaterals

Conclusion

1. According to the eight principles:
   Channel-collateral pattern, cold, and a combination of deficiency and excess.

2. According to etiology:
   Invasion of pathogenic wind and cold.

3. According to theory of channels and collaterals:
   Invasion of yang brightness channels and collaterals by wind-cold.

4. According to theory of qi, blood, and body fluids:
   Qi and yang deficiency.

Treatment principle

1. Tonify the qi and remove obstruction from the channels and collaterals.

2. Warm the yang and strengthen the Spleen.

Explanation of treatment principle

In the clinic various methods can be used to remove obstruction from the channels and collaterals. Where there is a pattern of excess in which a pathogenic factor blocks the channels and collaterals, the practitioner may choose to expel the pathogenic factor, regulate the qi, or remove the obstruction from the blood. Where there is a pattern of deficiency involving poor qi and blood circulation in the channels and collaterals, one must tonify the qi or nourish the blood.

In this case there is a combination of deficiency and excess. Both the invasion of the pathogenic factors and the deficiency of antipathogenic factors are associated with cold, thus the basic treatment principle is to use heat. One should warm the channels, collaterals, and yang qi of the body, remove the obstruction, and strengthen the antipathogenic factors. Strengthening the Spleen can help the antipathogenic factors in removing the pathogenic factors; the Spleen in this case was therefore strengthened, despite the fact that there was no Spleen deficiency.

Selection of points

GB-20 *(feng chi)*
jia cheng jiang (M-HN-18) [right side]
ST-7 *(xia guan)*
LI-4 *(he gu)*
ST-6 *(jia che)*
CV-12 *(zhong wan)*
LI-20 *(ying xiang)* [right side]
ST-36 *(zu san li)*

Explanation of points

GB-20 *(feng chi)* is used in treating exterior and interior wind patterns, which is fitting in light of the fact that the word wind *(fēng)* occurs in its name, along with *chí*, which means pool. Here *chí* means depression or hollow, referring to the point's location, which is in the depression between the insertions of the sternocleidomastoid and trapezius muscles. This point removes external or internal wind, disperses exterior patterns, and clears symptoms from the head. It can be used to treat many different types of head and facial disorders, as well as various wind patterns, including external and internal patterns. In this case the point is used for dispersing pathogenic wind and cold. This is the meeting point of the leg lesser yang channel and the yang linking vessel *(yáng wéi mài)*. Using the yang linking vessel in particular is helpful in removing exterior patterns when treating symptoms like aversion to cold and fever. In this case, while the main disorder is in the yang brightness channels, this point was chosen to capitalize on the ability of the lesser yang channels and yang linking vessel to expel the pathogens from the yang brightness channels. This is a very common clinical practice.

ST-7 *(xia guan)*. The word *xià* means below and *guān* means not only gate, but also critical junction. Here it implies something important, like a key or trigger. The point is located below the zygomatic arch, and serves an important function, hence its name. ST-7 *(xia guan)* disperses wind, clears pathogenic heat, and promotes the functioning of the joints and mind. In this case both sides are needled in order to regulate the yang brightness channels on both sides, and to help expel the pathogenic factors.

ST-6 *(jia che)*. In ancient times the mandible was called *jiá chē*. The name of this point refers to its location in the middle of the mandible. It promotes the functioning of the joints, removes obstruction from the channels and collaterals, alleviates pain, and relieves local swelling. In this case the point is used only on the right side as a local point.

LI-20 *(ying xiang)*. *Yíng* means to receive, and *xiāng* means fragrance. One of the functions of this point is to treat a diminished sense of smell or abnormal olfaction, hence the name. The point disperses pathogenic wind, clears heat, promotes the functioning of the nose, removes nasal obstruction, regulates qi, and removes obstruction from the channels and collaterals. It is a very important point for treating disorders of the face. Besides treating disorders of the nose (e.g., nasal obstruction, abnormal olfaction, nose bleeds), it can also be used to treat a wide variety of facial symptoms and disorders, including deviation of the mouth, facial pain, rashes, and muscular spasm. Here it is used as a local point to remove local obstruction and soothe the pain.

jia cheng jiang (M-HN-18) is a pair of miscellaneous points located 1 unit lateral to CV-24 *(cheng jiang)*, the terminal point of the conception vessel. These points disperse pathogenic wind, remove local obstruction, and assist the functioning of the channels and collaterals. They are used as local points to treat facial and trigeminal neuralgia, muscular spasms (facial tic), and ulcers of the gums. In clinical practice one or both sides may be used. These are very common points for symptoms in the lower area of the face, and especially for assisting the qi of the yang brightness channels in order to remove obstruction from these channels. In this case only the right side is used.

LI-4 *(he gu)*. *Hé* means joining and *gǔ* means valley; here the two words refer to an accumulation of muscles. The point is located in the middle of the first and second metacarpals, hence the name. It is the source point of the arm yang brightness Large Intestine channel and serves several very important functions:

- Removes pathogenic wind and relieves exterior patterns. It is very effective for treating the common cold, whether from wind-cold or wind-heat.
- Alleviates pain. This is an excellent point for removing obstruction from the channels and treating many types of painful patterns, including headache, toothache, facial, arm, and abdominal pain. It is also very commonly used in acupuncture anesthesia.
- Distant point. Besides treating disorders around the body in general, it can also treat disorders that follow the paths of the channels. It is especially good for facial complaints. It is therefore one of the four principal points, and one of the most commonly used acupoints in clinical practice.

The left arm yang brightness channel approaches the head from the left side and passes beneath the nose, then continues to the right-side LI-20 *(ying xiang)* where it terminates. The right arm channel proceeds in the opposite direction. When used as a distant point, one must determine on which side the disorder is located. For example, for a complaint on the right side of the face, use the left-side LI-4 *(he gu)* and vice versa.

   In this case all three functions of the point are employed in order to expel the pathogenic factors, alleviate the pain, and treat the facial problem. Although the disorder occurred in the right side of the face, the point is needled on both sides because of the patient's general condition, exposure to pathogenic cold, and both qi and yang deficiency.

CV-12 *(zhong wan)* is the alarm point of the Stomach and one of the eight meeting points of the yang Organs. It regulates the Organs of the middle burner, dispels blood stasis, and regulates qi. Because the point is primarily used to treat qi and yang deficiency, the tonifying needling method is utilized.

ST-36 *(zu san li)*. The word *zú* means leg or foot, *sān* means three, and *lǐ* means city or town, that is, a meeting place. *Lǐ* can also be a unit of measurement, roughly equivalent to one-third of a mile. The overall meaning of this point name is an accumulation of qi on the leg channel. (This contrasts with *shou san li* (LI-10), which means an accumulation of qi on the *arm* channel.) The word "three" refers to the location of the point three units below the kneecap or patella. This is the lower sea point of the leg yang brightness channel. It regulates and promotes the function of the Spleen and Stomach. It tonifies the antipathogenic factors, strengthens the basal qi of the body, and removes obstruction from the channels and collaterals. Like LI-4 *(he gu)*, it is one of the four principal points, and is especially well known for its ability to treat disorders of the Stomach and digestive system. It is one of the most commonly used points in clinical practice, and has shown particularly good results in treating disorders of the middle burner, such as stomachache, nausea, vomiting, abdominal distention, diarrhea, rumbling in the stomach, anorexia, food retention, and constipation. In this case the point is used to strengthen the Spleen and Stomach, treat the deficiency in the middle burner, and assist the body in expelling the pathogenic wind and cold from the channels and collaterals.

Combination of points

GB-20 *(feng chi)* and ST-7 *(xia guan)*. The first of these points is situated on the leg lesser yang channel, and its principal function is to remove wind and expel exterior patterns. It can also clear pathogenic factors from the head and eyes. The second point can be found on the leg yang brightness channel. It removes obstruction and stagnation from the channels and collaterals, and is very effective for treating local symptoms in the vicinity of the point. The function of this particular combination is to draw on the qi from the two channels to expel pathogenic factors and remove obstruction from the face and head.

ST-6 *(jia che)*, LI-20 *(ying xiang)*, and *jia cheng jiang* (M-HN-18). This compact group of points is used to treat disorders in the lower part of the face. ST-6 *(jia che)* and LI-20 *(ying xiang)* are both on yang brightness channels, the former on the Stomach channel, the latter on the Large Intestine channel. Because these two channels are rich in both qi and blood, these two points, together with *jia cheng jiang* (M-HN-18), serve as very strong local points. Together they regulate the qi and blood in the lower part of the face. This combination can treat nose, mouth, cheek, and tooth disorders, including such symptoms as pain, numbness, muscular spasms, or paralysis.

Follow-up

Because of the age of this patient, and the difficulty she experienced in coming to the clinic, the preferred plan of treating her three times a week was reduced to a more manageable regimen of once a week. After the first treatment the facial pain was considerably relieved, but she belched a lot (reversal of the Stomach qi), and the shortness of breath was obvious. The needling method for CV-12 *(zhong wan)* was accordingly changed to one of an even movement thereafter in order to treat the reversal of the Stomach qi. After two weeks' treatment the facial pain had more or less disappeared. The belching had likewise stopped, and the shortness of breath was improved, although there was still a feeling of breathlessness. CV-17 *(shan zhong)* was added to regulate the qi in the upper burner, promote the functioning of the Lung, and improve the shortness of breath. It was suggested that the patient control her diet to reduce her weight. She was asked to limit her intake of sugar and not eat much greasy food.

Another five treatments were given, once a week or once every other week. By then her weight had declined by almost 17.5 pounds (8 kilograms), the shortness of breath had disappeared, and there was no more facial pain. She experienced pain in her face only twice during this period, and both times it lasted only a very short time: once when she had diarrhea owing to food that disagreed with her while eating out, and again when she caught a head cold and the right side of her lips became a little painful. Both the diarrhea and the head cold cleared up quickly, and everything returned to normal. She was very satisfied with the treatment. Not long afterwards she moved and could not be followed up.

CASE 7: **Female, age 28**

Main complaint

Paralysis on the right side of the face and muscular tic

History

The disorder began three weeks after the patient gave birth. While she was breast feeding she suddenly developed a headache, an aversion to wind and cold, and discomfort and numbness on the right side of the face. She found that she could not close her right eye properly, and that it was dry and uncomfortable. The muscles in her face felt very tense. Her right ear was more sensitive than the left, and her mouth became deviated to the left. She felt that her sense of taste had diminished. However, there were few systemic problems. The exam revealed that the wrinkles on the right side of her forehead and the right nasolabial groove had disappeared. When she closed her eyes there was a 3mm gap between the eyelids of her right eye. When she was asked to show her teeth, two and a half could be seen on the right side, and five on the left. The right mastoid process was tender.

Tongue

Pale, with a thin, white coating

Pulse

Floating and tight

Preliminary diagnosis

At this stage, the diagnosis was right side peripheral facial paralysis. Because she was breast feeding, no conventional medicine was administered. There was not much improvement after three weeks, and the patient therefore turned to acupuncture (see below). After two weeks of treatment the facial paralysis was greatly alleviated. She came to the clinic twice thereafter, with long intervals between visits. The condition of the facial muscles continued to improve, and the movement of the muscles was almost back to normal.

Three months later the patient felt trembling in the muscles on the right side of her face and returned to the clinic. She had experienced this sensation for a week by the time she arrived. These muscles were very uncomfortable and tense. She also reported that she had involuntary muscular trembling, of varying duration, around the lateral side of the right eye, several times a day. She found that fatigue due to inadequate rest, physical exhaustion, or exposure to the cold to be precipitants. There was no local pain or swelling, and no redness.

Because of the time and energy she devoted to caring for her baby, she neither rested enough nor slept soundly at night. During the day she frequently felt dizzy and sometimes had palpitations, but because she felt that the symptoms were not very severe, she did not bother with treatment. Her appetite was normal, and she had no feeling of thirst. Her urination was normal, and her stools were slightly dry. She had one bowel movement every two or three days. Her complexion was pale, and the muscular force on both sides of her face was equal. The right palpebral fissure was slightly smaller than the left, an after effect of the facial paralysis.

Tongue

Pale, with a thin, white coating

Pulse

Thin

Analysis of symptoms

1. Occurrence of onset three weeks after childbirth—deficiency of blood.
2. Acute onset, accompanied by aversion to wind and cold—invasion of external pathogenic factor.
3. Right-side facial paralysis and deviation of the mouth and eye—obstruction of channels and collaterals.
4. Abnormal hearing and taste—malnourishment of the sensory orifices.
5. Discomfort and tension in the facial muscles, and trembling at the side of the eye during the past week—disturbance of internal wind caused by blood deficiency.
6. Occasional dizziness and palpitations—malnourishment of the spririt caused by blood deficiency.
7. Absence of thirst and normal urination—no retention of pathogenic heat.
8. Dry stools and bowel movements once every 2 to 3 days—failure of body fluids to moisten the Large Intestine.
9. Pale face and tongue—malnourishment caused by blood deficiency.

10. Thin, white tongue coating and floating pulse—disorder in the superficial part of the body.

11. Thin pulse—blood deficiency.

Basic theory of case

In Chinese medicine facial paralysis *(miàn tān)*, or paralysis of the facial muscles on one side of the face, is a mild form of windstroke. The channels and collaterals are invaded by wind, which means that the wind, or the wind plus cold, has invaded the superficial part of the channel and collateral system. This is known as a collateral or channel pattern. The symptoms are generally very localized, such as simple deviation of the mouth and eye, or an abnormal sensation in a localized area, such as numbness, slight weakness, or motor abnormality. The collateral type is the mildest category. The collaterals, which are branches of the channels, are most closely associated with the superficial parts of the body, and are thus most vulnerable. (A more detailed discussion can be found in the chapter on windstroke in *Acupuncture Patterns & Practice*.)

In China facial paralysis is one of the most commonly seen disorders in the traditional Chinese medical clinics, especially those clinics that specialize in acupuncture and moxibustion. Overall, the results of treatment are excellent. Most patients recover in a matter of weeks and there are basically no sequelae. However, some patients develop a muscular tic after recovering from their first onset of facial paralysis. This manifests as an episodic, involuntary trembling of the facial muscles, often at the side of the eye or mouth, or both. Precipitating factors include physical and mental stress, lack of rest, or exposure to wind and cold.

The typical cause of such a muscular tic is that, although the patient has recovered from a previous disorder, the pathogenic factor lingers in the body and in the channels; this can lead to other symptoms, which are different from the previous ones. Another cause is a situation in which the pathogenic factor has been removed but the antipathogenic factors (qi and blood) in the channels and collaterals have not recovered completely and are therefore not strong enough to ward off a *new* attack by a pathogenic factor. Or, the weakened state of the antipathogenic factors has led to malnourishment of the channels and collaterals, giving rise to internal wind.

Since the pathogenic factor is obstructing the channels and collaterals, and there is also deficiency of the antipathogenic factors, the treatment principle here is different from that of facial paralysis. Not only must the pathogenic factor be expelled, the antipathogenic factors must also be strengthened. The latter is the main treatment principle if the deficiency of the antipathogenic factors has resulted in internal wind.

Fig. 2-5

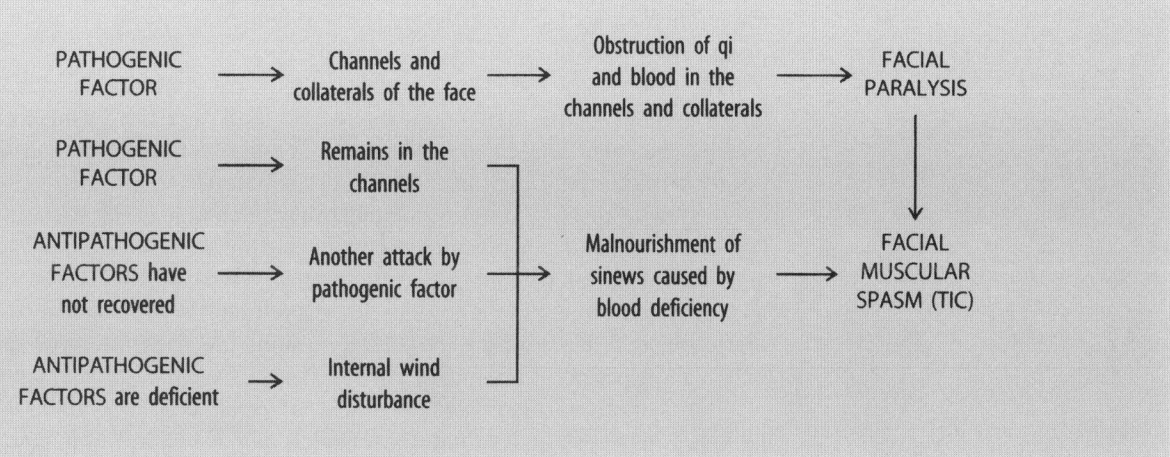

Cause of disease

1. Pathogenic wind

2. Deficiency of antipathogenic factors

The patient's initial onset was acute and accompanied by an aversion to wind and cold. The tongue coating was thin and white, and the pulse was floating and tight. All of these signs and symptoms are characteristic of an attack by pathogenic wind from the external environment.

While the main symptom of the second onset was a facial muscular tic, which may also be associated with pathogenic wind, this time the culprit was internal wind. Thus, although both onsets are associated with wind, it was a different type of wind each time.

Because wind is changeable, the symptom is also changeable. The accompanying general symptoms of dizziness, palpitations, dry stools, pale face and tongue, and thin pulse indicate that a deficiency of antipathogenic factors also played an important role in the development of the disorder.

Site of disease

Channels and collaterals

In the first stage of the disorder there was deviation of one side of the mouth and an eye, and the wrinkles on the right side of the forehead and the right nasolabial groove disappeared. There were few general symptoms. In the second stage there was facial muscular tension with trembling at the side of the right eye. All of this is evidence of a disorder of the channels and collaterals.

Pathological change

There are two groups of symptoms in this case. The first is associated with the initial occurrence, and the second with the subsequent disorder that arose three months later when the facial paralysis had almost been resolved.

The initial occurrence began three weeks after the patient gave birth to her baby. At this stage the antipathogenic factors (qi and blood) had not fully recovered from the rigors of childbirth, and, because of the insufficiency of protective qi, pathogenic wind easily invaded the surface of the body and occupied the channels and collaterals of the face. This disrupted the local circulation of qi and blood, which deprived the skin and muscles of nourishment. There was thus a loss of strength in the muscles on one side of the face, such that the patient was unable to fully close her lips and one eye, and her mouth was deviated toward the healthy side. Because the muscles and skin had become slack, the wrinkles on the affected side of the forehead and the ipsilateral nasolabial groove disappeared.

The sudden headache and tenderness in the mastoid process was due to the obstruction in the channels and collaterals caused by the invasion of pathogenic wind. The inability of the eyelid on the affected side to properly close has exposed the eye, which has become dry and uncomfortable. The poor circulation of qi and blood in the channels and collaterals has led to malnourishment of the ear and tongue, which accounts for the patient's hypersensitivity in the right ear, and her diminished sense of taste.

The pale tongue indicates blood deficiency, caused by childbirth, and the thin, white tongue coating and floating pulse suggest that the pathogenic factor has invaded the superficial level of the body. The tight nature of the pulse is evidence of an obstruction of qi in the channels and collaterals.

In view of these symptoms, the pathological change at the initial occurrence of this disorder mainly involved pathogenic wind invading the channels and collaterals. Apart from the pale tongue, there are few symptoms that would suggest a pattern of blood deficiency. The disorder is confined to the superficial level of the body, and is also very localized. This explains the patient's rapid recovery after only a short period of treatment.

The symptoms associated with the second occurence three months later included dizziness and palpitations, which suggest blood deficiency leading to malnourishment of the head and Heart spirit. The dry stools and infrequent bowel movements also indicate blood deficiency leading to a lack of body fluids to moisten the Large Intestine. Because the deficient blood cannot circulate properly to the upper part of the body, both the face and tongue appear pale, and because the blood does not fill the vessels as it should, the pulse is thin.

The reason for these symptoms is that the deficiency of blood following childbirth was aggravated by the patient's constant state of stress and exhaustion owing to lack of sleep and the continual attention required by her baby. This condition, on top of the previous right-side facial paralysis, led to the development of the episodic muscular tic. This time, however, there was no accompanying deviation of the mouth and eye. We can therefore conclude that the second disorder was not caused by an obstruction of the channels and collaterals, but by blood deficiency leading to malnourishment of the channels and collaterals.

The patient's facial paralysis was on the right side of the face, as was the subsequent muscular spasm. This is because the yin and blood deficiency which led to the malnourishment affected the already weakened part of the body. The absence of local pain, swelling, or redness means that there was no local obstruction of the channels and collaterals, nor was there a battle between the pathogenic and antipathogenic factors. The normality of the patient's appetite is evidence that the site of disease is not the middle burner. Moreover, the absence of thirst, the normal urination, and the white tongue coating reflect the absence of heat.

This analysis of the symptoms associated with the second occurrence underscores the differences between the pathological changes this time and that which occurred before. Although the two occurrences are related, the nature of the illness has changed in that there is no invasion by a pathogenic factor in the second occurrence.

Fig. 2-6

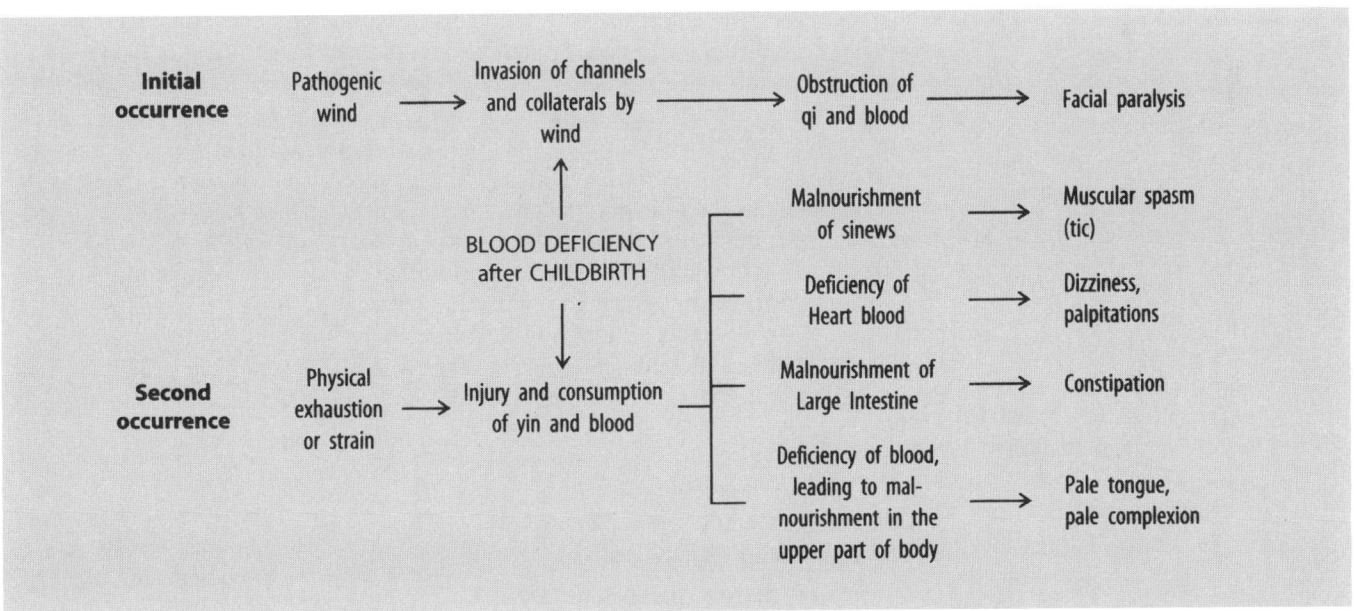

Pattern of disease | First onset:

The invasion of the collaterals on the body surface by pathogenic wind at the first onset pertains to a disorder of the channels and collaterals, and, according to the eight principles, to an exterior pattern. It is therefore a channel-collateral pattern.

The absence of fever, thirst, and heat symptoms, with a white tongue coating and a pulse that is not rapid, indicates a pattern of cold.

Since there is no evidence of symptoms that would indicate deficiency of the antipathogenic factors, we may conclude that the pattern is one of excess.

Second onset

There is no recent history of invasion by pathogenic factors, and no pathological change or corresponding symptoms involving external pathogenic factors residing in the channels and collaterals. It is thus an interior pattern.

The absence of local redness or swelling, the lack of thirst, the yellow color of the urine, and the pale tongue with a white coating are all indicative of a cold pattern.

The facial muscular tic as well as the symptoms involving the head, face, and Heart spirit may all be attributed to blood deficiency and the body's loss of proper nourishment. These symptoms are characteristic of deficiency.

Additional notes

1. Is there any evidence of invasion by external pathogenic factors during the second onset of the disorder?

While the patient has an episodic muscular tic on the right side of the face, there is no facial paralysis, reduction in strength, or pain. Hence there is no evidence of a pathological change that would be associated with the retention of an external pathogenic factor in the collaterals on the superficial level of the body, or with an obstruction of the channels and vessels. Since there is no record of exposure to external pathogenic factors in the history, we can rule out an invasion by external pathogenic factors in the diagnosis.

The muscular tic is the main symptom, a problem associated with wind, which can be either external or internal. Because of the obvious blood deficiency, however, it is this condition that accounts for the wind disturbance, and we may thus conclude that the wind in this case is of internal origin.

2. What is the main difference between this case and case 5?

While both cases are concerned with problems of blood deficiency, the pathological changes are different. In case 5, pathogenic cold obstructed the circulation of qi and blood, resulting in malnourishment of the channels and collaterals, which were deficient of blood. The symptoms in that case included an abnormal sensation on the face (numbness), a feeling that the skin was thicker than normal, a tingling sensation, and diminished sensitivity. In the present case, however, the deficiency of blood has led to malnourishment of the sinews, which has given rise to a disturbance of (internal) wind, with involuntary muscular spasms on the face.

Thus, while nourishing the blood is an essential principle of treatment in both cases, in case 5 it was necessary to remove the obstruction from the channels and collaterals, whereas in this case we must extinguish the wind in order to soften the sinews and facilitate their functioning. In other words, the treatment principle in both cases is similar, but the treatment methods are quite different.

Conclusion

First onset:

1. According to the eight principles:
   Channel-collateral pattern, cold, excess.

2. According to etiology:
   Invasion of external (pathogenic) wind.

3. According to theory of channels and collaterals:
   Invasion of the collaterals by external (pathogenic) wind.

Second onset:

1. According to the eight principles:
   Interior, cold, and deficiency.

2. According to etiology:
   Wind disturbance (internal wind).

3. According to theory of qi, blood, and body fluids:
Wind disturbance caused by blood deficiency.

Treatment principle

First onset:

1. Dispel external pathogenic wind.

2. Remove the obstruction from the collaterals.

Second onset:

1. Nourish the blood.

2. Extinguish the internal wind.

Explanation of treatment principle

In treating a disorder caused by external pathogenic wind, one must expel the pathogenic factor, as explained above. For treatment of internal wind, however, the patient's condition and diagnosis must be considered further. In most cases it is necessary to strengthen the antipathogenic factors. In this case, the second onset was due to (internal) wind disturbance. Because internal wind is associated with deficiency, the primary method of treatment here is to tonify the antipathogenic factors.

The basic pathological change is that the wind disturbance was caused by blood deficiency, and the sinews are accordingly malnourished. In Chinese medicine the Liver governs the sinews and is regarded as the "sea of blood." Patients with blood deficiency often have a deficiency of Liver blood; the emphasis in treatment is therefore often on nourishing the Liver blood. If the sinews can be nourished by Liver blood, the spasms, tension, and other symptoms associated with internal wind will be spontaneously relieved.

Results from tonifying the antipathogenic factors in the treatment of deficiency disorders do not take effect as quickly as the results of expelling pathogenic factors; the period of treatment is accordingly longer. Moreover, even after the symptoms have been relieved, a certain amount of additional treatment is required to strengthen the body so as to secure the result.

Selection of points

First onset prescription:

GB-20 *(feng chi)*
TB-23 *(si zhu kong)*
ST-7 *(xia guan)*
ST-4 *(di cang)*
GB-14 *(yang bai)*
ST-5 *(da ying)*
LI-20 *(ying xiang)*
LI-4 *(he gu)*

Second onset prescription:

GB-20 *(feng chi)*
ST-4 *(di cang)*
yu yao (M-HN-6)
CV-12 *(zhong wan)*
TB-23 *(si zhu kong)*
CV-4 *(guan yuan)*
GB-3 *(shang guan)*
ST-36 *(zu san li)*
LI-20 *(ying xiang)*
LR-3 *(tai chong)*

Explanation of points

GB-20 *(feng chi)* dispels pathogenic wind and obstruction from the channels and collaterals. Here the point is used primarily to dispel the external wind, and is therefore punctured only superficially. Its effect is to remove the pathogenic wind and cold from the surface of the body. The reducing method is used.

ST-7 *(xia guan)* dispels pathogenic wind, regulates qi, and removes obstruction from the joints and collaterals. In this case the point is used to expel wind and remove obstruction. It serves as a local point.

GB-14 *(yang bai)* is a meeting point of the Gallbladder channel and yang linking vessel, hence the word *yang* in the Chinese name. Because the point is used for treating various eye disorders, the word *bai* ("brightness") is also a part of the name. The point can be used to dispel pathogenic wind, promote the functioning of the eyes, and improve and strengthen the functioning of the Gallbladder. It is used in the treatment of such disorders as headache, vertigo, dizziness, paralysis of the eyelid muscles, muscular spasms, and night blindness. Here it is used to treat the dysfunction in opening and closing of the eyelid caused by the facial paralysis.

LI-20 *(ying xiang)* is the terminal point of the Large Intestine channel and a connecting point of both the arm and leg yang brightness channels. It is a very popular point for improving the sense of smell. It serves to dispel pathogenic wind, remove obstruction from the channels and collaterals, and promote the functioning of the nose. In practice it is commonly used to treat symptoms of facial paralysis (deviation of the mouth and disappearance of the nasolabial groove), facial pain and itchiness, nasal congestion, epistaxis, and poor or abnormal olfaction.

TB-23 *(si zhu kong)*. *Sī zhú* means very thin bamboo, and *kōng* means a depression on the surface of the body—a picturesque description of the location of this point, which is in a very shallow depression at the lateral end of the eyebrow. The point is used for treating pathogenic wind, alleviating pain, promoting the functioning of the head, clearing the eyes, and for disorders involving headaches, dizziness, red and sore eyes, and paralysis or tic of the eyelid. Horizontal puncturing is mainly used at this point.

ST-4 *(di cang)*. *Dì* means lower and *cāng* means a container for storing food. This point is located at both corners of the mouth, and is thus named because food enters the Stomach—where it is stored—via the mouth. The point serves to dispel pathogenic wind and remove obstruction from the channels and collaterals. It is very commonly used for treating facial paralysis, especially deviation of the corners of the mouth. It can also be used to treat facial pain or muscular tic (spasm).

ST-5 *(da ying)*. The word *dà* means big and *yíng* means abundance. These terms may be applied to this point, which is very rich in qi and blood. The point is located in the lower part of the face in an area through which the artery passes. This point serves to clear heat, dispel pathogenic wind, and resolve local swelling and pain. It is a very effective local point that can be used to treat deviation of the mouth, facial paralysis and muscular spasms, trismus, swelling of the cheeks, and toothache, among other disorders of the face. Besides serving as a local point, it can also be used as a distant point in the treatment of goiter in the neck, abdominal pain, and intestinal infections.

LI-4 *(he gu)* is the source point of the Large Intestine and a very important point for treating facial disorders. It serves to dispel pathogenic wind, relieve exterior patterns, clear obstruction from the channels and collaterals, and is very effective in alleviating pain. It yields excellent results when used in the treatment of facial disorders. It is very commonly used as a distant point.

Yu yao (M-HN-6) is located in the middle of the eyebrow, which is thought to be shaped like a fish, thus the name "fish waist." This point serves to remove obstruction, alleviate pain, clear the head and promote the functioning of the eyes. It is a commonly used miscellaneous point for facial and head disorders such as headache, eye diseases, facial paralysis affecting the eyes, muscular tic, toothache, and trigeminal neuralgia.

GB-3 *(shang guan)*. The word *shàng* means upper or above, referring to the location of this point, which is above the zygoma. *Yá guān* means "pass of the teeth." This point serves to remove obstruction from the joints, improve the functioning of the face, regulate the qi, and calm the spirit. It is very effective for treating migraine, deafness, tinnitus, deviation of the mouth and eyes, convulsions, and toothache.

CV-12 *(zhong wan)*. The *Great Compendium of Acupuncture and Moxibustion (Zhen jiu da cheng)* states that this is a meeting point of four channels: the arm greater and lesser yang channels, the leg yang brightness channel, and the conception vessel. This point serves to regulate the functioning of the middle burner, regulate the qi, and dispel blood stasis. Here it is used to regulate the qi and blood in order to help nourish the blood and dispel the wind.

CV-4 *(guan yuan)*. In this point name, *guān* means pivot or key, and *yuán* refers to basal qi. This is the alarm point of the Small Intestine and a meeting point of the conception vessel and the three leg yin channels. It serves to tonify the Kidney, strengthen basal qi, and nourish the blood. It can be used to treat various gynecological disorders such as irregular periods, excessive leukorrhea, disorders following childbirth, as well as patterns of deficiency. In this case there was a disturbance of internal wind due to childbirth that has resulted in blood deficiency. The point is used here to nourish the blood in order to extinguish the wind.

ST-36 *(zu san li)*. The *Classic of Nourishing Life with Acupuncture and Moxibustion (Zhen jiu zi sheng jing)* states that this point can be used to treat various deficiency patterns, especially those in which there is significant weight loss, or severe deficiency occasioned by a long-term illness. It is a very important point for treating general deficiency. It serves to regulate both qi and blood, strengthen the Spleen, harmonize the functions of the middle burner, and can thus assist the internal Organs in producing essence after childbirth (postnatal essence). It can also be used to strengthen the antipathogenic factors and basal qi, increasing the individual's ability to resist disease.

LR-3 *(tai chong)*. The word *tài* means very or big, and *tài chōng* means very important pass. It was given this name because it is a source and river point that is very rich in energy from the local vessels. This is the source point of the Liver channel. It serves to regulate the blood and spreads Liver qi. It is used to treat blood or yin deficiency leading to ascendant Liver yang or Liver wind. There is a very wide range of indications associated with this point, which basically consist of symptoms and disorders related to a dysfunction of the Liver in governing the free-flowing of qi, as well as a preponderance of Liver yang.

Combination of points   TB-23 *(si zhu kong)* and GB-14 *(yang bai)* are both located on lesser yang channels: the former is the terminal point of the arm lesser yang channel, the latter is on the leg lesser yang channel. Both points are very close to the eye. GB-14 *(yang bai)* is situated one unit above the midpoint of the eyebrow. When used in treating facial paralysis, the point is punctured horizontally, threading towards the upper eyelid. TB-23 *(si zhu kong)* is also punctured horizontally, but the direction is posterior and inferior. Both points are very capable of regulating qi, removing obstruction from the channels and collaterals, and improving the functioning of the sinews. In the treatment of facial paralysis, both are frequently used in treating paralysis of the muscles around the eyes, that is, when the eyelid cannot be closed. The two points can also be used in treating muscular spasms of the face.

TB-23 *(si zhu kong)* and *yu yao* (M-HN-6). The latter is a miscellaneous point located in the middle of the eyebrow. It can be used to relieve symptoms of the head, improve the functioning of the eyes, and to treat a variety of eye disorders and symptoms including both tic and paralysis of the eyelid. The puncturing method at this point must be gentle but quick, as this is a very sensitive point on the face.

 The functions of this combination are basically the same as that of the previous combination. This combination yields better results than the previous one for treating muscular tic of the eyelid. By contrast, GB-14 *(yang bai)* in the earlier combination is threaded a longer distance (through part of the frontals and upper part of the orbicular muscle of the eye, then into the upper eyelid) and is therefore an excellent choice for treating facial paralysis, as the needling can affect quite a large area of the muscles. Although the needling area is not as extensive, *yu yao* (M-HN-6) can be punctured perpendicularly or horizontally toward TB-23 *(si zhu kong),* and can bring very good results for treating muscular tic around the eyelid.

CV-12 *(zhong wan),* CV-4 *(guan yuan),* ST-36 *(zu san li),* and LR-3 *(tai chong).* This combination of four points serves to tonify the Liver and Kidney, tonify the qi, and nourish the blood. It is used in the treatment of several different types of deficiency. It can also be used to regulate the blood and disperse Liver qi or Liver wind. It is a very effective combination for treating a pattern involving both qi and blood deficiency, or qi and blood deficiency together with internal wind. These points are frequently combined and used in clinical practice, as they affect several Organs (Liver, Kidney, Small Intestine, Stomach, Spleen and Uterus) and channels (the arm greater and lesser yang channels, leg yang brightness, conception, and three leg yin channels). The combination is used primarily for treating disorders in the middle and lower burners, and for many different indications, including disorders of the digestive system, urinary system, menstruation, and genitals.

Herbal formula

During the later stage of the second onset (see below), the prepared herbal remedy Eight-Treasure Pill to Benefit Mothers *(ba zhen yi mu wan)* was prescribed. It is composed of the following ingredients:

Radix Rehmanniae Glutinosae Conquitae *(shu di huang)*
Radix Angelicae Sinensis *(dang gui)*
Herba Leonuri Heterophylli *(yi mu cao)*
Radix Paeoniae Lactiflorae *(bai shao)*
Radix Ligustici Chuanxiong *(chuan xiong)*
Radix Codonopsitis Pilosulae *(dang shen)*
Rhizoma Atractylodis Macrocephalae *(bai zhu)*
Sclerotium Poriae Cocos *(fu ling)*
Radix Glycyrrhizae Uralensis *(gan cao)*

Explanation of herbal formula

The function of this remedy is to tonify the qi and nourish the blood. Here it was used to assist the acupuncture treatment in nourishing the blood, extinguishing wind, and removing obstruction from the channels.

Follow-up

The first acupuncture prescription was used for the patient's initial disorder involving facial paralysis. She was treated once daily, six times a week. After two weeks the symptoms were largely alleviated: muscular tension was reduced, and the disability in closing the right eyelid and the deviation of the mouth had both resolved. Her hearing sensitivity and diminished sense of taste had likewise returned to normal.

When, after three months, the patient returned with the facial tic, the second acupuncture prescription was used. After four weeks of twice weekly treatments, the symptoms began to improve, the frequency of spasms associated with the tic around the lateral corner of the eye decreased, and the right side of the face became much more relaxed than before.

Acupuncture was continued for another three weeks, and the herbal remedy was introduced at this stage. The result was very good, but the patient caught a cold with a cough, nasal obstruction, and clear nasal discharge, which lasted for a week. There was no improvement in the muscular tic during this time. Use of the herbal remedy was temporarily stopped, but acupuncture continued. The cupping method was used at BL-12 *(feng men)* once daily for two days to dispel the wind and cold, warm the channels, and remove the external pathogenic factor.

When the cold symptoms had disappeared, acupuncture and herbs were used together for another three weeks, after which the symptoms had more or less disappeared. Acupuncture was terminated, but the herbal remedy was continued for another week. The patient was advised to return for a checkup if she decided to have another child within the next year or two.

One year later she did have a second pregnancy and came for a checkup. None of the symptoms recurred, and everything was normal after that childbirth.

CASE 8: **Male, age 48**

Main complaint

Pulling pain on the left side of the face and head

History

Three months ago the patient suddenly began to suffer from paralysis on the left side of the face. He was given acupuncture and herbs. After one month the symptoms more or less disappeared, and treatment was accordingly terminated, leaving him with only slight deviation of the mouth and left eye.

Thereafter he began to experience episodic pain with a pulling sensation, of short duration, on the left side of the face and head. At first the pain occurred only very occasionally and he paid little attention to it, but during the past week the attacks became more frequent and he came to the clinic for treatment. The attacks occur on a very irregular basis and there seems to be no precipitant. Because the pain is not too severe, the patient can tolerate it. During the attacks there are very slight muscular spasms on the left side of the face; during the intervals the muscles in the face and head remain tense and stiff, and there is some discomfort. The patient himself performs local massage.

The patient often suffers from dizziness or headaches, and sometimes experiences low frequency tinnitus, blurred vision, and numbness in the limbs. His appetite is normal. His mouth is dry and he tends to drink a lot of liquids. He does not sleep very soundly, often finds it difficult to fall asleep, and, when sleep finally comes, it is dream-disturbed. Bowel movements and urination are both normal.

Tongue

Red, with a thin, slightly yellow coating

Pulse

Sunken and wiry

Analysis of symptoms

1. History of facial paralysis on the left side—retention of pathogenic factor in the local channels and collaterals.
2. Episodic pulling pain on the left side of the face and head, stiffness and discomfort in the muscles—malnourishment of the sinews.
3. Muscular spasms on the left side of face during attacks of pulling pain—disturbance by Liver wind (internal wind).
4. General dizziness and tinnitus—malnourishment of the sensory organs.
5. Blurred vision and numbness in the limbs—insufficiency of yin and blood.
6. Dry mouth and thirst—deficiency of body fluids.
7. Unsound and dream-disturbed sleep—disturbance of Heart spirit.
8. Red tongue with slightly yellow coating—heat pattern.
9. Sunken pulse—interior pattern.
10. Wiry pulse—dysfunction of Liver qi.

Basic theory of case

Pain is a very common symptom and is often encountered in the clinic. When diagnosing pain, it is essential to note its location (orientation) and nature (qualitative analysis). By accurately locating the pain, one can determine its source. For example, a headache can be traced to a problem in a particular channel or collateral. Pain in the back, epigastric area, chest or stomach is often associated with a particular Organ. In order to judge the nature of pain, one must determine the reason for it. For example, a cold pain generally follows an invasion of pathogenic cold, and a burning pain may be encountered in the presence of pathogenic heat.

A pulling pain is one in which the skin feels as if it were being pulled or torn away; the local area also feels tense and constricted. The pain can be mild or very severe, and the attacks are episodic, coming at irregular intervals. This type of pain can be caused by malnourishment of the sinews, which are directly connected with the muscles and bones. The sinews rely on nourishment from the yin and blood to maintain their normal flexibility and contraction, and, when functioning correctly, they contribute to the body's agility. If any factor injures the yin or blood, the sinews will become malnourished, resulting in spasms that pull the tissues and muscles, causing a pulling pain and, in some cases, involuntary spasms and movement in the muscles.

In Chinese medicine the Liver stores the blood and is responsible for the sinews; sufficiency of Liver yin and blood is essential for the proper nourishment and functioning of the sinews. A pulling pain, spasms, trembling, numbness, and disability in movement of the limbs can all be caused by disorders of the sinews, owing to a lack of nourishment from deficiency of Liver blood or yin.

Fig. 2-7

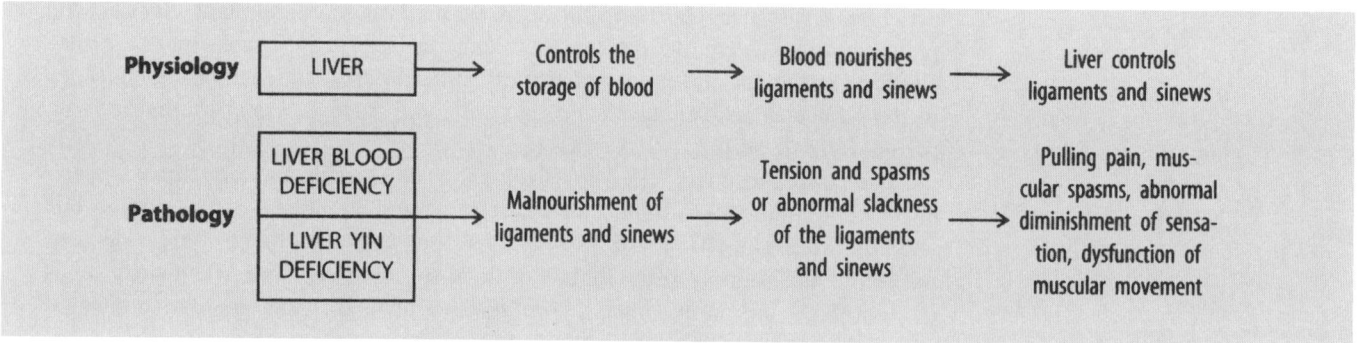

Cause of disease

Deficiency of yin and blood

The patient's episodic pulling pain on the face and head, and mild muscular trembling, are caused by abnormal contractions of the sinews resulting from deficiency of yin and blood. The dizziness, tinnitus, blurred vision, and numbness in the limbs are also evidence of malnourishment of the tissues.

Site of disease

Sinews and Liver

The patient has an episodic pulling pain on the left side of the face, together with local tension, discomfort, and muscular spasms. This is the main evidence to suggest a disorder of the sinews.

The blurred vision, tinnitus, and numbness of the limbs point to the Liver as the focus of the problem.

Pathological change

The sinews have a close relationship with the channels and collaterals. The twelve primary channels connect with them through the channel sinews *(jīng jīn)*. This means that the channels and collaterals allow the qi and blood to circulate into the sinews so that they can perform their activities throughout the body. A disorder of the channels and collaterals can affect the functioning of the sinews.

Here the patient has a previous history of paralysis on the left side of the face. This has left a very mild deviation of the mouth and left eye, which indicates an injury to the channels and collaterals. This history made the patient vulnerable to further injury caused by a variety of factors. At present the attacks of pain occur on the same side of the face as the paralysis; the pulling pain, muscular spasm, and tension indicate abnormal constriction of the sinews. This means that, besides the injury to the channels and collaterals, there is also malnourishment of the sinews, as well as a disturbance of wind. Because the pain is not very severe, in all probability the pattern is one of deficiency. The muscular spasms and tension indicate an interior disturbance of Liver wind.

With regard to the other symptoms, the frequent dizziness suggests malnourishment of the head and sensory orifices. The Gallbladder channel goes up, around, and through the ear before reaching the eye; the Liver channel rises and opens to the eye. The low frequency tinnitus and blurred vision suggest deficiency of yin and blood in the Liver and Gallbladder channels, leading to malnourishment of the ears and eyes. The numbness in the limbs is evidence of a lack of nourishment in the sinews, owing to deficiency of Liver yin and blood.

In summary, the basic pathological change in this case can be attributed to deficiency of Liver yin and blood.

The dry mouth and thirst indicate injury to the body fluids. The insomnia, dream-disturbed sleep, and difficulty in falling asleep result from a disturbance of spirit caused by fire from deficiency blazing upward. The red tongue and slightly yellow coating indicate a pattern of heat. The sunken, wiry pulse results from the imbalance of yin and yang in the Liver, which has disrupted the Liver qi.

Pattern of disease

This disorder was not caused by external pathogenic factors. The basic pathological change is that a dysfunction of the Liver yin and blood resulted in malnourishment of the sinews. The pattern is therefore interior.

The dry mouth, thirst, dream-disturbed sleep, red tongue, and yellow coating are evidence of heat.

The deficiency of yin and blood lead to malnourishment of the body. Because the symptoms in this case are mild, and in the absence of any evidence of an invasion or retention of pathogenic factors, we may safely conclude that this is a pattern of deficiency.

Additional notes

1. Why is it that external pathogenic factors were not involved in this case?

In practice, facial pain and abnormal sensations on the face are often caused by external pathogenic factors invading the channels and collaterals (see cases 5 and 6). Such cases are usually characterized by significant pain.

In this instance the pain is not very severe, which indicates that there is no specific obstruction in the channels and collaterals. Also the symptoms occur on an irregular basis, and there is no apparent precipitating factor. This suggests that the cause of the disease is not from the external environment. The fact that the patient has a pulling pain but not a cold pain indicates that cold has not been retained in the channels and collaterals; the symptoms are typical of malnourishment of the sinews. Thus, there is no evidence in this case of an invasion by external pathogenic factors.

2. Is there blood or yin deficiency?

Deficiency of Liver blood and deficiency of Liver yin can cause similar facial symptoms, as well as generalized symptoms around the body. What distinguishes these two patterns, that is, blood deficiency and yin deficiency, is the presence or absence of heat symptoms. A pattern of heat is associated with yin deficiency, but not with blood deficiency.

In this case the patient's mouth is dry, he tends to drink a lot, his sleep is dream-disturbed, and he has a red tongue with a yellow coating. These are all signs of heat from deficiency, thus Liver yin deficiency leading to internal wind is the problem. This also distinguishes this case from case 7, in which the wind disturbance is attributed to blood deficiency *(Fig. 2-8)*.

Fig. 2-8

	LIVER BLOOD DEFICIENCY	LIVER YIN DEFICIENCY
SIMILAR SYMPTOMS	Dizziness, tinnitus, insomnia, diminished or poor vision, trembling or muscular spasms either in the hands or feet, or generalized; thin pulse	
DISTINGUISHING SYMPTOMS	Absense of generalized heat, no thirst, pale complexion without normal luster	Tidal fevers or hot sensation, night sweats, restlessness, hot sensation in the chest, palms, and soles, dry mouth, malar flush
TONGUE and PULSE	Pale tongue with thin, white coating, thin or wiry and thin pulse	Red tongue with reduced moisture, thin and yellow coating, thin and rapid pulse or wiry, thin, and rapid pulse

Conclusion

1. According to the eight principles:
   Interior, heat, and deficiency.

2. According to etiology:
   Internal wind disturbance.

3. According to Organ theory:
   Liver yin deficiency and Liver wind disturbance (yin deficiency leading to internal wind).

Treatment principle

1. Nourish the yin and ease the Liver.

2. Nourish the sinews and soothe the spasms and pain.

Explanation of treatment principle

One of the Liver's functions is to store the blood, and the characteristics of this Organ are softness and gentleness. These pertain to the yin aspect. The Liver also governs the free-flowing of qi; the Liver qi function has the characteristic of rising and of being active. These characteristics pertain to the yang aspect. Thus, according to Chinese medicine, the Liver is said to have a combination of yin and yang aspects.

Liver disorders often manifest as deficiency of yin and blood; the Liver loses its yin-yang balance such that there is an excess or preponderance of yang and qi, that is, hyperfunction. This can result in disorders such as Liver qi attacking the Organs of the middle burner, ascendant Liver yang, or disturbance of internal Liver wind. This means that the Liver has lost its soft and gentle characteristics and has become hard.

The basic treatment principle is to nourish the yin and blood and balance the yang aspect of the Liver, that is, to control the preponderance of Liver yang or Liver qi, and to allow the Liver to recover its soft and gentle characteristics. In Chinese this procedure is referred to as softening or easing the Liver *(róu gān)*.

When Liver yin regains its effectiveness, the sinews will be properly nourished, and the general and facial symptoms will be spontaneously soothed.

Selection of points

GB-20 *(feng chi)*
TB-8 *(san yang luo)*
SI-18 *(quan liao)*
LR-6 *(zhong du)*
ST-4 *(di cang)*
LR-3 *(tai chong)*
GB-8 *(shuai gu)*

Explanation of points

GB-20 *(feng chi)* expels external and internal wind, removes exterior patterns, and clears symptoms and disorders from the head and eyes. This point is very effective for extinguishing internal wind, removing obstruction from the channels and collaterals, and relieving muscular spasms.

SI-18 *(quan liao)*. In Chinese, *quán* (as in *quán gǔ*) means zygoma, and *liáo* means a gap or space between the bones. This point is located in the depression below the zygoma, hence the name. The point serves to dispel pathogenic wind, reduce spasms and swellings, and relieve swelling. It is one of several important points for treating such facial disorders as deviation of the mouth and eyes, eyelid tic, toothache, and swelling of the face. In the ancient classic *Illustrated Manual on the Points for Acupuncture and Moxibustion as Found on the Bronze Figure (Tong ren shu xue zhen jiu tu jing)* it is mentioned that this is a meeting point of the arm lesser yang Triple Burner channel and the arm greater yang Small Intestine channel. This point can thus use the qi from both of these channels to treat different types of disorders of the face. The interior wind in this case can be attributed to deficiency of terminal yin. Because the lesser yang channel is both exteriorly and interiorly related to the terminal yin channel, this point makes use of the lesser yang channel to extinguish the internal wind and thus eliminate the facial tic.

ST-4 *(di cang)*. *Dì* means earth and by connotation "low," while *cāng* means a container for storing food. This point is located just beside the mouth, through which food must pass to enter the Stomach. It serves to remove obstruction and stagnation from the channels and vessels, expel pathogenic wind, and treat disorders of the lower part of the face, such as deviation of the mouth, soreness and swelling of the lips, excessive saliva, muscular tic around the corners of the mouth and/or eyelid, and facial pain. In this case it is used as a local point.

GB-8 *(shuai gu)*. The word *shuài* means commander, and *gǔ* in this context means mountain valley. The point is located above the ear, on the highest part of the bone, hence the name. The point promotes the function of the Liver in governing the free-flowing of qi, extinguishes Liver wind, promotes the function of the Gallbladder, clears heat, and dispels wind. Besides being used for treating a pattern of generalized wind, it can also treat disorders on the lateral side of the head, such as migraine. It is commonly prescribed for such problems as childood convulsions, restlessness and fullness in the chest and abdominal region, vomiting, and nausea. Here the point is used to help clear heat, extinguish wind caused by the Liver yin deficiency, regulate the qi, alleviate the pain on the lateral side of the head, eliminate the muscular tic, and relieve the tension.

TB-8 *(san yang luo)* is associated with the three arm yang channels, hence its name, which literally means three yang connection. It serves to promote the qi and blood, remove obstruction from the channels and collaterals, extinguish wind, and relieve pain. Besides acting as a local point, it can also serve as a distant point for the treatment of disorders on the side of the head. Here it is used as a distant point to regulate the qi and blood, clear the heat, and extinguish the wind.

LR-6 *(zhong du)*, or "middle place," is located on the medial aspect of the tibia. It is the accumulating point of the leg terminal yin channel. Apart from being used for treating acute patterns and disorders involving the Liver and Gallbladder, it is also used for regulating Liver qi and Liver blood. This function is employed here to treat the deficiency of Liver blood, which has caused the internal wind.

LR-3 *(tai chong)* is the source and stream point of the Liver channel. It serves to dispel Liver wind, control convulsions, drain heat, and regulate the blood. It is one of the most commonly used points in clinical practice, and is frequently used to treat disorders associated with the Liver and Gallbladder. It can be used as a distant point, and is very effective in the treatment of headache, dizziness, vertigo, seizures, manic disorders, and pain. Here it is used to ease the Liver and extinguish the Liver wind in order to treat the pain and muscular spasms.

Combination of points

SI-18 *(quan liao)*, ST-4 *(di cang)*, and GB-8 *(shuai gu)*. The first point is associated with the arm greater yang channel, ST-4 *(di cang)* with the leg yang brightness channel, and GB-8 *(shuai gu)* with the leg lesser yang channel. This group of points is used only for the treatment of face and head disorders. The points use the qi from the different yang channels to regulate the qi and blood in the face, and to remove obstruction from the channels and collaterals. GB-8 *(shuai gu)* is located on the upper part of the head, SI-18 *(quan liao)* in the middle of the face, and ST-4 *(di cang)* on the lower part of the face. Even though there are only three points, they are distributed over a relatively large area and are therefore very effective for treating facial disorders. All three points are punctured perpendicularly. Because SI-18 *(quan liao)* is in the middle of the face, it can be punctured to a depth of between 0.8 to 1 unit, and the reducing method is used to dispel the wind, eliminate the pain, and relieve the muscular spasms. ST-4 *(di cang)* can be punctured only to a depth of 0.3 to 0.5 units. Because GB-8 *(shuai gu)* is close to the bone, it must be punctured to a depth of only 0.2 to 0.3 units.

LR-6 *(zhong du)* and LR-3 *(tai chong)* are both on the Liver channel. The former is the accumulating point, and the latter the source point, of the channel. Both are excellent for calming Liver qi or Liver yang, and also serve to dispel internal wind. They are especially helpful in treating internal wind caused by Liver yin and Liver blood deficiency. However, because the cause of internal wind pertains to deficiency, we must be very cautious and avoid strong stimulation, which could further injure the Liver. In this case, even, balanced manipulation of the needle is used at both points. However, if the points are used for treating wind in a pattern of excess, the intensity of the needling may be increased. In other words, the method of needling is based on the nature of the disorder.

Basic herbal formula

Linking Decoction *(yi guan jian)* was originally prescribed for the treatment of Liver yin deficiency, or Liver yin deficiency accompanied by disharmony between the Liver and Spleen (Stomach). The formula contains the following ingredients:

Radix Rehmanniae Glutinosae *(sheng di huang)* 30g
Tuber Ophiopogonis Japonici *(mai men dong)* 10g
Fructus Lycii *(gou qi zi)* 12g
Radix Angelicae Sinensis *(dang gui)* 10g
Radix Adenophorae seu Glehniae *(sha shen)* 10g
Fructus Meliae Toosendan *(chuan lian zi)* 5g

The indications of this formula include pain in the intercostal , hypochondrial, epigastric, and abdominal regions, dry mouth and throat, poor appetite, dry and red tongue, and a thin, wiry pulse. The pathology associated with this pattern is yin and blood deficiency leading to dysfunction of the Liver in governing the free-flow of qi, which transversely affects the function of the middle burner.

Explanation of basic herbal formula

In this formula a fairly heavy dosage of Radix Rehmanniae Glutinosae *(sheng di huang)* is used, since here it serves as the chief herb. It is sweet and cold, associated with the Liver and Kidney channels, and nourishes Liver and Kidney yin. Fructus Lycii *(gou qi zi)* and Radix Angelicae Sinensis *(dang gui)* are the deputy herbs. The former is sweet and neutral, is associated with the Liver and Kidney channels, and nourishes the yin of the body. The latter is sweet and warm, is associated with the Liver and Spleen channels, and nourishes the blood. These two herbs assist in softening (easing) the Liver.

Radix Adenophorae seu Glehniae *(sha shen)*, Tuber Ophiopogonis Japonici *(mai men dong)*, and Fructus Meliae Toosendan *(chuan lian zi)* serve as both assistant and envoy herbs. The first two are sweet and cold, and assist the chief and deputy herbs in nourishing the yin of the body. A very small dosage of Fructus Meliae Toosendan *(chuan lian zi)* is included. It is bitter and cold, is associated with the Liver and Stomach channels, and promotes the function of the Liver in governing the free-flow of qi.

Modified herbal formula

Radix Rehmanniae Glutinosae Conquitae *(shu di huang)* 30g

Fructus Tribuli Terrestris *(bai ji li)* 10g

Fructus Lycii *(gou qi zi)* 15g

Flos Chrysanthemi Morifolii *(ju hua)* 10g

Radix Angelicae Sinensis *(dang gui)* 12g

Bombyx Batryticatus *(jiang can)* 6g

Lumbricus *(di long)* 6g

Explanation of modified herbal formula

Because there is yin deficiency and malnourishment of the sinews in this case, Linking Decoction *(yi guan jian)* is used as the basic formula, with modifications, in order to nourish the Liver yin.

We are mainly concerned with Liver yin and blood deficiency in this case, and there is no disharmony between the Liver and Spleen (Stomach). However, because the main symptoms involve spasms (tic) caused by malnourishment of the sinews, three of the herbs in Linking Decoction *(yi guan jian)* appear in the modified formula. These are the herbs that nourish the Liver and Kidney yin, although Radix Rehmanniae Glutinosae *(sheng di huang)* is replaced by Radix Rehmanniae Glutinosae Conquitae *(shu di huang)* in order to strengthen the function of nourishing the yin and blood. Four new herbs are added to extinguish the wind and relieve the spasms. All four herbs are associated with the Liver channel, and, combined with those for nourishing the yin, they soften (ease) the Liver and regulate the Liver qi while relieving the spasms in the sinews. The purpose here is to treat the manifestations and the root of the disorder together.

Follow-up

Because this patient was very busy at work he was given just one acupuncture treatment, followed by the herbal remedy. After acupuncture the pulling pain in the face disappeared and the patient said that he was very happy with the result. He was then asked to take one dose of the herbal remedy, divided into two half doses, every day for two weeks in order to deal with the yin and blood deficiency. Afterwards the patient experienced no more pain in the face, and the numbness in the limbs and dizziness were greatly alleviated. The herbal remedy was continued for another two weeks, and taken in the same manner. By then, all the symptoms had disappeared and the treatment was terminated. In a one-year follow-up there were no further occurrences of the symptoms.

In clinical practice the combination of herbal remedies and acupuncture is very common. This combination is often likened in Chinese medical literature to "walking on two legs." In this case, because the patient was too busy at work and could not regularly come to the clinic to receive acupuncture (even though it relieved the symptoms), he did take the herbal remedy, which was a good decision, since it also treated the root of the disorder. Cases like this are frequently encountered in China. If a patient is old, has problems with mobility, or cannot afford lengthy treatment, the combination of acupuncture and herbs can reduce the burden on the individual and still treat the disease very well.

Diagnostic Principles for Facial Disorders

Facial pain frequently occurs independently, although it sometimes accompanies or is related to facial spasms or paralysis. Because these conditions have similar causes and pathologies, they can affect each other.

Cause of disease

The most common cause of facial pain is an invasion by one or more of the six external pathogenic factors, of which pathogenic wind is the main one. As wind is a yang pathogenic factor, it tends to affect the yang aspects of the body, causing disorders of the upper part of the body, head, or face. When wind invades the skin, interstices, and pores *(zòu lǐ)* and resides in the superficial channel and collateral system, it can obstruct the normal circulation of qi and blood, causing facial pain. Because wind moves quickly and is changeable by nature, disorders caused by pathogenic wind attack suddenly, and exhibit rapidly changeable symptoms. There can thus be sudden attacks of facial pain when pathogenic wind obstructs the channel and collateral system. Although the affected area may be relatively limited, quite often patients are unable to pinpoint the exact spot and can only indicate the general area

As mentioned elsewhere, wind, in Chinese medicine, is the principal pathogenic factor *(bǎi bìng zhī zhǎng)*. Because other pathogenic factors frequently combine with wind, one may see wind combined with cold or dampness invade the body, causing facial pain. This is a common occurrence in the clinic.

Cold constricts, thus wind combined with cold can constrict the channels and collaterals, and the pain is usually rather severe. Dampness is characteristically heavy and turbid. When wind-dampness invades the channel system, facial pain with a heavy, distending quality results. Wind-heat (or wind-fire) is another common cause of facial pain. Heat or fire can injure the channels and collaterals and consume the body fluids, resulting in a burning pain, or a purely burning sensation, accompanied by dry mouth and throat, or even dry skin.

Besides the six external pathogenic factors, another cause of facial pain is deficiency of antipathogenic factors, especially of qi and blood in the channel and collateral system. Deficiency of antipathogenic factors on one hand means that external pathogenic factors can easily invade the channel and collateral system; on the other hand, it can be the direct cause of the disorder. Deficiency of yin and blood is most commonly encountered. This causes malnourishment of the channels, collaterals, sinews and muscles, which results in facial spasms or pain. This condition is also frequently seen in patients who develop facial pain after a history of facial paralysis.

Site of disease and pathological change

The site of disease for facial pain is the superficial level of the channel and collateral system. In certain cases the deeper levels of the channel system, or even the sinews and muscles, may be affected. The basic pathological change is either excess or deficiency. An invasion by an external pathogenic factor will lead to a pattern of excess whereby the pathogenic factor obstructs the passage of qi and blood in the channels and collaterals, which results in pain. Thus, treatment involves expelling the pathogenic factor in order to remove the obstruction from the channels and collaterals.

On the other hand, yin and blood deficiency can result in a pattern of deficiency, because the channels and collaterals do not receive sufficient nourishment from yin and blood. Deficiency also causes poor circulation, and thus poor nourishment of the sinews and muscles. Internal wind, which results from a condition of deficiency, causes facial disorders. For deficiency it is necessary to nourish the yin and blood, and extinguish the internal wind.

Deficiency of antipathogenic factors is the cause of malnourishment of the channels and collaterals, which, combined with an invasion by pathogenic factors, can lead to a combined pattern of deficiency and excess. In such cases, not only is there deficiency of qi and blood, but also obstruction of the channels and collaterals. When this occurs, treatment must focus on both aspects *(Fig. 2-9)*.

Diagnostic procedure

In most cases, we can determine whether the nature of a disease is deficient or excessive based on the history. Patterns of excess generally show a history of exposure to pathogenic factors; the disorder only occurs anew and lasts a short while. A pattern of deficiency, on the other hand, usually lasts a long time, or the facial pain is secondary to some other disorder. See *Fig. 2-10*.

Fig. 2-9

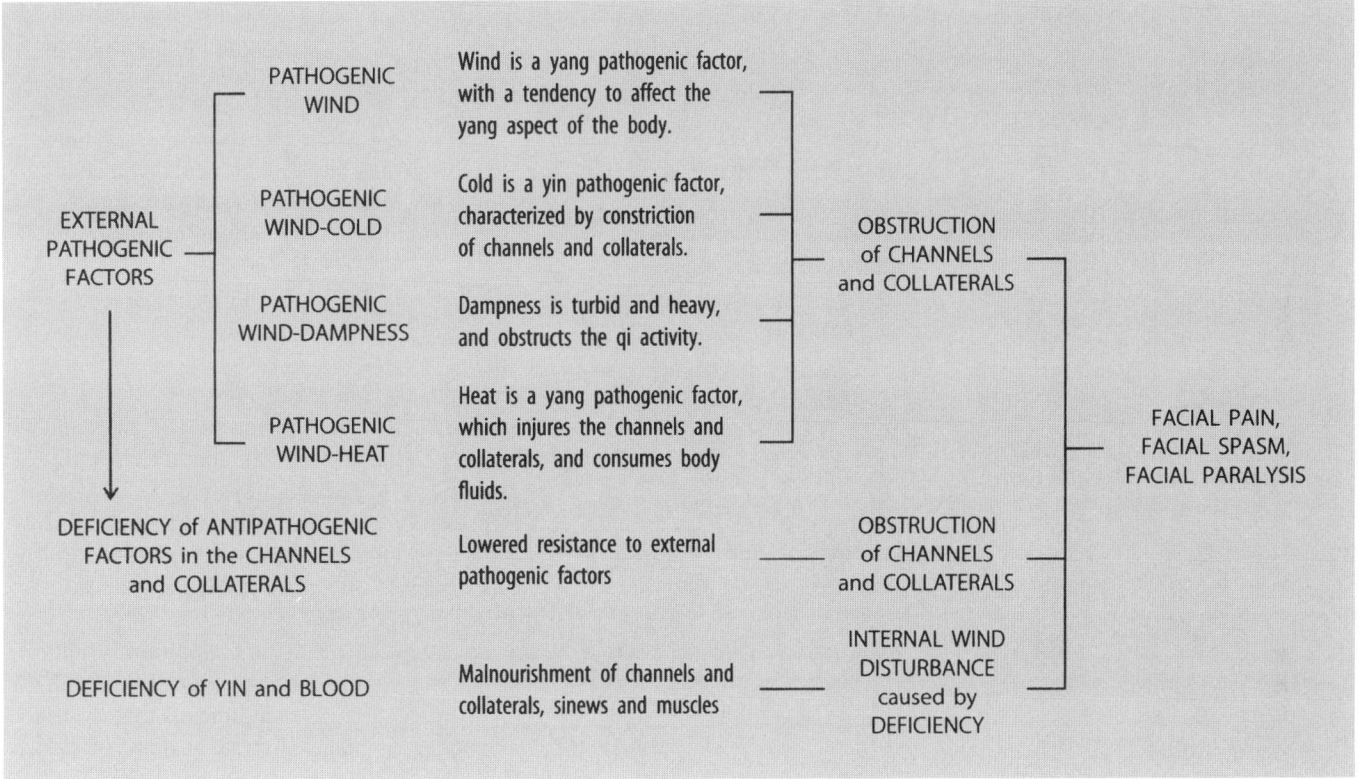

Fig. 2-10

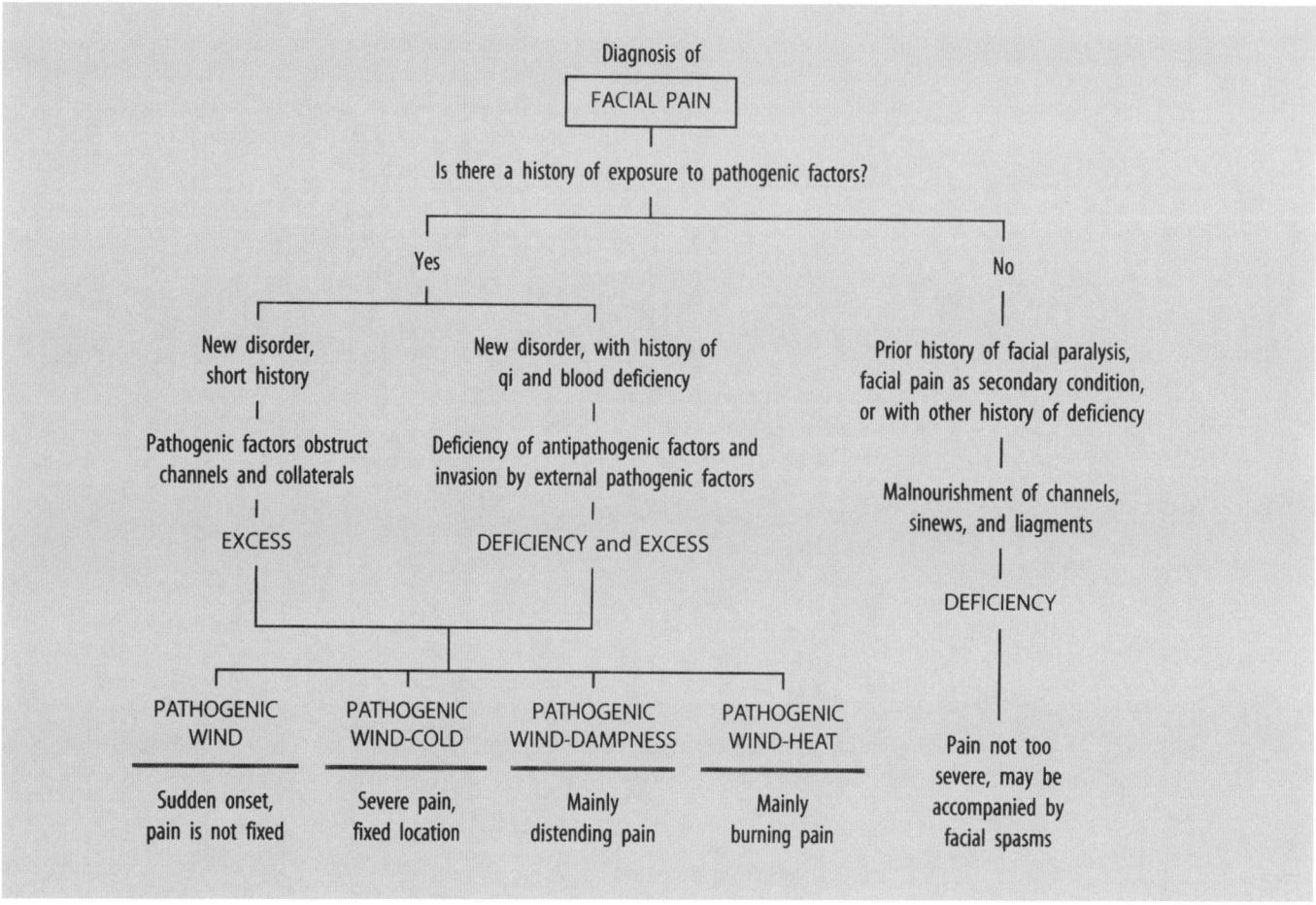

Diagnosis of

FACIAL PAIN

Is there a history of exposure to pathogenic factors?

Yes

No

New disorder,
short history

New disorder, with history of
qi and blood deficiency

Prior history of facial paralysis,
facial pain as secondary condition,
or with other history of deficiency

Pathogenic factors obstruct
channels and collaterals

Deficiency of antipathogenic factors and
invasion by external pathogenic factors

Malnourishment of channels,
sinews, and liagments

EXCESS

DEFICIENCY and EXCESS

DEFICIENCY

PATHOGENIC
WIND

PATHOGENIC
WIND-COLD

PATHOGENIC
WIND-DAMPNESS

PATHOGENIC
WIND-HEAT

Sudden onset,
pain is not fixed

Severe pain,
fixed location

Mainly
distending pain

Mainly
burning pain

Pain not too
severe, may be
accompanied by
facial spasms

Poor Appetite

CASE 9: **Male, age 48**

Poor appetite

The patient reported that his poor appetite started two-and-a-half years ago. It began when he experienced a very strong emotional upset following a period of intense anger. He felt a distended sensation and pain in the intercostal and hypochondrial regions, and a noticeable decrease in appetite. He suffered from indigestion after he ate. Initially he would have one to three bowel movements a day, but the quantity of stool was always very small. His stools were not loose and he passed a lot of gas. He frequently belched. A conventional medical checkup revealed no organic disorder. At that time he underwent one acupuncture treatment; his bowel movements improved initially, but later the symptoms returned. He then tried an herbal remedy, but the results were not very satisfactory, and the treatment was discontinued.

When he returned to the clinic on this occassion, he complained that his appetite was still poor. He was never hungry and felt that the abdominal distention after eating had become worse. He tended to drink a lot of water. His sleep was sometimes good and sometimes bad. He often had difficulty falling asleep. His energy level was very poor, and he felt very weak physically. He had not worked for over a year. He said that he had the belching problem for over twenty years. At one stage he had used a Chinese herbal tonic, but the digestive symptoms became worse and he therefore stopped taking it. The quantity of his urine tended to be less than normal, and was sometimes yellowish in color. His stools are slightly dry and contain particles of undigested food. He feels weak and sore in the lower back. During the past two weeks he has been suffering from a bad cold, and still has a slightly productive cough.

Dark with a red tip, slightly swollen body, and a thin, slightly yellow coating

Sunken, wiry, and slippery. The left pulse is thin and forceless, especially at the left proximal position.

1. Onset of illness after emotional upset (anger)—qi stagnation.
2. Poor appetite, poor digestion, and abdominal distention after eating—disruption of the Spleen's transportive and transformative functions.

3. Stifling sensation in the chest, distention in the abdominal and hypochondrial regions, belching, and excessive passing of gas—stagnant qi.

4. Poor energy and fatigue—qi deficiency.

5. Undigested food in the stools—dysfunction in the transportation and transformation of food.

6. Dark tongue with swollen body—poor circulation of qi and blood.

7. Sunken, wiry pulse—stagnant qi.

8. Thin, forceless pulse on the left—deficiency of antipathogenic factors.

Basic theory of case

According to Chinese medicine the Spleen and Liver are closely related physiologically and pathologically. A disorder of the Liver can affect the Spleen, and vice versa. In the next chapter, abdominal pain associated with disharmony between the Liver and Spleen will be discussed. In this chapter we will focus on some symptoms associated with the digestive system and appetite.

The Spleen and Stomach are responsible for the transportation and transformation of food, that is, for digestion. However, the activities of the two Organs differ. As the Spleen is responsible for the ascent of clear yang, it follows that the normal directional movement of Spleen qi is upward. Conversely, the Stomach is responsible for the descent of turbid yin, and the normal directional movement of Stomach qi is accordingly downward. The purpose underlying the harmonious activity of these two Organs is to digest food, and to transform both food and water into essence, which can then be transported to all the Organs. After digestion, waste must be removed from the body. The basic process of metabolism is to absorb and dispense nutrition on the one hand, and to remove waste from the body on the other. When the metabolic system is working normally, one will have a good appetite, normal digestion, and good physical and mental energy. Bowel movements will occur with normal frequency, and stools will be of a normal quantity.

The Liver is responsible for the free-flow of qi, and also for balancing and regulating the qi activity of the entire body, including the ascending and descending activities of the Spleen and Stomach. If the Liver's function in regulating the free-flow of qi is impaired, it could interfere with the Spleen's activities, such that food will not be transformed into essence, which nourishes the Organs. Thus the patient will develop symptoms relating to a change of appetite and digestion. When Liver dysfunction interferes with the Stomach's activity in the downward-movement of turbid yin, after digestion the feces and gas will not be released from the body in a timely manner, causing waste to accumulate in the body. If this condition worsens, the Stomach qi can reverse and the patient will have symptoms like hiccups, belching, nausea, regurgitation, vomiting, and foul breath with a smell of undigested food.

Fig. 3-1

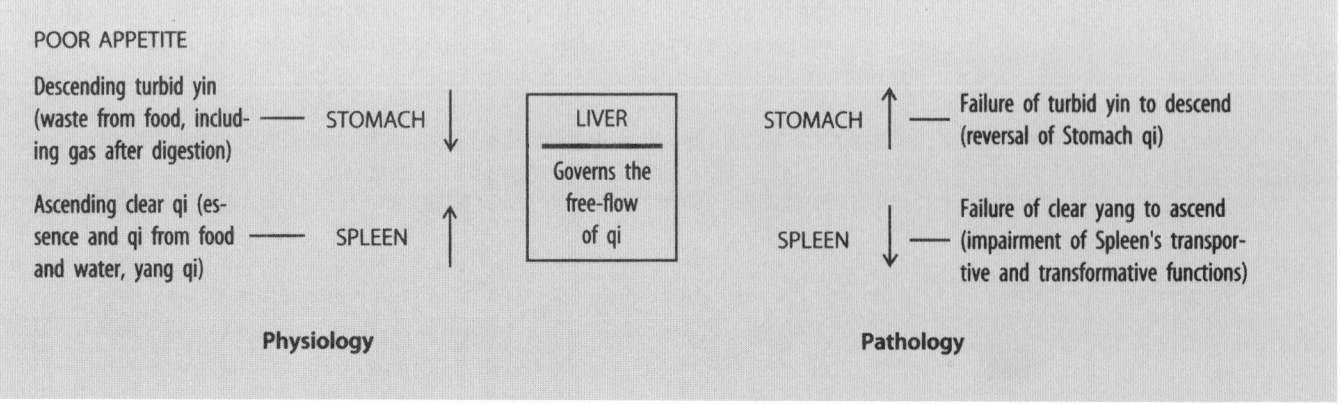

POOR APPETITE

| Physiology | | Pathology |

Descending turbid yin (waste from food, including gas after digestion) — STOMACH ↓

Ascending clear qi (essence and qi from food and water, yang qi) — SPLEEN ↑

LIVER
Governs the free-flow of qi

STOMACH ↑ — Failure of turbid yin to descend (reversal of Stomach qi)

SPLEEN ↓ — Failure of clear yang to ascend (impairment of Spleen's transportive and transformative functions)

Cause of disease	Emotional upset

The patient's history of illness commenced after a period of intense anger. This strong emotional upset led to a disorder of the qi activity and functions of the Organs. Emotional upset is therefore the apparent cause of the illness.

Site of disease	Spleen, Liver, and Stomach

The patient has a poor appetite, abdominal distention, indigestion, and stools containing undigested food, all of which is evidence of a Spleen disorder.

That the problem arose after a bout of intense anger, and there is pain and distention in the hypochondrial and intercostal regions, is indicative of a Liver disorder.

Belching for such a long period of time suggests a Stomach disorder.

Pathological change

The Liver helps regulate the emotions. A strong emotional upset may affect the normal circulation of qi and blood, impairing the Liver's ability to maintain the free-flow of qi, and leading to stagnation of Liver qi. This will usually affect the area around the Liver itself, and those areas through which the Liver channel passes. Thus the hypochondrial and intercostal regions may be affected by Liver stagnation, manifested as a distended, painful sensation in these areas.

Liver qi stagnation can also affect the Spleen and Stomach, disrupting the ascending and descending of qi, and impairing the Spleen's ability to transform and transport food. One may then experience reduced appetite, abdominal distention (especially after eating), and poor digestion. When the functions of the Spleen and Stomach are impaired, food cannot be digested properly, and the absorption of nutrients is interrupted. Food simply passes through the Intestines and is evacuated from the body. The frequency of bowel movements thereby increases, and stools will contain particles of undigested food.

Similarly, disruption in the downward movement of Stomach qi will prevent the turbid yin and qi from moving out of the abdomen. Instead, it will accumulate in the Stomach, and in a severe case will reverse in an upward direction, causing frequent belching and the passing of an excessive amount of gas.

Fig. 3-2

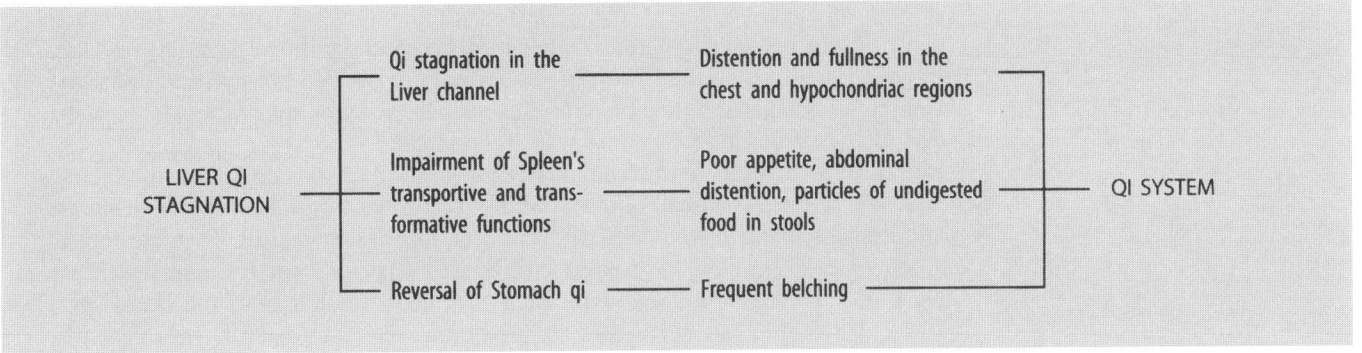

As a result of the prolonged illness in this case, the production of qi and blood has declined, causing a deficiency of qi. Malnourishment of the limbs, muscles, and Organs has led to physical fatigue, and to soreness and weakness in the lower back. The patient's sleep is very unstable—sometimes good, sometimes bad. This is a reaction to the undernourished Heart spirit.

From an analysis of the symptoms we may conclude that the main pathological change is in the qi system. And because of the interrelationship between qi and blood, the disruption in the circulation of blood can be attributed to the impaired circulation of qi as well. The tongue is dark and only slightly swollen, indicating that qi deficiency is the main problem, and that the blood has not been severely affected.

The weakness of the Spleen in transforming and transporting food has led to a diminished appetite. With less food entering the Stomach, there is no severe retention of food there. The main problem is qi stagnation. This explains why the tongue coating is not very thick, a condition found in many patients with digestive problems.

The sunken, wiry pulse indicates a dysfunction in the Liver's ability to regulate the free-flow of qi, and a resulting disruption in qi activity. The left pulse is thin and forceless, indicating deficiency of qi and blood, such that the vessels cannot be properly filled.

The patient's emotional state appears to have stabilized. The main problem is the dysfunction in the digestive system, and the diagnosis therefore points toward a disorder in the Spleen and Stomach. Yet the impaired ability of the Liver to regulate the free-flow of qi also has some bearing on the patient's condition.

Pattern of disease

This is an interior pattern. Apart from the slight cough and small amount of phlegm resulting from the patient's cold two weeks ago, there are no other symptoms of an exterior pattern at this time. All the main symptoms point to the interior.

Although the patient likes to drink a lot of liquids, his urine is yellow at times, and the tip of his tongue is red, these symptoms are very mild. One should therefore not be too concerned about the heat in this pattern; it is not enough to constitute a typical heat pattern. Qi stagnation is the main problem. It is neither a pattern of heat nor cold.

The patient's condition arose from qi stagnation, which pertains to excess; this is still the main problem. Because it is long-term, the antipathogenic factors have already been affected. The body is malnourished to a certain degree, and there are thus signs of deficiency. We may therefore conclude that this a combined pattern of both deficiency and excess.

Additional notes

1. What is the relationship between the deficiency and excess in this case?

A combination of deficiency and excess often occurs in clinical practice. In this type of case it is very important to determine which is more severe. That is to say, is there deficiency within excess, or excess within deficiency? Here the patient felt distention in the abdominal, intercostal, and hypochondrial regions in the early stages of the illness, which worsened after eating. He also belched and had other symptoms associated with a pattern of excess. These symptoms suggest that in the early stages the excessive pattern was predominant.

By the time the patient came to the clinic, however, the antipathogenic factors had been affected by the long-term illness. He now suffers from fatigue, weakness and soreness in the lower back, and has a thin, forceless pulse, all of which suggest a pattern of deficiency. He has poor physical energy and cannot even face daily work. He also has symptoms associated with malnourishment of the Heart spirit and Kidney deficiency (including the problem in the lower back). Thus, the earlier problem (Liver qi stagnation leading to qi stagnation of the middle burner) has progressed over time to qi deficiency of the Spleen and Stomach. The symptoms of deficiency are now more apparent, and deficiency has become the predominant disorder. We may therefore conclude that this case is one of excess within deficiency.

2. Why did the herbal tonic aggravate the symptoms?

In Chinese medicine this type of patient is referred to as one who is deficient but cannot tolerate tonification (*xū bú shòu bǔ*). This means that although the patient has a problem of deficiency, it is difficult for him to deal with the effects of a tonic. Chinese materia medica that function as tonics are generally heavy, rich, and cloying in nature, and thus put an extra burden on the middle burner. This makes digestion more difficult and increases the workload of the Spleen and Stomach. A patient whose transformative and transportive functions (in the metabolism of food and water) are impaired can expect poor digestion. Tonics can aggravate the qi deficiency in the Spleen and Stomach, causing the symptoms to worsen. Tonics are difficult to tolerate in such patients. Thus, the main treatment principle is to ensure the normal functioning of the Spleen and Stomach.

3. What is the cause of the heat symptoms?

There are very mild heat symptoms in this case, and little consideration has been given them in the diagnosis. However, the patient does tend to drink a good deal, his urine is occasionally yellowish, his stools can be dry, the tip of his tongue red, and the tongue coating slightly yellow. According to the history, the patient caught a cold two weeks previous; these symptoms are leftovers from the external heat. The symptoms are most commonly associated with wind-heat, but it is not a major problem at this time.

4. Is there any retention of dampness?

A slippery pulse is indicative of dampness, which can be produced when the Spleen's metabolism of water is impaired. In this case, however, there is no other evidence supporting a diagnosis of retention of dampness.

Conclusion

1. According to the eight principles:
   Interior, neither heat nor cold (or very slight heat), combination of excess and deficiency (excess within deficiency).

2. According to etiology:
   Emotional upset.

3. According to theory of qi, blood, and body fluids:
   Combination of qi deficiency and stagnation.

4. According to Organ theory:
   Disharmony between the Liver and Spleen;
   Spleen and Stomach qi deficiency.

Treatment principle

Strengthen the Spleen and tonify the qi while regulating the qi.

Explanation of treatment principle

In general, the basic principle for treating disharmony between the Spleen and Liver is to regulate the Liver qi to remove the obstruction; the qi stagnation in the middle burner will thereupon resolve itself. In this case, however, the long history of illness has led to a combination of deficiency and excess (excess within deficiency), and it is now the deficiency of Spleen and Stomach qi that is the main problem. For this reason, a strong (that is, reducing) method cannot be used to remove the obstruction and regulate the qi; rather, tonification is indicated as the basic treatment. Yet because this patient has little tolerance for tonics, it is important that tonification not be overdone. We should proceed in two steps. First, try to strengthen and regulate the qi of the Spleen and Stomach to improve the transformative and transportive functions, and thereby put the body in good order. In other words, use a method for regulating qi while at the same time use a gentle method to tonify the qi. This is how to combine tonification and regulation of qi. Caution must be exercised to avoid injuring the antipathogenic factors. Second, as the Spleen and Stomach functions improve, gradually increase the ratio of tonification to regulation.

Selection of points

First group:

PC-6 (*nei guan*)	CV-11 (*jian li*)
SP-4 (*gong sun*)	LI-10 (*shou san li*)
LR-5 (*li gou*)	ST-36 (*zu san li*)

Second group:

PC-6 *(nei guan)*   GV-12 *(shen zhu)*
SP-4 *(gong sun)*   BL-20 *(pi shu)*
LR-5 *(li gou)*   BL-21 *(wei shu)*

Explanation of points

PC-6 *(nei guan)* is a connecting point of the arm terminal yin Pericardium channel. It serves to regulate qi, alleviate pain, and is very effective for relieving qi stagnation in the upper and middle burners. It also settles the Heart spirit and calms restlessness and anxiety. It is an excellent choice for treating symptoms associated with psychological and mental disorders, such as insomnia, depression, and insanity. In this case, the point is used to regulate qi and remove the stagnant qi.

SP-4 *(gong sun)* is the connecting point of the Spleen channel, which is associated with the Stomach channel. In ancient times, according to the order of the different Organs, the Liver, which is associated with wood, was regarded as the grandfather *(gōng)*, the Heart was said to belong to the next generation, and the Spleen, which is associated with earth, was regarded as the grandson *(sūn)*. This is a connecting point between the Spleen and Stomach channels, and is also a confluent point associated with the penetrating vessel. It is an important point for regulating the functions of the Spleen and Stomach. It can be used to harmonize the Spleen and Stomach, regulate the functioning of the Intestines, alleviate pain in the chest and epigastric regions, and treat poor digestion, abdominal pain, and diarrhea. It serves to regulate qi and blood, especially qi. In this case the point was selected to promote the functioning of the Spleen and Stomach, improve the patient's appetite, regulate qi, and remove the qi stagnation.

LR-5 *(li gou)*. The word *lí* means woodworm, and *gōu* means a small hollow or depression. Among the functions of this point, which is located in the depression on the edge of the tibia, is to relieve itchiness—which is likened to the feeling of small crawling insects—around the genitals, hence the name. This is a connecting point of the Liver and Gallbladder channels. It is used to promote the Liver function of governing the free-flow of qi. In this case the reducing method is used at this point, the purpose being to remove the obstruction from the channels and Organs, and the qi stagnation from the Liver. When the latter purpose is accomplished, there will be no further disharmony between the Liver and Spleen. And when the obstruction is removed, the channels and collaterals will resume their normal functioning, alleviating the fullness and distention in the chest, intercostal, and hypochondrial regions. This point also serves to relieve the hypofunction of the Liver, so that it does not overact against the Spleen.

CV-11 *(jian li)* regulates the Organs, especially the Spleen and Stomach. Its Chinese name, which literally means to construct or build up the interior, refers to regulating the functions of the Organs, usually by means of tonification. Like most other conception vessel points, when this point is used to regulate the Organs, the emphasis is on the yang Organs. It is used to harmonize the middle burner Organs, regulate qi, remove food retention, and promote digestion. In this case there is a combination of deficiency and excess—Spleen and Stomach qi deficiency, interfering with the transportation and transformation (metabolism) of food—and thus the patient has a poor appetite, and suffers from abdominal distention and poor digestion. The purpose served by this point is to strengthen the Spleen and Stomach. It is used as a local point, and is tonified. Needling this point often causes subcutaneous bleeding, and, in some cases, there may be local subcutaneous swelling due to hemorrhage. Although this is not serious, patients will naturally become anxious. Puncturing this point must therefore be done very gently. A strong throbbing-and-lifting method is not recommended; gentle tonification with rotation is most suitable.

LI-10 *(shou san li)*. The word *shŏu* means hand or arm, *sān* means three (referring to its location three units below LI-12), and *lĭ* means a gathering place or city. This point is the upper body analog to ST-36 *(zu san li)*. It regulates the qi in the channels and collaterals, and regulates the functioning of the Large Intestine. In this case the point has been selected to regulate the qi in the middle burner. Even (balanced) needle manipulation is recommended.

ST-36 *(zu san li)* regulates the Spleen and Stomach, promotes the antipathogenic factors, and removes obstruction from the channels and collaterals. Here it is used to relieve qi deficiency in the middle burner. In view of the fact that the patient has qi stagnation, an even needle manipulation is recommended.

GV-12 *(shen zhu)* is a point located between the scapulae which can provide strong support for the body, hence its name, which means column of the body. This point serves to promote the movement of qi (especially in dispersing) in the upper burner, settle the Heart spirit, and calm restlessness. In this case the tonification method is used to promote the functioning of the upper burner and nourish the Heart spirit. The use of this point is an example of the method of promoting the functioning of the Heart through the governing vessel.

BL-20 *(pi shu)*. This point *(shū)* is very close to the Spleen *(pĭ)* and is located where the qi from the Spleen channel accumulates in the back; it is thus the back associated point of the Spleen. It serves to strengthen the Spleen, harmonize the Stomach and Spleen, and resolve dampness. It can help promote the transportive and transformative functions of the middle burner, relieve qi stagnation, and reduce abdominal distention.

BL-21 *(wei shu)*. This point *(shū)* is located close to the Stomach *(wèi)*, where the qi of the Stomach accumulates in the back, and hence is the back associated point of the Stomach. It promotes the functioning of the Spleen and Stomach, especially the Stomach's downward-moving (descending) action, and harmonizes the qi in the middle burner. This point can be used to alleviate the symptoms associated with the Stomach, and is also very effective in removing obstruction from the chest and hypochondrial regions. Thus in this case, besides alleviating the symptoms in the middle burner, it can also be used as an assistant point to remove the qi stagnation, which is the source of the fullness and distention in the chest, intercostal, and hypochondrial regions.

Combination of points

PC-6 *(nei guan)*, SP-4 *(gong sun)*, LR-5 *(li gou)*. There are two pairs in this small group of connecting points. The first pair is comprised of PC-6 *(nei guan)* and SP-4 *(gong sun)*, both of which are associated with the eight confluent points, which are used to regulate the qi of the Stomach, Heart, and chest. They are especially useful in alleviating the qi stagnation and painful symptoms in the upper and middle burners. This combination is very effective in promoting the transportive and transformative functions of the middle burner. The second pair is comprised of PC-6 *(nei guan)* and LR-5 *(li gou)*, both of which are connecting points on the arm and leg terminal yin channels. These points stimulate the qi and yin when they have reached the end of the channel circulation system, removing the old and promoting the new. They are therefore suitable for patients with deficiency of qi or yin, and can be used together in treating deficiency patterns and to promote the antipathogenic factors.

All of these are connecting points, each of which is associated exteriorly and interiorly with two channels. This is an example of using a minimum number of points to access a maximum number of channels. Because connecting points are very effective in removing qi stagnation, regulating the qi, and harmonizing the circulation of qi, they are good choices for treating patterns of qi stagnation. Here the points were chosen because the qi stagnation involves the middle burner and Liver.

LI-10 *(shou san li)*, ST-36 *(zu san li)*. This combination was discussed in previous cases. Both the arm and leg yang brightness channels are utilized to regulate the Stomach and Intestines. This is a good combination for regulating qi.

BL-20 *(pi shu)*, BL-21 *(wei shu)*, GV-12 *(shen zhu)*. The back associated points of the Spleen and Stomach are used to promote the functioning of the middle burner, and to regulate the Spleen and Stomach. GV-12 *(shen zhu)* is very effective in promoting the yang qi of the body through the governing vessel, settling the Heart, and alleviating symptoms in the upper burner, where it promotes the dispersing function of qi, and also settles the Heart spirit. It is used in combination with the back associated points here for treating the main problem in the middle burner, and the accompanying symptoms in the upper burner.

Follow-up

Three points in the two groups of acupoints are the same, and three are different. The first group emphasizes the regulation of qi and the elimination of qi stagnation, while the second group, besides regulating qi, places a certain amount of emphasis on the promotion of the transportive and transformative functions of the Spleen and Stomach. Both groups include points for tonification. Thus both groups can regulate qi and tonify deficiency; they can both be used for the qi deficiency and stagnation in this case, that is, the combination of deficiency and excess. Planning these two different groups of points is important for this case, as they focus on different aspects of the treatment.

For the first three weeks of treatment, the first group of points was used as the primary group, and the second as the secondary group. The patient was treated once daily, mainly with the first group of points; the second group was used only once or twice a week. After three weeks the fullness, distention, and pain around the chest and hypochondrial regions was largely alleviated, the patient's appetite started to improve a little, and the abdominal distention decreased. Although the patient was able to eat a little more than before, he still did not feel very hungry. This indicates that the functioning of the middle burner had not yet returned to normal, which also explains his lack of physical energy at this stage.

After three weeks the second group of points was used most of the time, alternating with the first group only once or twice a week, depending on the patient's condition. Moxibustion was used at GV-12 *(shen zhu)*. Treatment was administered every other day (three times a week). After a month there was improvement in the patient's general energy, and, during this period, he gradually regained his appetite, the abdominal distention continued to decrease, he began to sleep better, and his emotions remained normal. He was very pleased with the treatment, and, because of the demands of his work, did not return to the clinic, although he was advised to do so if the symptoms recurred. Six months later, a checkup revealed that the symptoms had not returned. The patient was in good health and only occasionally experienced some discomfort in the abdominal region, but this affected neither his life nor his ability to work.

CASE 10: **Female, age 82**

Main complaint

Poor appetite and lack of energy

History

The patient complained of a decrease in appetite one week before. She didn't feel hungry and ate very little. When she ate a little more than her fill, she suffered discomfort in the abdominal and gastric regions, but no frank pain. She belches frequently but does not vomit or experience nausea. Her energy is poor, her limbs are weak, and her hands and feet are numb. Quite often she suffers mild dizziness, but has no sensation of things spinning around her, and there is no imbalance when she walks. She is not thirsty, and her sleep and urination are normal. Her stools are dry and she has had no bowel movement for the past week.

Tongue

Slightly red (normal) with a thick, white, and moldy coating

Pulse

Wiry and slippery

Analysis of symptoms

1. Poor appetite and reduced intake of food—impairment of the Spleen's transportive and transformative functions.
2. Discomfort in the abdominal and gastric regions when she overeats—obstruction of qi activity.
3. Excessive belching—reversal of Stomach qi.
4. Lack of energy, weakness in the limbs, and dizziness—dysfunction in ascending of clear yang.
5. Dry stools and no bowel movement for one week—qi obstruction in the yang Organs.
6. Thick, white, and moldy tongue coating—retention of food.
7. Slippery pulse—retention of food.

Basic theory of case

In Chinese medicine the Spleen is responsible for the muscles as flesh because the Spleen and Stomach are the source of qi and blood. (The contraction of the muscles is a function of the sinews, which are governed by the Liver.) The flesh of the body is dependent for its nourishment upon the essence of food and water, which emanate from the middle burner. With the nutrients from the middle burner, the muscles are able to develop and thereby maintain the body in a healthy condition. That is why, in Chinese medicine, strong, healthy limbs and muscles are associated with the health of the transportive and transformative functions of the middle burner. If these functions of the Spleen and Stomach become impaired, the muscles can lose their shape and become weak and emaciated (their flesh aspect). Of course, this process will also diminish their strength and force.

The Spleen is also responsible for the upward-movement (ascending) of clear yang. This is also an important supporting function for the limbs and muscles. In the chapter on dizziness in *Acupuncture Patterns & Practice* we noted that clear yang ascends to the head where it keeps the mind clear and maintains the normal functioning of the head and brain. Similarly, the upward-movement of clear yang supports, provides nutrition for, and promotes the functioning of the limbs and muscles. This idea is expressed in the adage, "The clear yang serves the four limbs *(qīng yáng shí sì zhī)*." The normal functioning of the limbs, which manifests in strength, agility, and freedom of movement, depends on the normal functioning of the Spleen in transforming and transporting food and nutrients (metabolism). It is normal that there be a certain amount of weight in the arms and legs; even though they are quite heavy, a healthy person will be unaware of this because the clear yang enables the body to move freely without any sensation of heaviness. If the Spleen's transportive and transformative functions are impaired, however, the upward-movement of clear yang will be interrupted, and the essence of food and water will not be dispersed through the body. When this occurs, one's strength will diminish and there will be a feeling of fatigue, weakness, or heaviness in the limbs.

Physiologically speaking, there are two aspects of Spleen function with respect to the muscles: one is yin and the other yang. The yin aspect mainly manifests as the supply of substance and replenishment of nutrients; the yang as the functional aspect of the muscles, including movement, agility, and flexibility. These two aspects balance and support each other; if one is injured, it may affect the other.

Fig. 3-3

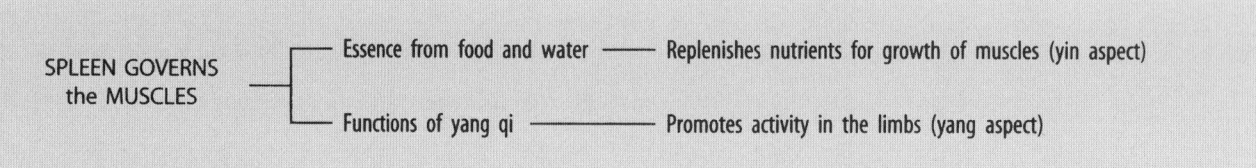

SPLEEN GOVERNS the MUSCLES
— Essence from food and water —— Replenishes nutrients for growth of muscles (yin aspect)
— Functions of yang qi —————— Promotes activity in the limbs (yang aspect)

Cause of disease	Qi stagnation

There is no history of invasion by external pathogenic factors in this case. The dysfunction in the digestive system suggests obstruction of the upward and downward movement (ascending and descending) of the qi of the middle burner. Thus, qi stagnation is the cause of this disorder.

Site of disease   Spleen and Stomach

The poor appetite, lack of energy, and discomfort in the abdomen after eating provide the main evidence of a Spleen disorder.
Belching is the main symptom implicating the Stomach.

Pathological change   Failure or impairment of the clear yang to ascend is an important pathological change in Chinese medicine. There are various causes, two of which are often encountered in the clinic. The first is deficiency of Spleen qi. Qi deficiency can impede the upward-movement of clear yang, preventing its dispersement through the body, including the limbs. The second cause is the obstruction of qi activity, which interferes with the ascending and descending of qi in the middle burner. The pathway of the clear yang is thereby obstructed. In this case, qi obstruction is the cause of the clear yang's inability to properly ascend.

The disorder here has lasted only one week, and the antipathogenic factors have therefore not been severely affected. Since there is stagnation of qi in the middle burner, impairment of the Spleen's transportive and transformative functions as well as the upward and downward movement of qi in the middle burner, the essence (nutrients) from food is not being properly transported throughout the body. Instead, food has accumulated in the Spleen and Stomach. The patient's appetite has therefore declined, and, if she eats any more than her fill, she feels discomfort in the abdominal region.

Food essence is the main substance for replenishing the clear yang. Qi stagnation in the middle burner can interfere with the delivery of food essence. As a result, the clear yang's ability to circulate throughout the body and limbs is impeded, and the patient may accordingly experience general fatigue, tiredness, and weakness in the limbs.

The dizziness in this case is caused by the interruption in the ascent of clear yang. And because it is unable to reach the head, the patient feels dizzy.

The Spleen and Stomach are responsible for balancing the upward and downward movement of qi in the middle burner. The coordination of these activities is very important in the maintenance of normal digestion. Because of the Spleen's inability to properly maintain the upward-movement of clear yang, the turbid yin in the Stomach does not descend properly; this causes an upward reversal in the movement of Stomach qi, and thus excessive belching. The dizziness can also be caused by the reversal of turbid qi.

Because the middle burner qi is not properly descending, the downward-movement of the Large Intestine's qi is likewise impaired, which interferes with the normal movement of the bowels. In this case the patient has had no bowel movement for a week.

Tongue coatings are normally caused by the rising of Stomach qi, which forms on the surface of the tongue. The particles on the surface of a normal tongue coating are very fine. A moldy coating has thick and very coarse particles, which are very loose and pile up in an irregular manner on the surface of the tongue. This indicates retention of an excessive pathogenic factor. In this case the upward and downward movement of qi in the middle burner is impaired. Turbid qi remains in the Stomach and also reverses upward, which accounts for the thick, moldy tongue coating. The wiry pulse reflects the impaired qi activity, and its slippery quality indicates retention of food.

Qi stagnation is found in both this and the previous case. The symptoms and site of disease are very similar, but in the previous case there is a tendency toward deficiency, whereas here there is a tendency toward excess. The diagnosis is therefore quite different in the two cases, as are the treatment principles and methods. In Chinese medicine successful treatment depends on the ability to properly distinguish among different patterns.

Fig. 3-4

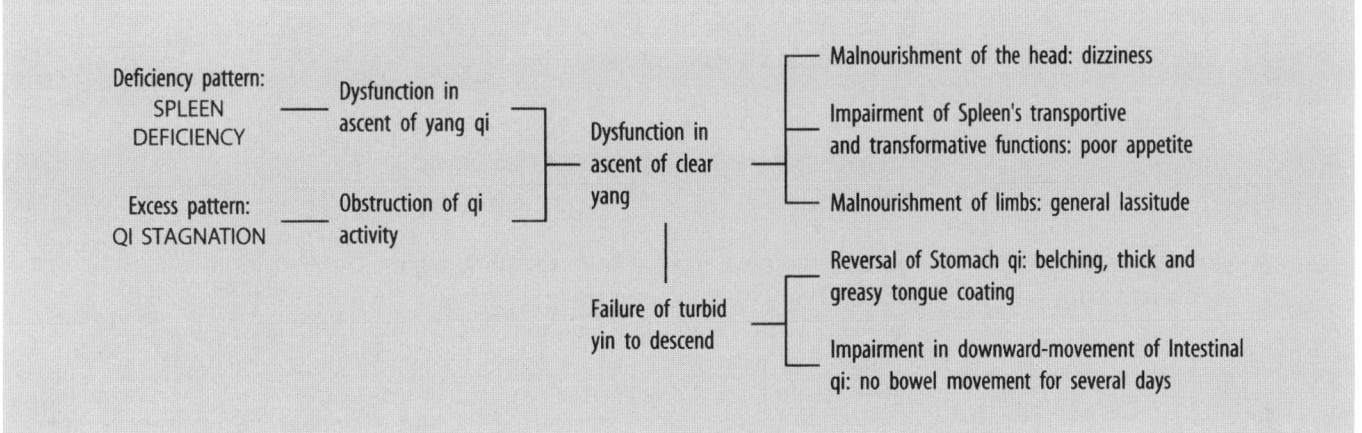

Pattern of disease

The disorder is located in the middle burner. The patient's appetite has diminished, she belches excessively, and there is no history of an invasion by an external pathogenic factor. It is therefore an interior pattern.

The patient does not feel hot or cold. She is not thirsty, her urine is not yellow, the tongue coating is white, and the pulse is not rapid. Thus, there is neither a heat nor a cold pattern here.

Qi stagnation has occurred in the middle burner, but the antipathogenic factors have not been affected. This is therefore a pattern of excess.

Additional notes

1. Is there deficiency or excess in this case?

This patient is quite elderly (82) and suffers from fatigue, dizziness, and a diminished appetite. It is easy to conclude that there is qi deficiency, and that the body is malnourished. But why has this case been diagnosed as a pattern of excess?

All the above symptoms are secondary to the obstruction of qi activity, and the impairment in the upward-movement of clear yang. They do not result from primary Spleen qi deficiency, and thus the diagnosis points to qi stagnation, which is a characteristic of excess, not deficiency. In the clinic it is impossible to determine whether the controlling pattern is one of excess or deficiency by examining just one or two symptoms. One must look for the cause of the symptoms. Only then is it possible to reach a reasonable conclusion, and make an accurate diagnosis.

2. What is the cause of the numbness in the hands and feet?

There are various causes for numbness in the hands and feet. The most common are qi stagnation and blood deficiency, the details of which are discussed in case 20 in *Acupuncture Patterns & Practice.*

3. Do the dry stools indicate a pattern of heat?

The general symptoms in this case reveal no obvious manifestations of heat, so this cannot be the cause of the dry stools. They are, in fact, caused by the obstruction of qi in the yang Organs. When the turbid yin is unable to properly descend, stool will remain in the Intestines too long, and moisture (that is, water) will be absorbed by the Intestines little by little. The longer the stool remains in the Intestines, the drier it becomes.

Conclusion

1. According to the eight principles:
   Interior, neither cold nor heat, excess pattern.
2. According to theory of qi, blood, and body fluids:
   Qi stagnation.
3. According to Organ theory:
   Qi stagnation in the Spleen and Stomach (inability of clear yang
   to ascend, and reversal of Stomach qi).

Treatment principle

1. Regulate the qi and remove the obstruction from the middle burner.
2. Promote the upward-movement of clear yang.
3. Promote the downward-moving actions of the yang Organs.

Explanation of treatment principle

Because of the stagnation of qi in the middle burner, the main principle should be the regulation of qi to remove the obstruction. But in view of the patient's age, the antipathogenic factors may be injured if the regulation is too strong. On the other hand, the patient has had no bowel movement for a week. Although this symptom results from the stagnation of qi, the obstruction of qi in the yang Organs can aggravate the stagnation of qi. Thus a very important treatment principle in this case is the regulation of qi in the yang Organs. If the obstruction of qi in the yang Organs can be alleviated, the symptoms associated with qi reversal will be resolved, the turbid qi will properly descend, the Spleen qi will ascend, the clear yang will be dispersed throughout the body, and all the symptoms will be resolved.

Selection of points

CV-10 *(xia wan)*
BL-57 *(cheng shan)*

Explanation of points

CV-10 *(xia wan)* is a meeting point of the leg greater yin and conception vessels. Its Chinese name means lower stomach cavity, which describes its location. The point serves to harmonize the Organs of the middle burner, regulate the qi, reduce food retention, and promote digestion. It regulates the qi in the middle burner, and is important for promoting the downward-moving functions of the Stomach. Here it is used as a local point, specifically for the removal of qi stagnation. The reducing method of needle manipulation is utilized.

BL-57 *(cheng shan)*. The word *chéng* means to hold or contain, and *shān* means mountain. Because the middle of the gastrocnemius muscle is big and puffy, it resembles a small mountain; the depression below it, which looks as if it could hold (or contain) the mountain, is the location of this point. The point is very effective locally in soothing problems related to the sinews, muscles, and vessels. It also has the important action of regulating the Organs and promoting the downward-moving functions of the Large Intestine. It is thus a good point for unblocking the Large Intestine, as it helps move the feces, regulate the qi, and improve the appetite.

Combination of points

The combination of the two points in this prescription regulates the qi and promotes its downward-moving action. It is therefore useful in resolving problems which manifest both in the upper part of the body, such as poor appetite, as well as the lower part, such as constipation.

Follow-up

The patient was given acupuncture once a day for two days, after which her bowel movements improved and she passed a lot of gas. Her appetite was also much improved, but she still belched a little. After an interval of three days, she was given one more treatment, after which the symptoms resolved. The patient then had a good appetite and no longer suffered from general lassitude. She was advised to avoid overeating in order to prevent food retention and qi stagnation.

Although this patient was quite elderly, her general health was not too bad. Her problem was qi stagnation, which relates to a pattern of excess. Because there was no particular heat or cold in this case, the main purpose of the treatment was to remove the qi stagnation. As soon as it was removed, all of the other symptoms disappeared of their own accord. In clinical practice many practitioners automatically use tonification in treating the elderly, but this is not always appropriate, as old age does not necessarily imply deficiency. The elderly often have complications arising from deficiency, but when an elderly person suffers solely from a pattern of excess—like the woman in this case—one must be brave but cautious. If the reducing method must be used during treatment to deal with a problem of excess, one must be positive in one's approach, yet treat carefully. In so doing, a very quick and effective result may be achieved, as in this case.

CASE 11: **Female, age 24**

Main complaint

Anorexia

History

The patient suffered from chronic cholecystitis for two years. She complained that, over the last few months, her appetite had gradually diminished to the point that she now could eat very little. She dislikes any kind of greasy or heavy food. She feels that her stomach is distended, but there is no pain or nausea. She is tired both physically and mentally. She is irritable and has a bad temper. She is restless and feels hot in the chest, but is not thirsty. Her sleep is disturbed by dreaming, and when she wakes in the morning her energy level is low. Her urine is yellow and her stools are loose. Her menstrual cycle is regular, but she bleeds more than usual. She sometimes has papulae on her face, but they are not itchy and there are no secretions.

Tongue

Red with a yellow, thick, and greasy coating

Pulse

Wiry, slippery, and rapid

Analysis of symptoms

1. Poor appetite and reduced food intake—Spleen's transportive and transformative functions are impaired.
2. Abdominal distention—obstruction of qi activity.
3. Fatigue and tiredness—exhaustion of antipathogenic factors.
4. Restlessness, hot sensation in the chest, and dream-disturbed sleep—Heart spirit disturbed by heat.
5. Irritability and bad temper—impairment of the Liver's control over the free-flow of qi.
6. Yellow urine and slightly increased bleeding during menstruation—pathogenic heat.
7. Loose stools—dampness.

8. Red tongue with a yellow, thick, greasy coating—damp-heat.

9. Slippery, rapid pulse—damp-heat.

10. Wiry pulse—impairment of the Liver's control over the free-flow of qi.

Basic theory of case

In Chinese medicine there is a very close relationship between the Liver and Gallbladder. In ancient times it was noted that the physical liver and gallbladder are contiguous organs, and their associated channels are related to one another interiorly and exteriorly. Physiologically, the Gallbladder stores bile, which in Chinese is called "essential juice" *(jīng zhī)*. Chinese medicine holds that, although it accumulates in the Gallbladder, bile is derived from the essence of the Liver. In a general sense then, bile may be regarded as one of several very important yin essences in the body. Together, the Gallbladder and Liver control the free-flow of qi, which is closely related to the upward and downward movement of Spleen and Stomach qi, in that dysfunction in one can affect the other. Thus, a healthy Liver and Gallbladder is essential to good digestion.

When food metabolizes, it first enters the Stomach, then moves to the Small Intestine; the waste is passed out of the body through the Large Intestine. Water enters the Stomach, moves to the Small Intestine and Triple Burner, and the waste is passed out of the body through the Bladder. These yang Organs are therefore not only responsible for transforming food and water into essence, but also for removing waste. The Gallbladder, however, is different: even though it stores bile, the bile cannot be removed as waste. For this reason the Gallbladder is referred to as a "special yang Organ with a unique function *(qí héng zhī fǔ)*."

Because of this unique characteristic of the Gallbladder, its associated disorders share many similarities with those of the Liver, including the etiology and pathogenesis of disease, as well as clinical symptoms. For example, a strong emotional upset may equally impair the free-flow of qi in the Liver as well as in the Gallbladder, and then affect the digestive system and function of the middle burner. In clinical practice these types of disorders are often said to exist in both the Liver and Gallbladder, thus the two Organs are often treated in accordance with the same principle, and with the same methods.

Fig. 3-5

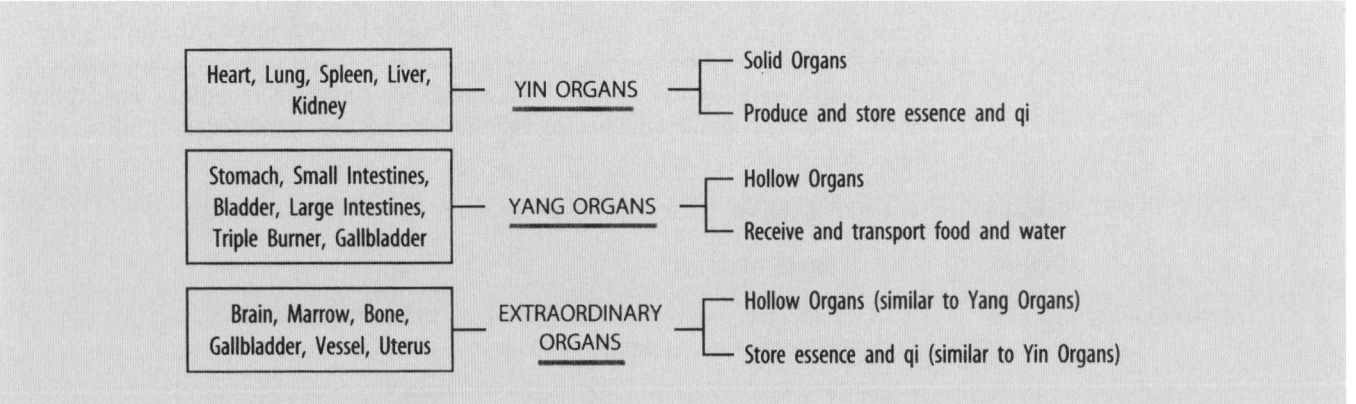

Heart, Lung, Spleen, Liver, Kidney	YIN ORGANS	Solid Organs
		Produce and store essence and qi
Stomach, Small Intestines, Bladder, Large Intestines, Triple Burner, Gallbladder	YANG ORGANS	Hollow Organs
		Receive and transport food and water
Brain, Marrow, Bone, Gallbladder, Vessel, Uterus	EXTRAORDINARY ORGANS	Hollow Organs (similar to Yang Organs)
		Store essence and qi (similar to Yin Organs)

Cause of disease

Damp-heat

The patient has a poor appetite and especially dislikes greasy and heavy foods. She has loose stools, a thick, greasy tongue coating, and a slippery pulse—evidence of dampness, which is a heavy, turbid pathogenic factor with a greasy nature. Dampness typically obstructs qi activity. We may conclude from these symptoms that there is retention of dampness in the body.

The patient also suffers from restlessness, insomnia, and irritability, and her urine is yellow. These symptoms are evidence that pathogenic heat is disturbing the Heart spirit and consuming the body fluids. When heat and dampness combine to cause illness, it is called damp-heat.

Site of disease

Spleen, Liver, Gallbladder

The patient suffers from anorexia, poor appetite, abdominal distention, and fatigue, all of which suggests a Spleen disorder.

She is irritable and is quick to anger, which reflects a disorder of the Liver and Gallbladder.

Pathological change

Chronic cholecystitis is the term used in biomedicine for inflammation of the gallbladder. In Chinese medicine, however, the Liver and Gallbladder are related interiorly and exteriorly, and if the patient's symptoms involve a dysfunction of the Liver and Gallbladder, then a Liver disorder will be diagnosed.

The free-flow of qi, which is controlled by the Liver, regulates the qi activity of the Spleen and Stomach in their upward- and downward-moving actions. If the qi activity becomes stagnant or obstructed, the free-flow of qi will be impeded, and the Spleen and Stomach's transportive and transformative functions will be compromised. That is what happened in this case.

This dysfunction of the Liver can result in the stagnation of Liver qi, which may give rise to internal heat. Heat may be a factor in such symptoms as irritability and bad temper. Pathogenic heat rises and disturbs the Heart spirit, affecting the mind. This explains why the patient is restless, feels discomfort in the chest, and has dream-disturbed sleep. The impediment to the Spleen's transportive and transformative functions has resulted in food accumulating in the middle burner. Because the food is not being transported properly from the Stomach through the Intestines, there is diminished appetite and abdominal distention. These symptoms are aggravated when the patient eats greasy or heavy food, since these types of food can increase the load on the digestive system. This accounts for the patient's aversion to heavy, greasy foods.

An analysis of the signs and symptoms, especially the tongue coating and pulse, leads to the conclusion that there is internal damp-heat, which has obstructed the qi activity and impaired the functions of both the Liver and Spleen. What is the source of the damp-heat? This question is difficult to answer. It is possible that the dampness was of external origin, or it could be that the inability of the Spleen and Stomach to transform and transport the body fluids has led to retention of dampness internally. With respect to the heat, it is likely that the stagnation of Liver qi has given rise to internal heat. The combination of heat and dampness, and the resulting retention of damp-heat, is reflected in such symptoms as the yellow urine and loose stools.

The tongue is red with a yellow coating, which indicates heat. The thick, greasy coating indicates retention of dampness. The slippery pulse indicates dampness, and its rapid quality indicates heat. The wiry quality is evidence that the free-flow of qi, which is governed by the Liver and Gallbladder, is impeded.

In addition to these symptoms, there are also abnormalities concerning menstruation and the skin. Heat accumulating in the body has stimulated the circulation of blood, causing the excessive menstrual bleeding. The facial papules indicate that heat has already entered the blood *(Fig. 3-6)*.

Pattern of disease

In this case there are disorders of the Liver, Gallbladder, and Spleen. In the absence of a history of invasion by a pathogenic factor, or of such symptoms as fever or aversion to cold, we may conclude that this is an interior pattern.

The patient is restless, irritable, has yellow urine, a red tongue with a yellow coating, and a rapid pulse. All of this is evidence of heat.

The presence of damp-heat, together with the obstruction of qi activity, indicate that the pathogenic factor is strong. It is therefore a pattern of excess.

Fig. 3-6

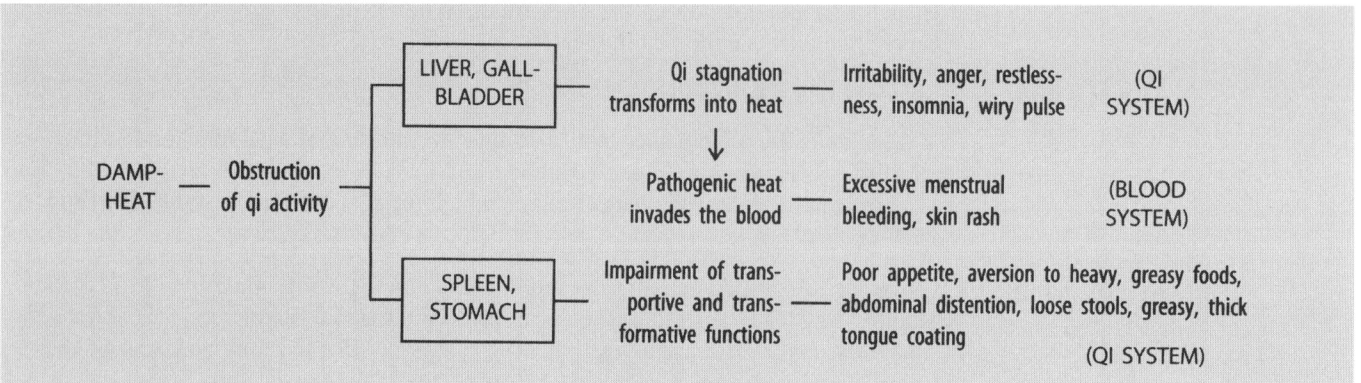

DAMP-HEAT — Obstruction of qi activity	LIVER, GALL-BLADDER	Qi stagnation transforms into heat ↓ Pathogenic heat invades the blood	Irritability, anger, restlessness, insomnia, wiry pulse (QI SYSTEM)
			Excessive menstrual bleeding, skin rash (BLOOD SYSTEM)
	SPLEEN, STOMACH	Impairment of transportive and transformative functions	Poor appetite, aversion to heavy, greasy foods, abdominal distention, loose stools, greasy, thick tongue coating (QI SYSTEM)

Additional notes

1. Is there deficiency in this case?

The patient has a poor appetite, lacks energy, and suffers from general lassitude. These symptoms are often associated with a pattern of Spleen qi deficiency. Why, then, has the pattern been diagnosed as one of excess?

The illness here has been caused by damp-heat, that is, two types of pathogenic factors. The diminished appetite results from dampness obstructing the qi activity, which affects the transformation and transportation of food as well as the upward- and downward-moving actions of Spleen and Stomach qi. This is therefore an excessive pathogenic factor, rather than deficiency. Fatigue or general lassitude is caused by stagnant heat in the body, which can consume or injure the antipathogenic factors. In this case the lack of energy, and the malnourishment of the limbs, is not caused by Spleen qi deficiency but by heat consuming the antipathogenic factors. Furthermore, there is no evidence of qi deficiency in the tongue and pulse signs.

2. Is there really a pattern of heat in this case?

The patient has yellow urine, and a red tongue with a yellow coating, all of which are symptoms of heat. Yet it is well known that heat often consumes the body fluids, causing thirst and dry stools—symptoms that are absent from this case. How can this be explained?

The reason for these contradictory symptoms is that there are two different pathogenic factors: dampness and heat. Unlike the normal body fluids, dampness does not provide the body with nourishment; it is a moist pathogenic factor. Retention of dampness can partly offset the effect of the heat, that is, the thirst caused by heat. Because dampness counteracts the symptom of thirst, patients with damp-heat generally do not feel thirsty, or, if they do, they don't want to drink very much. Similarly, patients with a heat pattern will often suffer from constipation. However, because dampness is a moist pathogenic factor with a tendency to descend through the body, dampness can flow into the Intestines, causing loose stools. This explains why there is no constipation in this case, but loose stools. Thus, despite the contradictory symptoms, there really is a pattern of heat in this case.

Conclusion

1. According to the eight principles:
   Interior, heat, excess.

2. According to etiology:
   Damp-heat.

3. According to Organ theory:
   Disharmony of the Liver (Gallbladder) and Spleen, with damp-heat in the Spleen.

Treatment principle

1. Clear the heat and remove the dampness.

2. Regulate the qi and promote the functioning of the Spleen.

Explanation of treatment principle

Because the retention of damp-heat in the middle burner is the main pathological change and also the cause of the obstructed qi, clearing heat and removing dampness is the basic treatment principle in this case. In fact, the heat is quite strong here, and clearing the heat will therefore be more important than removing the dampness. Because it is the Spleen that is responsible for transforming and transporting fluids, when the Spleen is functioning properly the qi activity will be smooth and the Spleen and Stomach's normal upward- and downward-moving actions will remove the dampness from the body. This is why regulating the qi and promoting the functioning of the Spleen is necessary for the removal of the retained dampness.

Stagnant qi has interfered with the Liver's ability to govern the free-flow of qi, and stagnant or obstructed qi leads to internal heat. Thus, regulation of the qi will not only remove the stagnant Liver qi, it will also help clear the heat.

Basic herbal formula

Three-Nut Decoction *(san ren tang)* is one of the formulas used to treat epidemic febrile diseases, especially those attributable to damp-heat during the summer. The original formula contains the following ingredients:

Semen Pruni Armeniacae *(xing ren)* 15g
Fructus Amomi Kravanh *(bai dou kou)* 6g
Semen Coicis Lachryma-jobi *(yi yi ren)* 18g
Talcum *(hua shi)* 18g
Medulla Tetrapanacis Papyriferi *(tong cao)* 6g
Semen Coicis Lachryma-jobi *(yi yi ren)* 6g
Herba Lophatheri Gracilis *(dan zhu ye)* 6g
Cortex Magnoliae Officinalis *(hou po)* 6g
Rhizoma Pinelliae Ternatae *(ban xia)* 10g

Explanation of basic formula

This formula can be used to clear heat and remove dampness—especially in those patterns in which dampness is stronger than heat—in epidemic febrile diseases. Common symptoms include headache, aversion to cold, soreness and heaviness throughout the body, stifling sensation in the chest, poor appetite, lack of thirst, a white, greasy tongue coating, and a soggy pulse. The basic pathological change is an invasion of external dampness and heat. Dampness blocks the qi activity, leading to an obstruction of qi in the channels, collaterals, body surface, and Organs, especially those of the middle burner (Spleen and Stomach). This results in such symptoms as soreness, pain, heaviness, and a stifling sensation.

In this formula, Fructus Amomi Kravanh *(bai dou kou)* is acrid and warm and is associated with the Lung, Spleen, and Stomach channels. It dries dampness, regulates qi, and promotes qi activity in the middle burner. It is especially good for removing qi stagnation and promoting the dispersal of qi. Here it serves as the chief herb.

There are two deputy herbs: Semen Pruni Armeniacae *(xing ren)* and Semen Coicis Lachrymajobi *(yi yi ren)*. The former is bitter and warm, and is used to arrest coughing and remove asthma. Here it regulates the Lung qi and promotes the downward-moving action of the qi activity in the upper burner. The latter herb is sweet, bland, and slightly cold. It is associated with the Spleen and Stomach channels and is used to strengthen the functioning of the Spleen, promote the metabolism of water, and promote the qi activity in the lower burner.

There are five assistant herbs: Cortex Magnoliae Officinalis *(hou po)*, Rhizoma Pinelliae Ternatae *(ban xia)*, Talcum *(hua shi)*, Medulla Tetrapanacis Papyriferi *(tong cao)*, Semen Coicis Lachryma-jobi *(yi yi ren)*, and Herba Lophatheri Gracilis *(dan zhu ye)*. Cortex Magnoliae Officinalis *(hou po)* is bitter, acrid, and warm, and Rhizoma Pinelliae Ternatae *(ban xia)* is acrid and warm. Together, these two herbs serve to regulate qi, dry dampness, and reinforce the actions of the chief and deputy herbs in promoting qi activity. Talcum *(hua shi)*, Medulla Tetrapanacis Papyriferi *(tong cao)*, Semen Coicis Lachryma-jobi *(yi yi ren)*, and Herba Lophatheri Gracilis *(dan zhu ye)* are sweet, bland, and cold. They act to clear heat, promote the metabolism of water, and remove dampness from the body.

The formula as a whole is acrid and warm in nature. Semen Pruni Armeniacae *(xing ren)*, Fructus Amomi Kravanh *(bai dou kou)*, and Semen Coicis Lachryma-jobi *(yi yi ren)* together regulate the qi through the upper, middle, and lower burners in order to promote qi activity and remove the obstruction of dampness.

Modified herbal formula

Herba Agastaches seu Pogostemi *(huo xiang)* 8g
Semen Coicis Lachryma-jobi *(yi yi ren)* 15g
Sclerotium Poriae Cocos *(fu ling)* 10g
Rhizoma Coptidis *(huang lian)* 5g
Cortex Moutan Radicis *(mu dan pi)* 8g
Semen Plantaginis *(che qian zi)* [boil in cotton gauze] 10g
Rhizoma Cyperi Rotundi *(xiang fu)* 6g
Cortex Magnoliae Officinalis *(hou po)* 6g
Herba Lophatheri Gracilis *(dan zhu ye)* 6g

Explanation of modifed formula

Damp-heat blocking the qi activity is the basic pathological change in this case, but the heat is stronger than the dampness, and there is also disharmony between the Liver and Spleen. Three-Nut Decoction *(san ren tang)* is generally used for regulating qi and removing dampness, but in this case we must reduce the quantity of dry and warm herbs.

In the modified formula, Herba Agastaches seu Pogostemi *(huo xiang)*, Sclerotium Poriae Cocos *(fu ling)*, and Semen Coicis Lachryma-jobi *(yi yi ren)* as a group replaces Fructus Amomi Kravanh *(bai dou kou)*, Semen Pruni Armeniacae *(xing ren)*, and Semen Coicis Lachryma-jobi *(yi yi ren)* in the original Three-Nut Decoction *(san ren tang)* formula. While the three herbs in the modified formula regulate qi activity through the upper, middle, and lower burners, their primary focus is the middle burner. They lack the warm and dry characteristics of the original combination in Three-Nut Decoction *(san ren tang)*. Another modification here is the omission of Rhizoma Pinelliae Ternatae *(ban xia)* and Medulla Tetrapanacis Papyriferi *(tong cao)*. Semen Plantaginis *(che qian zi)* replaces Talcum *(hua shi)*. As the functions of these two herbs are very similar, one can be substituted for the other. We have chosen Semen Plantaginis *(che qian zi)* because, as the weaker of the two, it is less likely to injure the Spleen and Stomach.

The second group of herbs, Cortex Magnoliae Officinalis *(hou po)*, Semen Plantaginis *(che qian zi)*, and Herba Lophatheri Gracilis *(dan zhu ye)*, is used to regulate the qi and promote the metabolism of water. Compared with the original formula, this function has not been altered very much.

A third group of herbs has been added: Rhizoma Cyperi Rotundi *(xiang fu)* regulates the Liver qi, Rhizoma Coptidis *(huang lian)* clears heat from the qi level, and Cortex Moutan Radicis *(mu dan pi)* is used for cooling the blood. These herbs were added in view of the primacy of heat in this case, and because the disorder is mainly in the qi level, and has also affected the blood to some degree.

Follow-up

Treatment in this case lasted two months. In the beginning, one package of the herbal formula was taken daily in two half-doses. Although there was little improvement at first, the patient was encouraged to continue the treatment for three weeks, at the end of which the restlessness and heat symptoms were largely alleviated. Her appetite was much improved, and she noticed that the quantity of her urine had increased. The herbal formula was continued for another two weeks, with minor alterations to accommodate the patient's condition. After this time the herbs were stopped for one week. The patient was much better, and the primary symptoms had all but disappeared. Treatment resumed for another two weeks, during which the dosage of some of the herbs was slightly increased to regulate the Liver qi. By the end of the fortnight, the symptoms were gone, and treatment was accordingly terminated.

The patient was reexamined one month and six months later. As there were no further symptoms and her appetite remained normal, no additional treatment was required.

When a disorder involves retention of dampness, because of its greasy quality, the duration of both the illness and treatment can be very long, and improvement is not always apparent at the beginning. This should not be interpreted to mean that the treatment is ineffective. If the practitioner is patient and perseveres, there will be gradual but definite improvement. This is a common occurrence in patterns of this nature.

CASE 12: **Female, age 62**

Main complaint

General lassitude and poor appetite

History

Two weeks ago the patient had an upper respiratory tract infection. She had a high fever continuously for one week, and her body temperature was about 39°C. Her temperature returned to normal, but she now feels very tired. She has no appetite and her energy is poor. She has a constant bland sensation in her mouth, and food has no taste. Her mouth is dry and she tends to drink a lot. At night she feels hot all over and has night sweats. All her joints are sore. She is fatigued and finds it hard to get motivated. Sometimes she experiences palpitations. There is no chest pain, no aversion to cold, and no more sore throat, cough, or nasal congestion. Her urine is yellow and her stools are dry. She has a bowel movement once every other day.

Tongue

Thin, red body with a dry, yellow coating

Pulse

Thin and rapid

Analysis of symptoms

1. Continuous high fever—retention of heat in the body.
2. Poor appetite, lassitude, and lack of taste—Spleen's transportive and transformative functions are impaired.
3. Dryness in the mouth and thirst—injury to body fluids.
4. Feeling hot at night, night sweats, and palpitations—accumulation of heat from deficiency in the body.
5. Soreness in all the joints, listlessness—malnourishment of the sinews.
6. Yellow urine and dry stools—heat pattern.
7. Red tongue with a thin body and yellow, dry coating—injury to the yin caused by heat.
8. Thin, rapid pulse—heat from deficiency.

Basic theory of case

In Chinese medicine there are two aspects to every Organ: yin and yang. The Spleen and Stomach likewise have their yin and yang aspects, which are associated with different parts of their functions or physiological make-up. The Spleen and Stomach's yang aspect is responsible for the transformation and transportation of food and water, that is, digestion. The Stomach yang and qi help in breaking food down into fine pieces, and with its storage in the Stomach. They also maintain the food at a certain temperature so that it can be absorbed by the body. The Spleen yang and qi extract nutrients from the broken-down food, and transform it into the essence of food and water, which will nourish the body. The waste is transported into the Large Intestine.

The yin aspect of the Spleen and Stomach nourishes and moistens the Organs. It also moistens and softens food in order to help in digestion and absorption. Thus the yin aspect of the Spleen and Stomach supports the metabolism of food and water.

The yin and yang aspects of these Organs are mutually supportive; if one aspect is lacking or dysfunctional, the other aspect cannot function properly either. In the clinic, yin deficiency of the Spleen and Stomach very often occurs in the late stages of a febrile disease, as pathogenic heat injures the body fluids and the yin aspects of the body.

Fig. 3-7

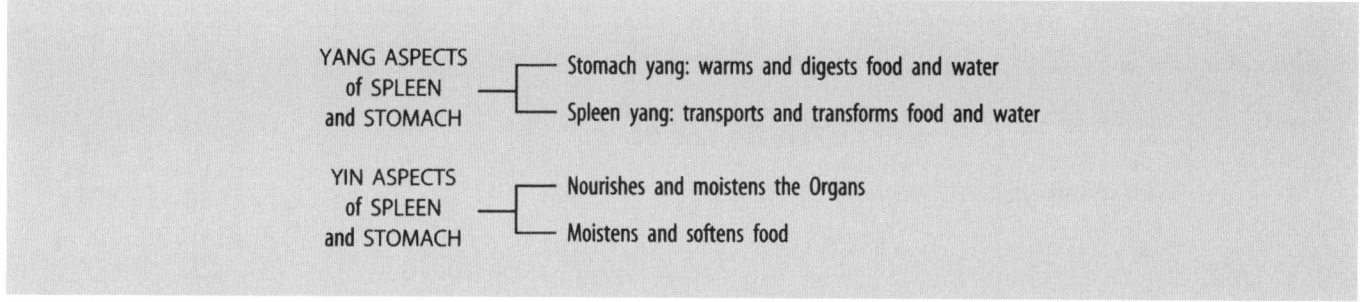

YANG ASPECTS of SPLEEN and STOMACH	Stomach yang: warms and digests food and water
	Spleen yang: transports and transforms food and water
YIN ASPECTS of SPLEEN and STOMACH	Nourishes and moistens the Organs
	Moistens and softens food

Cause of disease   Warm-heat

Two weeks ago, before her present illness, the patient had a continuous fever. The fever left her with symptoms involving the Spleen and Stomach, and evidence of an invasion by pathogenic warm-heat, which has consumed the antipathogenic factors and injured the body fluids.

Site of disease   Spleen and Stomach

Poor appetite, lack of taste, and dry stools indicate that the Spleen and Stomach are the site of the disorder.

Pathological change   Warm-heat is a yang pathogenic factor which can consume the qi and injure the body fluids. If it is very strong it will also injure the yin aspects of the body. Proper treatment in clearing heat can expel the heat from the body, but if the body fluids and yin aspects of the body have been injured, they will often not recover quickly. Thus, deficiency of yin or body fluids, with malnourishment of the body, is a common pattern found in the later stages of a febrile disease.

The injury to the yin of the Spleen and Stomach has affected their transportive and transformative functions, such that the patient has a very poor appetite, bland sensation in her mouth, and inability to taste food. The deficiency of body fluids accounts for her thirst and lack of moisture in the Intestines, causing dry stools. The lassitude and poor energy are the result of heat consuming the body's qi during the fever. Normal qi levels have yet to be restored.

The patient feels hot during the night, suffers from night sweats and palpitations, and her urine is yellow. These symptoms indicate that some heat still remains in the body, but this is not the warm-heat that resulted from the invasion of pathogenic heat. Rather, it is heat from deficientcy that has accumulated in the body, which was caused by a deficiency of yin and fluids. This type of heat is not very severe. The sensation of feeling hot all over usually occurs in the afternoon or at night. In Chinese medicine these are called tidal fevers *(cháo rè)*. The patient is also prone to episodic or night sweats, and palpitations.

In Chinese medicine the joints are referred to as the dwellings of the sinews. This means that the sinews are gathered around the joints. The flexibility of the joints is dependent upon the body fluids, which provide nourishment and moisture. When pathogenic heat is severe, it will injure and consume the body fluids. Deprived of their normal nourishment, the joints become sore and inflexible, affecting the patient's activity and agility.

Fig. 3-8

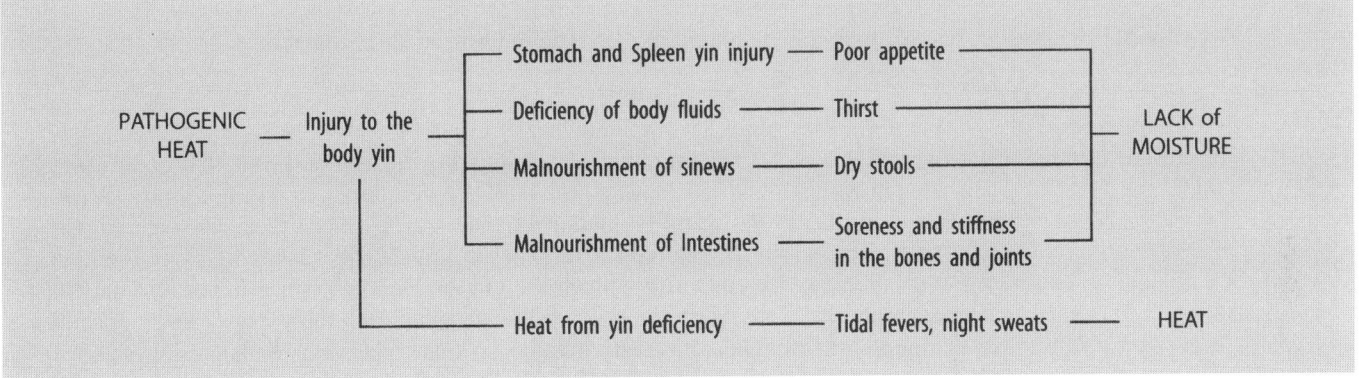

The red tongue reflects the presence of heat, and the thin body suggests deficiency of yin and body fluids. The tongue has lost its normal shape because of the yin deficiency. The yellow tongue coating, which lacks moisture, likewise suggests the presence of heat in the body, and the deficiency of body fluids. The thin, rapid pulse is a sign of internal heat and yin deficiency; the pulse is thin because the vessels are not being properly filled, and rapid because of the presence of heat.

Pattern of disease

This is an interior pattern. Although there was an invasion of warm-heat two weeks before, all the symptoms of an exterior pattern have now disappeared, and those associated with an interior pattern remain.

The patient suffers from deficiency of yin and body fluids, and heat (or fire) from deficency has accumulated inside her body. She feels hot at night and suffers from night sweats, her urine is yellow, and she has dry stools, all of which suggest heat. Accordingly, this is a heat pattern.

When the qi and yin are both injured the patient will have a poor appetite, general lassitude, a thin tongue body, and a thin pulse, all part of a pattern of deficiency.

Additional notes

1. Are there any signs of Kidney yin deficiency in this case?

In the late stages of a febrile disease the yin of the body can be affected. In clinical practice, yin deficiency can occur in the Kidney, Spleen, Stomach, or Liver. Yin deficiency of all kinds have many similar symptoms. What about Kidney yin deficiency in this case? The symptoms here, which are not very severe, are mostly associated with digestion. The duration of the illness is also very short. Thus the main yin deficiency is to be found in the Spleen and Stomach, and there is no concrete evidence to suggest Kidney yin deficiency.

2. In which category of pathogenic factor does warm-heat belong?

In Chinese medicine, warm-heat is a general term used to describe wind-heat, damp-heat, dry-heat, epidemic toxic factors, and other warm-heat type pathogenic factors in the external environment. The common characteristic of these pathogenic factors is that they invade the body from the outside and cause a rapid emergence of disease, with very obvious symptoms of heat. Different pathogenic factors will appear in different seasons: in spring, there are wind-heat or spring-warmth, and in summer, summer-heat or summer-dampness. The patient in this case had a continuous high fever, but the season is not recorded in her history. All we can say, therefore, is that there is warm-heat.

Conclusion

1. According to the eight principles:
   Interior, heat, deficiency.

2. According to Organ theory:
   Spleen and Stomach yin deficiency.

Treatment principle

1. Nourish the yin and body fluids in the Spleen and Stomach.
2. Clear the heat.

Explanation of treatment principle

Yin deficiency often accompanies heat from deficiency; therefore, treatment frequently involves nourishing the yin and clearing the heat at the same time. It is not enough to just clear the heat. Because of the deficiency of yin and body fluids, there will be a relative preponderance of yang qi. If only the heat is cleared, the yang qi can easily be injured in the process, which will adversely affect both the yin and yang. Thus, nourishment of the yin is obligatory, since increasing the yin and body fluids will restore the normal balance between the yin and yang. It is still important that the heat be cleared, however, since otherwise the heat will continue to consume the yin of the body. The point is that, when clearing the heat, one must not be too aggressive, since the internal heat (or fire) is from deficiency, and not from excess.

Selection of points

GV-13 *(tao dao)*
LU-7 *(lie que)*
KI-6 *(zhao hai)*
BL-20 *(pi shu)*
jia ji (M-BW-35) at the 12th thoracic vertebra

Explanation of points

GV-13 *(tao dao)*, the "kiln pathway," is an important point for clearing heat, calming the spirit, and relieving panic attacks and convulsions. It clears heat in both exterior and deficiency patterns. This serves as the main point in this case, since the patient is showing heat from deficiency subsequent to an invasion of (external) pathogenic heat. There are also signs of disturbance of the spirit and palpitations, which this point can help relieve. It draws on energy from the qi, especially in the governing vessel, to calm the spirit.

LU-7 *(lie que)*. The name of this point means a small, narrow seam or depression. The point is located on the upper part of the styloid process of the radius, where there is a small, narrow seam. It is the connecting point of the arm greater yin channel and the arm yang brightness channel, and also the confluent point of the conception vessel. It promotes the dispersing function of the Lung, removes wind, and regulates the conception vessel. It is very effective in regulating the qi. In clinical practice, LU-7 *(lie que)*, in combination with certain other points, can be used to treat patterns of either excess or deficiency. Examples of excess would be those patterns involving pain, such as in the head, neck, back of the shoulders, and nape of the neck, or involving a sore and swollen throat. Where there is a pattern of deficiency, LU-7 *(lie que)* can be used for yin deficiency, especially the heat associated with such deficiency, as in this case.

KI-6 *(zhao hai)*, or "sea of brightness," is the confluent point of the yin heel vessel. It nourishes the yin, strengthens the functions of the Kidney, calms the spirit, settles the emotions, and soothes the throat. The body fluids and yin have been injured in this case from the heat of the febrile disease, and the patient suffers from palpitations and night sweats. This point, in combination with the first two, is a good choice, even though there is no specific Kidney yin deficiency here. It is used not only for nourishing the Kidney yin, but also for nourishing the body yin in general, and for promoting the functioning of the limbs. Because of its connection with the yin heel vessel, it can help regulate the motor function, and promote the circulation of protective qi. And since protective qi circulates into the yin heel channel, use of this point can help the patient sleep well.

BL-20 *(pi shu)* is the back associated point of the Spleen. It tonifies the Spleen, harmonizes the Stomach and Spleen, and removes dampness. In this case, because the Spleen and Stomach are injured, this point is used for strengthening the middle burner and promoting the Spleen's transportive and transformative functions. The tonification method of manipulation is used.

Jia ji (M-BW-35). This group of points is also known as *huá tuó jiā jǐ*. Hua Tuo is the name of a famous doctor in ancient times. The word *jiā* means to press from both sides, and *jǐ* is the Chinese word for spinal column. This name is given to seventeen pairs of points evenly distributed on both sides of the spinal column, from the first thoracic vertebra to the fifth lumbar vertebra. One may select several points, or just one pair. Each of the points looks as if it were "pressed" from both sides of the spinal column, hence the name. The particular pair of points chosen in this case is at the level of the 12th thoracic vertebra, which is at the same level as, and is used instead of, BL-21 *(wei shu)*, the back associated point of the Stomach. Most of the *jia ji* (M-BW-35) points around the lower part of the back are used for promoting the functions of the Stomach and Intestines. They are especially used to regulate the middle burner, helping to restore function to the Spleen and Stomach by promoting the transportation and transformation of food essence.

Combination of points

GV-13 *(tao dao)*, LU-7 *(lie que)*, KI-6 *(zhao hai)*. In this combination, the latter two points are confluent points. LU-7 *(lie que)* is the confluent point of the conception vessel and is used to regulate the blood, while KI-6 *(zhao hai)* is associated with the yin heel vessel and is used to nourish the yin and promote the functioning of the limbs. Together, these two points are very suitable for patterns involving the late stage of a febrile disease. GV-13 *(tao dao)* here is used to reduce heat, especially heat from deficiency caused by the depletion of the yin and body fluids. Thus the combination is used to reduce heat, balance the yin and yang, nourish the yin of the body, and clear the heat from deficiency.

BL-20 *(pi shu)*, 12th thoracic *jia ji* (M-BW-35). This is an example of a back associated point and a *jia ji* (M-BW-35) point used in combination. In clinical practice, the needling sensation from a back associated point is, generally speaking, not as strong as that of a *jia ji* (M-BW-35) point. As the latter has the advantage of being closer to the governing vessel, it can draw on the qi from the governing vessel to strengthen the functioning of its related Organ. Thus, combined with the back associated point BL-20 *(pi shu)*, this combination is used to strengthen the middle burner and alleviate the digestive system symptoms.

Basic herbal formula

Glehnia and Ophiopogonis Decoction *(sha shen mai men dong tang)* is a formula that is commonly used for the treatment of febrile diseases.

Radix Adenophorae seu Glehniae *(sha shen)* 9g

Rhizoma Polygonati Odorati *(yu zhu)* 6g

Tuber Ophiopogonis Japonici *(mai men dong)* 9g

Folium Mori Albae *(sang ye)* 5g

Semen Dolichoris Lablab *(bian dou)* 5g

Radix Trichosanthis Kirilowii *(tian hua fen)* 5g

Radix Glycyrrhizae Uralensis *(gan cao)* 3g

Explanation of basic herbal formula

This formula is mainly used for patterns involving pathogenic dryness injuring the Lung, or for the late stage of an epidemic febrile disease. At this stage, the pathogenic heat has already been cleared, but not before injuring the body fluids in the Lung and Stomach. The symptom picture in both patterns includes low fever, thirst or a dry cough, yellow urine, dry stools, a red and dry tongue, and a thin, rapid pulse. The pathological change is that pathogenic dryness, or pathogenic heat, injures the body fluids in the Lung and Stomach, causing malnourishment of the body.

In this formula, Radix Adenophorae seu Glehniae *(sha shen)* is sweet and cold, and is associated with the Lung and Stomach channels. It nourishes the yin and clears heat from the Lung. It also strengthens the Stomach functions and promotes the body fluids in the Stomach. It serves as the chief herb in this formula.

There are four deputy herbs. Tuber Ophiopogonis Japonici *(mai men dong)* is sweet and cold, and Rhizoma Polygonati Odorati *(yu zhu)* is sweet and neutral. Both are associated with the Lung and Stomach channels, nourish the yin, and help with the production of body fluids. Folium Mori Albae *(sang ye)* and Radix Trichosanthis Kirilowii *(tian hua fen)* are both bitter, sweet, and cold in nature, are associated with the Lung channel, and serve to clear heat from the Lung and Stomach.

There are two assistant herbs: Semen Dolichoris Lablab *(bian dou)*, which is sweet and warm, and strengthens the functions of the Spleen, and Radix Glycyrrhizae Uralensis *(gan cao)*, which is sweet and neutral, and strengthens the Stomach.

This formula can be used for treating deficiency as well as injury to the yin and body fluids that occurs in the late stages of various disorders.

Modified herbal formula

Radix Pseudostellariae Heterophyllae *(tai zi shen)* 10g
Radix Dioscoreae Oppositae *(shan yao)* 15g
Radix Adenophorae seu Glehniae *(sha shen)* 10g
Tuber Ophiopogonis Japonici *(mai men dong)* 6g
Cortex Moutan Radicis *(mu dan pi)* 5g
Radix Glycyrrhizae Uralensis *(gan cao)* 5g

Explanation of modified herbal formula

The patient is in the late stage of a febrile disease, owing to the deficiency of yin and body fluids in the Stomach and Spleen. Glehnia and Ophiopogonis Decoction *(sha shen mai men dong tang)* is used as the basic formula to nourish the body fluids and strengthen the yin of the body.

In the modified formula that was used in this case, the herbs in the original formula that affect the Lung have been omitted, leaving only those that nourish the Spleen and Stomach. Radix Pseudostellariae Heterophyllae *(tai zi shen)* and Radix Dioscoreae Oppositae *(shan yao)* are substituted for Semen Dolichoris Lablab *(bian dou)* and Rhizoma Polygonati Odorati *(yu zhu)*, not only to nourish the yin, but also to gently tonify the qi. This is appropriate in this case where both the qi and yin (especially the yin) have been injured in the late stage of a febrile disease. Cortex Moutan Radicis *(mu dan pi)* has also been added to clear the heat from deficiency so as to prevent further injury to the yin and body fluids.

Follow-up

The patient was given only two acupuncture treatments, with a day off in between. The herbal formula was taken daily, with one package divided into two half-doses, for one week. During this time the symptoms were alleviated: her appetite improved, the night sweats disappeared, she recovered her energy, and her joints became less sore. Since by the fifth and sixth days the symptoms had more or less disappeared, and as the patient was otherwise in good health, the treatment was terminated.

This particular type of pattern frequently occurs during the recovery phase after a high fever. While many patients may recover from such an illness without treatment, the duration of this stage of the illness may often be protracted, especially if the patient is advanced in years (over 60). The disorder may consume too much of such a patient's energy, and, in this condition, one is vulnerable to various infections. Proper treatment can shorten the duration of the illness, strengthen the body's resistance, and improve the constitution. Treatment in such cases generally does not last very long, and there is no real need for long-term follow-up.

Diagnostic Principles for Poor Appetite

Abnormal appetite comprises several different disorders including diminished or poor appetite (even anorexia), excessive appetite (overeating), abnormal taste, and parorexia (pica). In clinical practice it is poor appetite that is most commonly encountered, especially as an aspect of other disorders. It may therefore involve a variety of pathological changes, but in general, the site of disease is the Spleen and Stomach.

In Chinese medicine the Spleen and Stomach are known as the "root of post-Heaven," and are the most important source for the replenishment of the antipathogenic factors. When the transportive and transformative functions of the Spleen and Stomach are normal, the appetite and digestion will be normal. A healthy person will have a good appetite, and an ill person with a good appetite can recover quickly. Appetite is thus an important diagnostic marker in Chinese medicine, and is also useful in judging the success of treatment. It is well known that poor appetite, although not recognized as an independent disorder, is a very significant factor in clinical practice, and this is why it is given special attention in this book.

Etiological and pathological change

The most common causes of diminished (poor) appetite are retention of dampness in the Spleen (either damp-cold or damp-heat) and deficiency of Spleen qi. Other causes encountered in the clinic include qi stagnation in the middle burner, food retention (from improper diet), and Spleen and Stomach yin deficiency *(Fig. 3-9)*.

Symptoms and differentiation

Retention of damp-cold in the Spleen involves symptoms such as poor appetite, coldness and pain in the epigastric and abdominal regions, nausea or clear vomitus, lack of thirst, heaviness in the limbs and body, clear urine, loose stools, a pale and swollen tongue with a white, moist coating, and a sunken and moderate pulse.

Fig. 3-9

Symptoms of damp-heat retention in the Spleen include poor appetite, a gener-

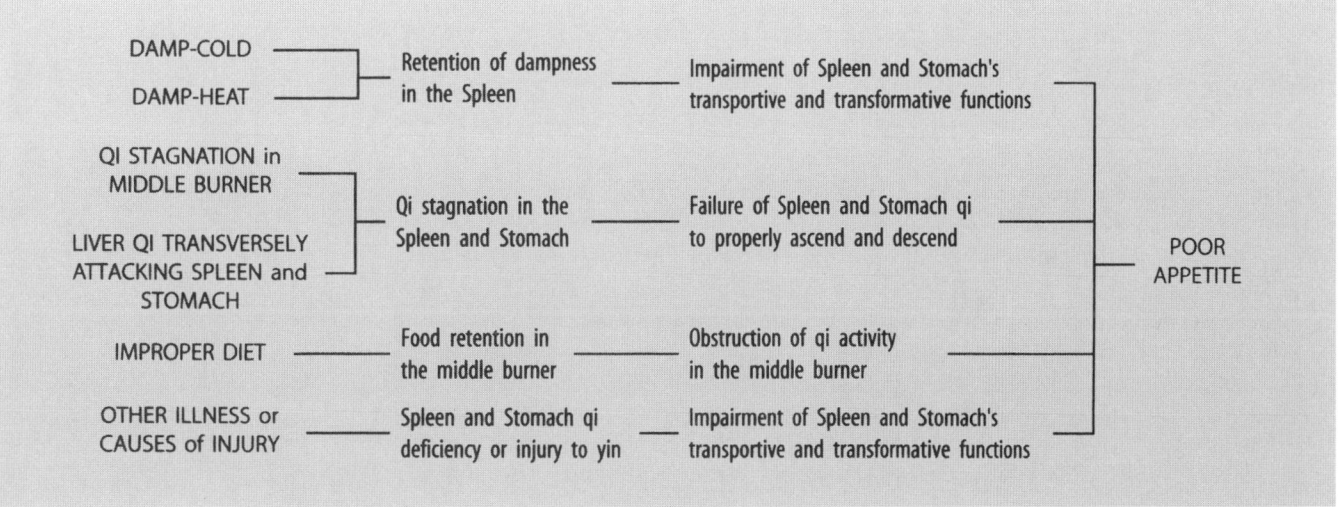

alized hot sensation in the body, distention in the epigastric and abdominal regions, nausea or sticky and yellowish vomitus, thirst but with little desire to drink, heaviness in the limbs and body, yellow urine, yellow and loose stools, which are sticky and difficult to pass, a red tongue with a yellow, greasy coating, and a slippery, rapid pulse.

Qi stagnation in the middle burner is characterized by poor appetite, distention and fullness in the epigastric and abdominal regions, frequent belching that may temporarily relieve the abdominal distention and fullness, and nausea or retching. If the Liver qi transversely attacks the Spleen and Stomach, there may be abnormal emotional changes, distention in the hypochondrial region, no obvious change in the condition of the tongue, and a wiry pulse.

Food retention in the Stomach is associated with a history of overeating. Symptoms include an aversion to food, pain and distention in the epigastric and abdominal regions which is aggravated by pressure, foul breath, regurgitation and vomiting, or diarrhea with very smelly stools containing particles of undigested food. The distention and pain are generally relieved after vomiting or diarrhea. The tongue coating is thick and loose, and the pulse is slippery.

Symptoms of qi deficiency in the Spleen and Stomach include poor appetite, distention and fullness in the epigastric and abdominal regions which worsens after eating, fatigue, general lassitude which is aggravated by physical activity, loose stools, a pale tongue with a white coating, and a forceless pulse.

Yin deficiency in the Spleen and Stomach frequently occurs in the late stage of febrile disease. Symptoms include poor appetite, or being hungry but with an aversion to eating, dull pain or discomfort in the epigastric and abdominal regions, dry mouth and throat, red and dry lips, diminished quantity of yellow urine, dry stools, a dry, red tongue with a thin body and little coating (or peeled coating), and a thin and rapid pulse.

It is important to remember that poor appetite is only one symptom. Apart from identifying the site of a disease, it can be difficult to determine its cause on the basis of appetite alone. In practice, therefore, one must also rely on the accompanying symptoms.

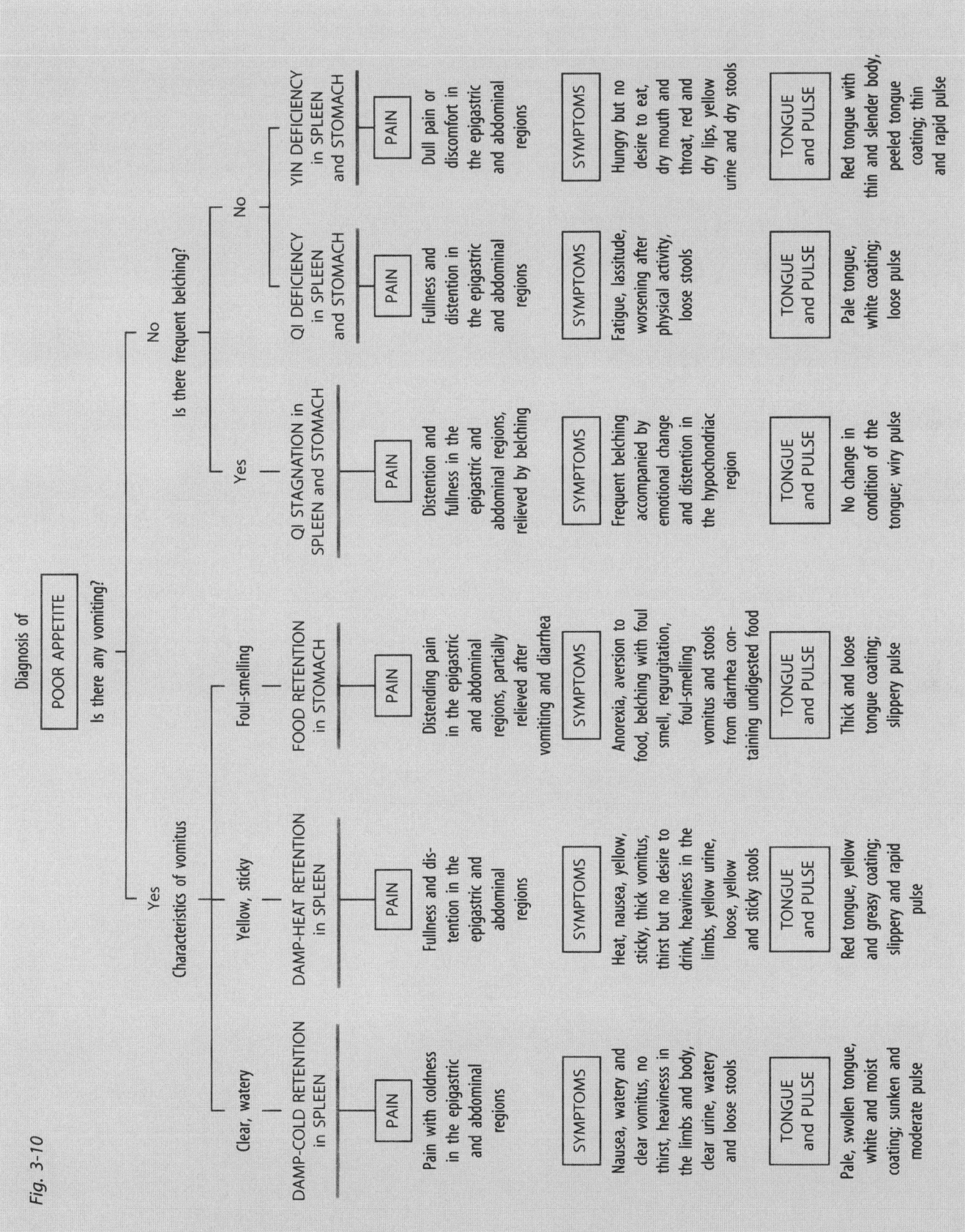

Fig. 3-10

Abdominal and Epigastric Pain

CASE 13: **Male, age 36**

Main complaint

Distention and pain in the epigastric region.

History

The patient first experienced distention and pain in the epigastric region three days ago for no apparent reason. He also complained of coldness in the same area. Sometimes the pain decreases. He has a poor appetite, and the distention worsens if he eats too much.

Belching somewhat relieves the distention. The patient also experiences general lassitude. He does not regurgitate food, however, and does not feel thirsty. His sleep and urination are both normal, and he has a bowel movement two to three times a day. The stools are not watery, and are without any blood or pus.

Tongue

Slightly red body, with a thin, white, and slightly greasy coating

Pulse

Slippery and slightly sunken on the left side

Analysis of symptoms

1. Distention and slight pain in the epigastric region—qi stagnation in the middle burner.
2. Localized coldness—dysfunction of yang qi in warming the body.
3. Poor appetite—impairment of the transportive and transformative functions of the middle burner.
4. Frequent belching—reversal of Stomach qi.
5. White and greasy tongue coating—damp-cold.
6. Slippery pulse—dampness.

Basic theory of case

The concept of qi activity is unique to Chinese medicine. It can be described as the directional pathways for the movement or circulation of qi through the body, such as up and down or in and out. Like qi itself, which has no particular form and is only manifested through various bodily functions, qi activity is also a functional concept and has no visible form or shape. Although invisible, the effects of qi activity on various physiological processes throughout life are very important. All the normal functions of the Organs, for example, the dispersing and downward-

Fig. 4-1

moving actions of Lung qi, are dependent upon qi activity, which must be free of obstruction.

In the clinic, a disorder related to the obstruction of qi activity is called qi stagnation.

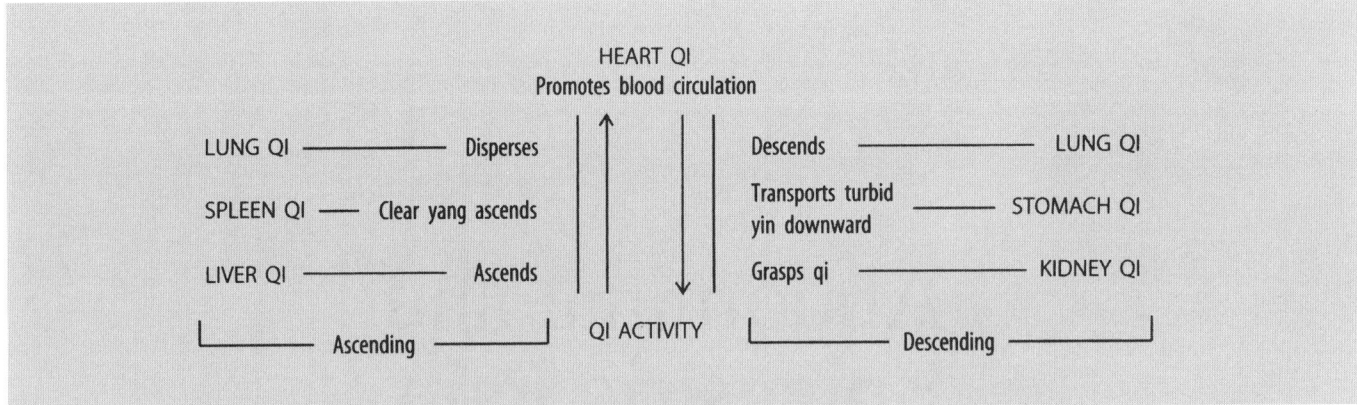

Qi stagnation can be traced to a variety of causes, but the basic pathological change is poor circulation (hence stagnation) of qi. Qi stagnation can adversely affect the local tissues, channels and collaterals, Organs, or even the entire body, and thereby give rise to a wide variety of clinical symptoms. In some cases stagnant qi can lead to the blockage of normal qi activity, resulting in such patterns as reversal of qi (also known as rebellious qi) or sinking of qi. The normal flow of qi—upward or downward—can be reversed, depending on which of the internal Organs is involved. Such patterns are very common.

Cause of disease

Pathogenic cold

Cold is a yin pathogenic factor which can injure or consume the body's yang qi, leading to a feeling of cold in the middle burner. In this case, the patient has a cold feeling in the epigastric region, and the tongue coating is thin, white, and slightly greasy. These symptoms are characteristic of cold, and pathogenic cold is thus the cause of the illness.

Site of disease

Stomach

The patient complains of distention and fullness in the epigastric region, and when he eats too much the distention becomes worse. This is the main indicator that the Stomach is the site of the disease.

Pathological change

Qi stagnation, whereby the circulation of qi is impeded, can be attributed to various causes. For example, it may be caused by an invasion of an exterior pathogenic factor, or by severe emotional upset, retention of phlegm, dampness, harmful water, or stasis of blood. Any one of these things can obstruct the pathway of qi. In this case, it was an invasion of pathogenic cold that caused the disease.

According to Chinese medicine, the yang of the body is the force underlying the activity of qi. Cold is a yin pathogenic factor which can consume or interfere with the yang qi. Cold is characterized by constriction, which can impede the circulation of qi and lead to stagnation.

In this case, qi stagnation has occurred in the Stomach, which feels distended. When the distention becomes severe there is pain. Because the yang qi of the Stomach is injured, a feeling of cold sets in. The stagnant qi interferes with the function of transporting food out of the Stomach, and the patient thus has a poor appetite. Over-eating increases the retention of food in the Stomach, and aggravates the feeling of distention. The normal movement of Stomach qi is downward; the frequent belching here is caused by a reversal (upward) in the directional movement of Stomach qi. This is a reaction of the Stomach qi as it encounters an obstruction to its normal downward movement. In other words, belching is a manifestation of the reversal in the normal flow of qi. As the Stomach qi reverses its direction and moves upward, the obstructed qi (and thus the abdominal distention) is relieved somewhat when the patient belches. There was no complaint of regurgitation, and the patient was not thirsty, both of which suggest the absence of heat.

The tongue is slightly red with a thin, white coating, which is a normal presentation for the tongue. This means that there is no apparent injury to the body's qi and blood. However, the tongue coating is also slightly greasy, and the pulse is slippery, both of which are signs of dampness. We can infer from this evidence that there was an invasion of pathogenic cold which interfered with the metabolism of body fluids, and that the dampness and harmful body fluids are now retained inside the body. The white coating on the tongue, and the absence of a rapid pulse, indicate that there is no heat or damp-heat in the system. We can therefore conclude that damp-cold was produced and retained interiorly; there was no invasion of pathogenic dampness.

The patient has two or three bowel movement a day, which can be attributed to dampness. The color and quality of the stools are normal, indicating that the damp-cold is not yet severe.

Fig. 4-2

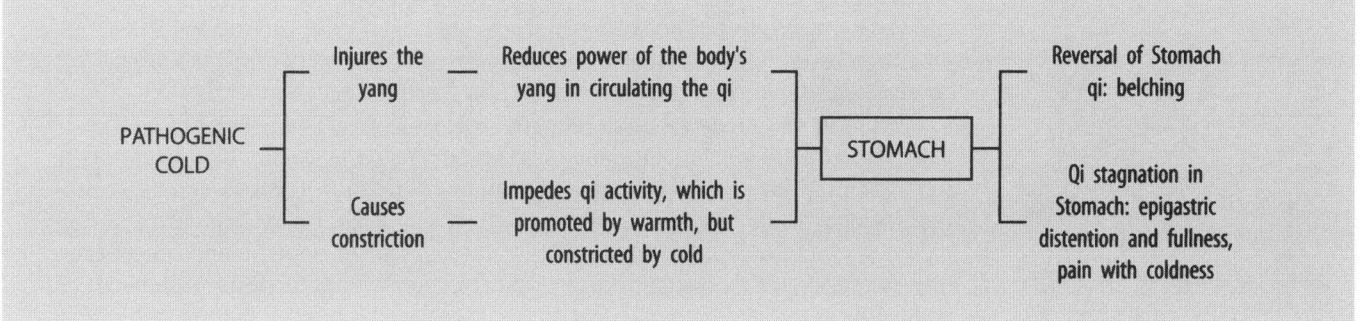

Pattern of disease

This is a disorder of the middle burner. In the absence of exterior pattern symptoms, we may conclude that this is an interior pattern.

The patient has a cold feeling in the epigastric region, a white tongue coating, and a pulse that is not rapid. These symptoms are evidence of a cold pattern.

There is poor qi circulation, and stagnation of qi in the middle burner, but no evidence of injury to the underlying antipathogenic factors. This is therefore a pattern of excess.

Additional notes

1. Is the cold here of internal or external origin?

Exterior cold occurs when pathogenic cold from the environment invades the body; interior cold is caused by a deficiency of yang qi. In this case the patient has no apparent history of catching cold or of invasion by any other pathogenic factor, and there is no definitive evidence to suggest yang deficiency. Analysis of the symptoms points to a pattern of excess, as the history is very short (only three days long). Therefore it is likely that the cold came from the external environment. Yet it did not enter the body through the skin; rather, it invaded the Stomach directly, for example, by means of the patient eating too much cold food, or not dressing warmly. That is why there are no symptoms of an exterior pattern (fever, aversion to cold). The evidence points very clearly to an interior pattern caused by a direct invasion of pathogenic cold.

2. Why is the pulse sunken on the left side alone?

A sunken pulse indicates an interior pattern, but in this case the pulse is only sunken on the left wrist. In fact, this is not related to the patient's general condition and therefore has no particular significance here.

Conclusion

1. According to the eight principles:
   Interior, cold, excess.

2. According to etiology:
   Invasion of pathogenic cold.

3. According to theory of qi, blood, and body fluids:
   Qi stagnation.

4. According to Organ theory:
   Qi stagnation in the Stomach.

Treatment principle

1. Warm the Stomach.

2. Regulate the qi.

Explanation of treatment principle

Because of the various causes of qi stagnation, the treatment principle may differ in each case. Here the qi disorder was caused by an invasion of cold. We therefore need to warm the body yang, because warmth will stimulate the movement of qi.

Warming the Stomach will help relieve the cold in the middle burner, and help the yang qi recover. As the qi activity (circulation) improves, the stagnation of qi in the Stomach will be relieved, and the symptoms will disappear: the distention and feeling of fullness in the Stomach will diminish, and as the Stomach qi resumes its proper movement downward, the belching will also cease.

In discussing treatment, no mention has been made of damp-cold. That is because in this case the damp-cold is secondary to the invasion of cold and injury to the yang qi, and therefore does not need direct treatment. Moreover, the symptoms of damp-cold here are not very severe. If we can warm the Stomach and regulate the qi of the middle burner so as to restore the transportive and transformative functions of the middle burner, the retention of damp-cold will itself be resolved.

Selection of points

PC-6 *(nei guan)*
SP-4 *(gong sun)*
CV-12 *(zhong wan)*
ST-21 *(liang men)*

Explanation of points

PC-6 *(nei guan)* is the connecting point on the lesser yin channel. This point regulates the qi and alleviates pain; it also calms the spirit. The draining or reducing method of needle manipulation is used here.

SP-4 *(gong sun)* is the connecting point on the Spleen channel. It regulates the Spleen and harmonizes the Stomach, regulating the functions of the Intestines. The draining method is used here to remove the qi stagnation from the middle burner and alleviate the pain. In Chinese medicine, when the obstruction is removed, the pain will be alleviated.

CV-12 *(zhong wan)* is the alarm point of the Stomach and one of the eight meeting points of the yang Organs. It regulates the qi in the middle burner and removes obstruction from the blood. It also resolves dampness in the middle burner. The draining method is used here: the needle is held perpendicularly when puncturing, and is maintained in this position throughout.

ST-21 *(liang men)*. The Chinese name for this point means "gate of food." It is only two units lateral to CV-12 *(zhong wan)*. This point serves to harmonize the

Stomach and remove the retention of food, thereby promoting the digestive functions of the Spleen and Stomach. The draining method is used to remove the obstruction caused by retention of cold. The point is punctured perpendicularly until qi is obtained. Then the angle of the needle is changed to a horizontal position, pointing toward the feet, so that the tip of the needle follows the direction of the Stomach channel. A rotating method is used for draining. If the tip of the needle is pointed in a direction contrary to the flow in the Stomach channel (that is, toward the head), this would also be consistent with draining. However, in this case strong draining is not required. Here, needle manipulation is used to drain, and needle direction is used to tonify. In this way the damp-cold is dispelled while the Stomach qi is protected.

Strong moxibustion is used at this point and at CV-12 *(zhong wan)*. The moxa box is used with two pieces of moxa stick, and the heavy method is applied for fifteen minutes. This removes the cold and alleviates pain, while promoting the qi in the middle burner.

Combination of points

CV-12 *(zhong wan)* and ST-21 *(liang men)* are local points which are mutually reinforcing. When used together, CV-12 *(zhong wan)* is often needled perpendicularly, while the needle is pointed in a downward direction at ST-21 *(liang men)*. These two points are effective in treating problems in the middle burner, and are important for alleviating epigastric pain.

PC-6 *(nei guan)*, SP-4 *(gong sun)*, and CV-12 *(zhong wan)* regulate the qi in the middle burner. This combination is comprised of two connecting points and one alarm point. Its use helps remove the obstruction to the qi in order to regulate the qi and thereby alleviate the pain.

Follow-up

After the first day's treatment the abdominal distention had noticeably diminished, and the patient felt a good deal less pain. The following day he was given the same treatment. He reported that the symptoms had disappeared, and that his appetite had been restored to normal. Treatment was therefore ended. The patient returned for a checkup a month later, and everything was normal.

CASE 14: **Female, age 50**

Main complaint

Distention, fullness, and pain in the epigastric and abdominal regions

History

Two weeks ago the patient experienced distention, fullness, and pain in the epigastric and abdominal regions. There was no apparent feeling of heat or cold in these areas. The pain was dull, and her appetite was not affected. The distention and pain did not become worse after eating. Very often the pain was most obvious after a bowel movement, and would ease slightly after eating a bit. She did not feel thirsty, nor did she belch or regurgitate. Her bowel movements and urination were normal.

Tongue

Pale body with a mottled yellow and white coating

Pulse

Wiry and slightly lax

Analysis of symptoms

1. Pain and distention in the epigastrium and abdomen—stagnation of qi in the Stomach and Spleen.
2. Relief of pain after eating—deficiency of antipathogenic factors.
3. Absence of hot or cold feeling in the abdomen—no deficiency or excess of yin or yang.
4. Pale tongue—malnourishment of qi and blood.
5. Wiry and slightly lax pulse—obstruction of qi activity.

Basic theory of case

Here it would be helpful to clarify the concept of excessive patterns. These result from an invasion or retention of excessive pathogenic factors. Qi stagnation is a pattern caused by the poor circulation of qi, whereby qi activity is obstructed. It is therefore classified as a pattern of excess. The causes of qi stagnation can be divided into two major groups: excessive or deficient.

As explained in a previous case, obstruction of qi activity may be caused by a pathogenic factor or by a strong emotional factor. Obstruction will eventually lead to stagnation of qi. This type of qi stagnation pertains to excess. On the other hand, when yang or qi deficiency lowers the overall level of energy, the movement of qi is slowed and lacks force. This can also lead to qi stagnation, which is regarded as a combination of deficiency and excess. In the absence of any apparent pathogenic factor, there is no pathogen to be removed. However, the draining method is still the proper means of removing the obstruction of qi. In addition, however, tonification should also be considered.

Whether due to excess or deficiency, qi stagnation can disrupt the movement of blood as well as the metabolism of water. This can lead to blood stasis, retention of harmful water, or phlegm. When this occurs the pathogenic factors are mixed together and influence each other, causing other complications that must be diagnosed and treated. That is why it is important to determine the relationship between the pathogenic factors and antipathogenic factors, as well as the severity of the pathogenic factors and the extent to which the antipathogenic factors have been injured. Only then will we be in a position to prescribe the correct method of treatment, tailored to the individual case.

Fig. 4-3

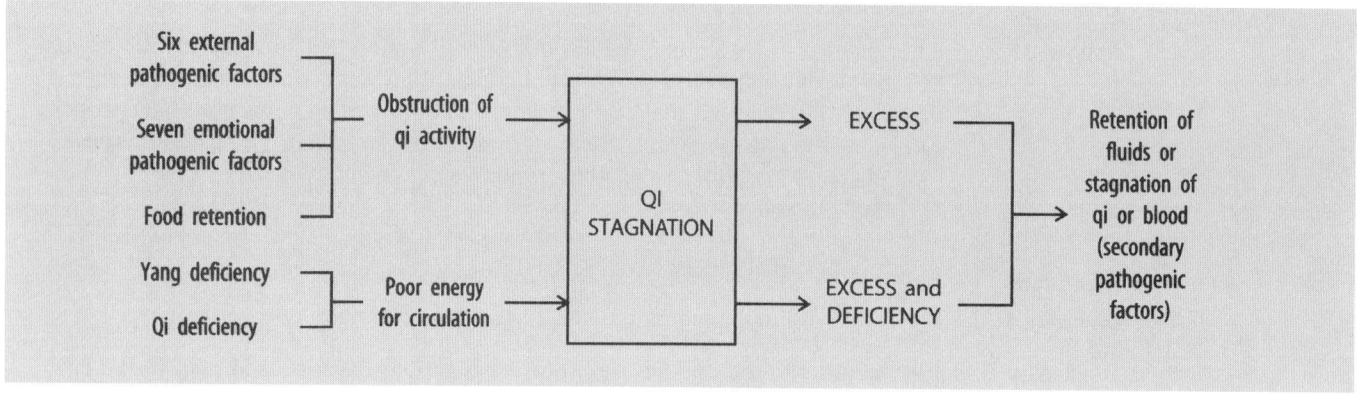

Cause of disease

Insufficiency of antipathogenic factors

The patient experiences a dull pain in the epigastric and abdominal regions, which is relieved somewhat after eating. The tongue is pale and the pulse lax. All of these signs suggest an insufficiency of antipathogenic factors. There is not enough evidence here to indicate an invasion by a pathogenic factor. The cause of the disease is therefore an insufficiency of antipathogenic factors.

Site of disease

Spleen and Stomach

Distention, fullness, and pain in the epigastrium and abdomen are the primary symptoms, indicating that the site of the disease is the Spleen and Stomach.

Pathological change

Localized distention, fullness, and pain is characteristic of qi stagnation. Here the symptoms are located in the epigastric and abdominal regions, indicating that the stagnation of qi has occurred in the Spleen and Stomach. Because there is no feeling of heat or cold, we can deduce that there is no significant imbalance of yin and yang.

The pain is very mild and dull, and is associated with eating and with bowel movements. Normally, bowel movements consume very little of the body's qi, but if a person has a pattern of qi deficiency, bowel movements can aggravate the deficiency of qi. When this happens the pain will increase after a bowel movement. Eating can relieve the pain to a certain extent because food can, at least temporarily, improve the body's energy level and lessen the deficiency of qi.

Fig. 4-4

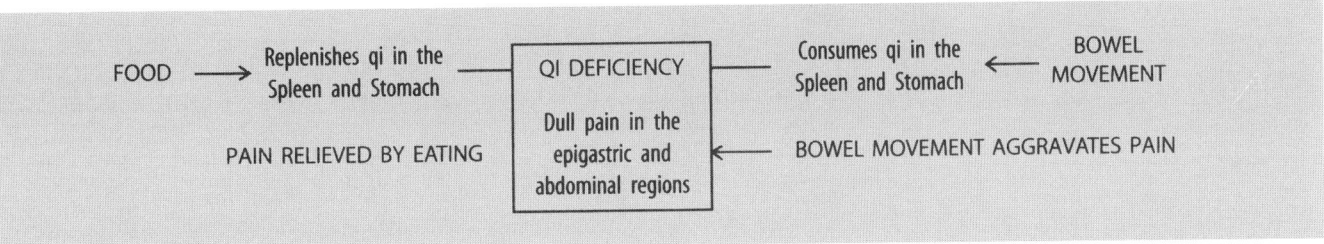

From the evidence of qi deficiency in this case we may conclude that the energy of the body is inadequate to circulate the qi, which has thereupon become stagnant in the Stomach and Spleen. Thus, the distention and fullness in the epigastrium and abdomen is caused by qi deficiency.

The history in this case is fairly short, and the symptoms are not too severe (the appetite, urination, and bowel movements are still normal); there is thus no apparent dysfunction in the digestive system. The patient does not belch or hiccup, and the symptoms are not aggravated by eating. This means that there is no retention of food in the Stomach. Furthermore, the patient is not thirsty and does not regurgitate, indicating that there is no heat.

The tongue is pale because the body of the tongue lacks nourishment from the blood. In this case it is due to qi deficiency, which lacks the force to properly circulate the blood through the upper part of the body.

The pulse is wiry, indicating an obstruction to the qi activity. Its lax quality results from qi deficiency in the Spleen and Stomach. These signs conform to our diagnosis of qi stagnation caused by deficiency of qi.

Pattern of disease

This is an interior pattern because the patient has qi stagnation in the middle burner (Spleen and Stomach) and there are no symptoms of an invasion by any pathogenic factor.

Cold or heat can be discounted in the absence of any feeling of cold or heat in the Stomach or epigastric regions, the absence of thirst or regurgitation, and the normal bowel movements and urination.

There is a combination of deficiency and excess. The qi stagnation in the middle burner, and the pain and distention in the epigastrium and abdomen, indicate a pattern of excess. And because the qi stagnation here is caused by qi deficiency, there is also deficiency.

Additional notes

1. What is the reason for the mottled yellow and white tongue coating?

In Chinese medicine a white tongue coating indicates the presence of cold, or at least the absence of heat. A yellow coating indicates the presence of heat. In this case there is no apparent imbalance of yin and yang. There are no heat symptoms of any kind. But the patient's tongue has both a yellow and white coating. The reason for this is that the qi has become stagnant in the middle burner, which can lead to heat from constraint. However, the heat is not very conspicuous, and we don't have enough evidence at this time to diagnose heat.

2. What is the cause of the deficiency in this case?

The deficiency here is one of most commonly encountered patterns in the clinic. A frequent cause of this pattern is a chronic or long-term illness which has consumed the antipathogenic factors. However, this diagnosis does not rely only on the duration of the illness, but mainly on the patient's presentation. The illness here has lasted only two weeks, but the clinical symptoms point to a pattern of deficiency. The cause of this deficiency could be that the patient has suffered from a mild insufficiency of Spleen and Stomach qi, mild enough that it never manifested in clinical symptoms. But recently there may have been an aggravating factor that caused the symptoms to appear. The deficiency and its accompanying symptoms may also be due to ageing, which has brought about a gradual degeneration in the body's antipathogenic factors.

3. How does one distinguish the cause of illness from the problem of deficiency or excess?

Both this and the previous case presented with abdominal distention, fullness, and pain. And in both cases the symptoms were not very severe, and the patients' bowel movements and urination were normal. Why, then, the different diagnoses? In the previous case there was retention of cold which caused the Stomach qi to stagnate; this is a pattern of excess. In the present case, by contrast, there is a combination of deficiency and excess: qi deficiency in the Spleen and Stomach, which has led to qi stagnation (excess). The main distinguishing points in these two cases include:

- The duration of the illness. The previous case lasted just three days; there were no Stomach disorders, and the antipathogenic factors had not been affected. Here, the illness has lasted two weeks, the patient is much older, and the antipathogenic factors are deficient.

- The nature of the pain. The abdominal distention in the previous case was aggravated by eating, and belching helped relieve the discomfort. This indicated that the pathogenic factor was strong. Here, eating relieves the discomfort, and the pain becomes worse after bowel movements. This evidence would suggest that the antipathogenic factors are deficient, and that the internal Organs are being deprived of their proper nourishment.

Readers are referred to case 15 for additional information.

Conclusion

1. According to the eight principles:
   Interior, neither heat nor cold, and a combination of excess and deficiency.
2. According to theory of qi, blood, and body fluids:
   Qi deficiency and stagnation.
3. According to Organ theory:
   Qi stagnation with qi deficiency in the Spleen and Stomach.

Treatment principle

1. Invigorate the functioning of the Spleen and strengthen the qi.
2. Regulate the qi and remove the obstruction.

Explanation of treatment principle

A pattern of qi stagnation means that the qi cannot move smoothly, that its circulation is obstructed. This is a pattern of excess that must be regulated, and the draining method is therefore indicated. On the other hand, qi deficiency means that the qi is not strong enough; a reinforcing or tonification method is required to increase the production of qi and to reduce the consumption or loss of qi.

The two patterns exist simultaneously; one must be drained, the other reinforced. But if the draining method is used for a deficiency pattern, it can further consume the qi; and if tonification is used in treating a pattern of excess, it can aggravate the obstruction of qi. Here the qi stagnation (excess) is caused by qi deficiency, thus tonifying the qi is the main method used to strengthen the circulation of qi and remove the obstruction from the middle burner. But since the use of tonification alone can increase the feeling of distention (caused by qi stagnation) in the middle burner, it is vital that the qi be regulated, either through herbs or acupuncture, because regulating the qi will facilitate the circulation of qi and thereby prevent any increase of discomfort in the middle burner.

Selection of points

ST-25 *(tian shu)*
SP-15 *(da heng)*
CV-12 *(zhong wan)*
LI-10 *(shou san li)*
ST-36 *(zu san li)*

Explanation of points

ST-25 *(tian shu)* is located in the abdominal region. It is the alarm point of the Large Intestine channel and is therefore associated with the yang brightness Organs (Large Intestine and Stomach). It is an important local point, and the main one for the treatment of epigastric and abdominal disorders. It can be used in treating excess, as it helps reduce qi stagnation, alleviate pain, promote the digestive functions, and reduce food retention. It can also be used in treating deficiency, such as Spleen and Stomach qi deficiency, with its attendant symptoms of abdominal distention and diarrhea. As this case involves a combination of deficiency and excess, the point is used to tonify the qi of the middle burner, regulate the qi of the digestive system, promote the functions of the yang brightness Organs, and alleviate pain. It is used as a local point.

SP-15 *(da heng)* is on the Spleen channel, and is located in the abdominal region, 4 units lateral to the umbilicus. It can warm the local area and regulate the qi of the Spleen and Intestines. Warming helps the qi to circulate, which thereby relieves the pain. Hence ST-25 *(tian shu)* and this point are selected on opposite sides: ST-25 *(tian shu)* on the right and SP-15 *(da heng)* on the left. The purpose is to reduce the number of needles, involve an additional channel, and thereby utilize these two points to the best advantage.

CV-12 *(zhong wan)* is the alarm point of the Stomach channel and an influential point for the yang Organs. It is an important point for regulating the qi of the middle burner, and for removing obstruction from the digestive system. It also tonifies middle burner qi and strengthens the functions of the Spleen and Stomach. Here the point is used not only for tonifying the deficiency, but also for regulating the qi. It serves as a local point.

LI-10 *(shou san li)* regulates and promotes the functions of the Large Intestine. It serves to regulate qi and alleviate pain. The *Great Compendium of Acupuncture and Moxibustion (Zhen jiu da cheng)* observes that this point can also be used for lower back pain when the pain makes it difficult to lie down. The lyrics of the late-Ming acupuncture song "Ode of Xi Hong" *(Xi Hong fu)* say that this point can be used for treating continuous pain in the upper part of the shoulder radiating to the area around the umbilicus. Clinically, the point is often used for abdominal pain, especially in the paraumbilical area, as well as lower back pain, vomiting, and diarrhea. Here it serves as a distant point.

ST-36 *(zu san li)* is an important point for regulating the Stomach and Large Intestine. It regulates the functions of the middle burner (Spleen and Stomach), removes obstruction from the channels and Organs, and alleviates pain.

Combination of points

ST-25 *(tian shu)* and SP-15 *(da heng)* are both situated very close to the umbilicus: ST-25 *(tian shu)* is 2 units from the umbilicus, and SP-15 *(da heng)* is just 4 units away. Although they are very close together, these points are associated with different Organs. ST-25 *(tian shu)* is associated with the yang brightness (Large Intestine and Stomach), SP-15 *(da heng)* with greater yin (Spleen). And although both points are located in the abdominal region, the former tends toward the yang aspect, the latter toward the yin. In combination they are used to regulate the Spleen and Stomach.

CV-12 *(zhong wan)* and ST-25 *(tian shu)* is one of the most frequently used combinations, important in the treatment of abdominal pain associated with qi stagnation. CV-12 *(zhong wan)* helps regulate and tonify the qi, and is an important local point. ST-25 *(tian shu)*, apart from its local function, is good for regulating the qi in the yang brightness channels and Organs. Thus one point is associated with two channels and two yang Organs (Stomach and Large Intestine).

LI-10 *(shou san li)* and ST-36 *(zu san li)*. LI-10 *(shou san li)* is situated close to the elbows, ST-36 *(zu san li)* to the knees. *Shǒu* in Chinese means hand, and *zú* means foot; both points are termed *sān lǐ* ("three miles"). These two points (bilaterally) are used to regulate the hand and leg yang brightness channels. The arm yang brightness is associated with the Large Intestine, and the leg yang brightness with the Stomach. Since both are yang brightness, they are often combined. Moreover, they have similar actions: both are used in treating qi stagnation of the Large Intestine and Stomach, and retention of food—very common causes of Stomach and abdominal pain. Together these points are very good for regulating qi. They are a good example of a distant combination. They are not only used for patterns of excess in the yang brightness Organs and channels, but in some cases can be also used in treating deficiency.

Follow-up   The patient was treated once a day for the first three days, after which the abdominal distention and pain had diminished. The pain following bowel movements also declined, and her appetite improved. Treatment was then changed to every other day. The same points were used, but with a gentle, even needle movement. After two weeks the abdominal pain disappeared and the distention was largely relieved. During the third week the patient was given only two treatments in order to consolidate the result of the first stage of treatment. After that, the epigastric problem was almost completely relieved.

Treatment was then stopped for two weeks. When the patient returned, there were no apparent symptoms. She very occasionally experienced abdominal distention. The patient was given two more treatments in the space of a week. She returned for a checkup three and four months later, and there were no further symptoms.

It can be gathered from a case like this that in clinical practice, there is, in fact, no fixed course of treatment. The duration of treatment depends entirely on the patient's response. Each patient recovers at their own pace and should not be compared with others. Moreover, the duration of treatment is not always shorter than the history of the disorder, as can be seen in this case. The treatment of a disorder entailing deficiency is very often longer than the history of the illness itself.

The Chinese have a saying: "Getting a disease is like a mountain falling down; getting rid of a disease is like reeling off silk *(dé bìng rǔ shān dǎo, qù bìng rǔ chōu sī).*" The general idea here is that when a person falls sick with a disease, it can feel like a quick catastrophe, a "mountain falling down," but the ensuing recovery can feel as long and slow as "reeling off silk" (from a cocoon). Everyone involved in the process can experience this, patient and practitioner alike. The onset of a disease can be very rapid, but this does not mean that the actual illness started at that moment. It may have begun long ago, but was hidden in the body. Only when an imbalance of yin and yang reaches a certain level does the illness manifest in symptoms. Thus, during treatment, patience and confidence are needed.

CASE 15: **Male, age 52**

Main complaint	Epigastric pain
History	Over the past five years the patient has experienced recurring attacks of epigastric pain. The diagnosis, in conventional biomedicine, was not clear, and the only medicine the patient took was pain killers when the pain became severe. The symptoms have worsened over the last two months. During this time he experienced frequent epigastric pain and indeterminate gnawing hunger (*cáo zá* — see below), a burning pain in the epigastric region, and frequent regurgitation. He has not felt any local coldness, nor has his appetite been affected. The pain he has experienced is not related to when he eats.

The patient has suffered from hypertension for the past eight years. He now often complains of a stifling sensation in the chest, shortness of breath, restlessness, insomnia, and, in particular, difficulty in falling asleep. His bowel movements and urination are normal. |
| **Tongue** | Normal color, thin coating, yellow and greasy in the middle |
| **Pulse** | Wiry, slippery, slightly forceless |
| **Analysis of symptoms** | 1. Epigastric pain—obstruction of the qi activity.
2. Burning pain with no local feeling of cold—interior heat.
3. Indeterminate gnawing hunger in the stomach—disturbance by pathogenic heat. (Indeterminate gnawing hunger (*cáo zá*) is a feeling of unease in the epigastrium as if it were empty, yet there is no desire to eat. The stomach feels hot, rough, and "peppery.")
4. Regurgitation—upward reversal of heat.
5. Restlessness and insomnia—disturbance of Heart spirit.
6. Yellow tongue coating—heat pattern. |
| **Basic theory of case** | In Chinese medicine the Stomach is regarded as the "sea" of food and water. This means that food enters the Stomach, where it is first stored and then transported away. Pathogenic factors from the outside can easily enter the Stomach with the food, causing Stomach disorders. For example, too much raw and cold food, such as fruit and salads, can lead to retention of pathogenic cold in the Stomach; or eating too much spicy food can lead to internal heat or retention of fire; or eating unclean foods can bring toxins into the Stomach. Thus, both heat and cold patterns are frequently found in Stomach disorders.

The common causes of Stomach heat include:

• Eating too many hot peppers or other spicy foods.

Hot peppers and spicy foods have the characteristic of heat. Over-indulgence in this type of food can easily lead to heat or fire in the Stomach, resulting in a pattern of Stomach heat.

   • Overeating what in Chinese is called "thick flavors (*hòu wèi*)." This refers to foods that are greasy, sweet, rich, heavy, and/or have a strong taste.

This type of food can be quite cloying and is not easily digested; it stays in the digestive system and lodges in the Stomach, obstructing the qi activity and leading to internal heat.

   • Qi stagnation leading to fire.

The function of the Stomach is to receive, digest, and transport food and water. Receiving, transporting, softening, warming, and "rotting" (digesting) the food are |

the functions of Stomach yang. Certain pathogenic factors like depression, emotional upset, and retention of food may cause stagnation of qi in the middle burner. This can accumulate with the yang qi of the Stomach, causing heat from constraint (or fire), which may result in a heat pattern in the Stomach. Heat from other Organs which affects the middle burner may also lead to Stomach fire.

Any one of these conditions can cause heat from excess, which is commonly encountered in the clinic. In addition, deficiency of yin and body fluids in the Spleen and Stomach, or chronic excessive heat, can injure the yin. These disorders can cause internal heat, and are classified as heat from deficiency (or "empty" heat) in the middle burner.

Fig. 4-5

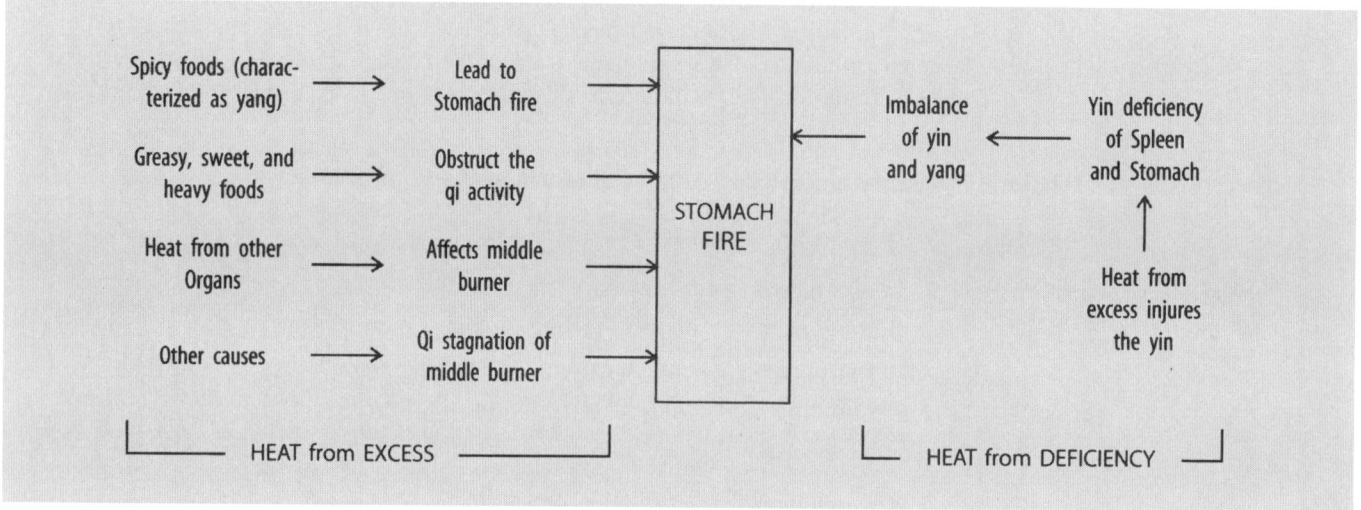

Spicy foods (characterized as yang) →	Lead to Stomach fire →		
Greasy, sweet, and heavy foods →	Obstruct the qi activity →		Imbalance of yin and yang ←	Yin deficiency of Spleen and Stomach
Heat from other Organs →	Affects middle burner →	STOMACH FIRE		↑
Other causes →	Qi stagnation of middle burner →			Heat from excess injures the yin
└── HEAT from EXCESS ──┘			└── HEAT from DEFICIENCY ──┘	

Cause of disease	Pathogenic heat
	The patient suffers from indeterminate gnawing hunger and a burning pain in the Stomach. He also experiences regurgitation, restlessness, and insomnia. All of these symptoms are evidence of heat, which is a yang pathogenic factor characterized by unsteadiness, upward-movement, disturbance of the Stomach, and over-acceleration of the circulation of qi and blood.
Site of disease	Stomach and Heart
	This patient has had recurrent attacks of epigastric pain over the past five years, indicating a Stomach disorder. She also suffers from restlessness, insomnia, and difficulty in falling asleep, which is evidence of Heart involvement.
Pathological change	Epigastric pain can result from either excess or deficiency, heat or cold. Here the patient has recurrent attacks of epigastric pain with a burning sensation. This would suggest retention of heat in the interior, which disturbs and obstructs the circulation of qi and blood, causing pain. Because heat is a yang pathogenic factor, the temperature is high in this case, which explains the absence of localized cold. The patient has indeterminate gnawing hunger in the epigastrium, resulting from the retention of heat in the Stomach, which disturbs the normal functioning of the middle burner, upsetting the qi and blood. When the heat rises upward, the movement of Stomach secretions reverses and travels upward toward the mouth, causing regurgitation. Heat in the Stomach results from excessive yang. Stomach yang normally serves to digest and transport the food; thus, a patient with pure Stomach heat usually does not have a poor appetite, and in some cases may even feel hungry after over-eating.

When heat in the Stomach is severe, the heat from the middle burner can rise up and affect the upper burner, causing a disturbance of the Heart spirit. This is manifested in symptoms like restlessness and insomnia. The patient here has difficulty in falling asleep, which is a characteristic of insomnia caused by heat disturbing the spirit.

Fig. 4-6

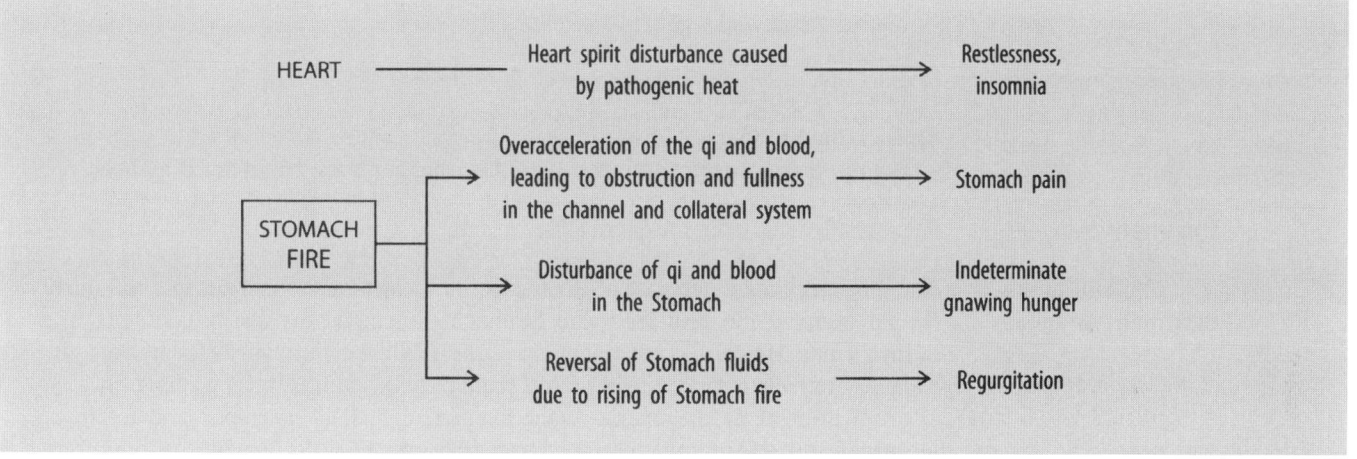

The middle of the tongue corresponds to the Spleen and Stomach. The coating in that area is yellow, indicating that there is heat in the middle burner (Spleen and Stomach).

Pattern of disease

The disorder here has lasted for several years. The problem is in the Stomach, which indicates an interior pattern.

The burning pain in the Stomach, restlessness, and insomnia are evidence of a heat pattern.

The pathogenic heat is intense, but there is nothing to indicate deficiency of antipathogenic factors; it is therefore a pattern of excess.

Additional notes

1. What is the reason for the greasy coating and the wiry, slippery pulse?

A greasy coating and slippery pulse are symptoms of dampness or retention of food. In this case the patient's appetite is not abnormal, but because the pathogenic factor is in the epigastric region, the digestive functions of the Spleen and Stomach can be affected, and we therefore cannot exclude the possibility of damp-heat or retention of food. However, they are not very severe yet, and do not need to be independently treated. The wiry pulse, which reflects obstruction of qi activity, is related to the qi stagnation and blood stasis in the Stomach.

2. Is there deficiency in this case?

The patient complains of a stifling sensation in the chest and shortness of breath, and has a forceless pulse. Are these not signs of deficiency? Because the history is very long, the antipathogenic factors are injured, and the pathogenic factor is in the Stomach, the qi and blood may both be affected, and there thus may be qi deficiency. However, at the present time the prevailing condition is one of excessive heat in the Stomach. The pathogenic heat disperses the normal qi, which has contributed to the present symptoms; but it is not heat from deficiency. In view of the fact that the dominant pattern is one of excess, we may therefore exclude deficiency from the diagnosis.

3. Is the Stomach disorder related to the hypertension in this case?

No. The patient's main complaint is a problem in the digestive system. The hypertension in this case is not associated with the Stomach disorder. Hypertension is a concept of conventional biomedicine; Chinese medical theory does not analyze blood pressure.

Many practitioners make the mistake of believing that Liver yang rising is equivalent to hypertension, but this is not correct. Here, for example, there are no symptoms of Liver yang rising.

Conclusion

1. According to the eight principles:
   Interior, heat, excess.

2. According to etiology:
   Retention of pathogenic Heat.

3. According to Organ theory:
   Heat in the Stomach combined with disturbance of the Heart spirit by heat.

Treatment principle

Remove the heat from the Stomach.

Explanation of treatment principle

The primary characteristic of this case is heat, thus the principle is fairly simple: remove the heat from the Stomach. Since the disease has affected the Stomach and Heart, the treatment principle could be removal of heat from the Stomach and Heart, or removal of heat from only the Stomach, as we have chosen.

The Stomach is the primary location where heat is produced and retained. Disturbance of Heart spirit is only a secondary result of Stomach heat; therefore, if the heat is removed from the Stomach, the heat in the Heart will simultaneously disappear. If the symptoms of insomnia are not too severe, in theory it is unnecessary to treat the Heart and Stomach together. Clinically, treatment of the Stomach heat is of primary importance. Treatment of the Heart heat, if necessary at all, is of secondary importance.

Selection of points

ST-34 *(liang qiu)*
PC-4 *(xi men)*
CV-12 *(zhong wan)*
ST-44 *(nei ting)*

Explanation of points

ST-34 *(liang qiu)* is the accumulating point on the leg yang brightness channel. It is a good choice for removing heat, and an excellent one for regulating qi, removing qi stagnation, and alleviating local or epigastric pain. This is one of the important points used in the treatment of acute Stomach problems. In this case the point is suitable for treating the interior, heat, and excess pattern. Because it is good for clearing heat, removing qi stagnation, and regulating qi, it can remove the heat from the chest and Stomach as well as from the muscles and skin. In this case, the Stomach heat has affected the Heart, and so this point is an ideal choice.

PC-4 *(xi men)* is the accumulating point on the arm terminal yin channel. It calms the emotions, promotes the functions of the Heart, and alleviates pain. It also removes heat from the blood. It is commonly used in treating palpitations and pericardium pain. It is also useful for nasal hemorrhage (epistaxis), hematemesis, and epilepsy. It clears heat from the middle and upper burners. In this case, the point is combined with ST-34 *(liang qiu)* to clear the heat, calm the emotions, regulate the qi in the pericardium channel, remove the pathogenic heat, and alleviate the pain.

CV-12 *(zhong wan)* is used as a local point. It is an alarm point of the Stomach, and a meeting point of the arm greater yang, arm lesser yang, and leg yang brightness channels with the conception vessel. Because of its association with the Small Intestine and Triple Burner, and because it can also regulate the qi, the even or draining method of needle manipulation is used at this point to clear the heat, regulate the middle burner, and reduce the retention of food. It is a very important point for treating epigastric pain.

ST-44 *(nei ting)* is a spring point and serves to remove heat from the qi level. It is located on the foot and has a strong distant action. It is very effective for clearing Stomach heat, alleviating pain, and regulating yang Organ qi. It is an important point for treating disorders in the yang brightness channel, and is thus used for treating such problems as toothache, sore and swollen throat, epistaxis, abdominal and epigastric pain, constipation, and diarrhea. Here it was chosen as a distant point to clear heat and alleviate pain.

Combination of points

ST-34 *(liang qiu)* and PC-4 *(xi men)*. The former point is located above the knee, the latter in the middle of the forearm. This is a combination of accumulating points, both of which can regulate yang Organ qi. The former tends more toward the qi and yang aspect, and the latter toward the blood and yin aspect. Together they are very good for regulating qi, clearing heat, and alleviating pain. This is an important combination for treating acute disorders in the middle and upper burners. These two points are used as distant points and are ideal for patients—such as children, or those with weak constitutions—who may be frightened of needles in the chest and abdominal region.

CV-12 *(zhong wan)* and ST-34 *(liang qiu)* are used in combination for treating abdominal pain. The first serves as a local point, and the second as a distant point. The use of the draining method at both points is recommended for treating excess, especially qi stagnation. Tonification should be used at the first point, and draining at the second, when the pair is used for treating a combination of deficiency and excess.

ST-34 *(liang qiu)*, PC-4 *(xi men)*, CV-12 *(zhong wan)*, ST-44 *(nei ting)*. This combination is very effective in treating acute epigastric pain. It has the advantage of requiring very few needles. It is useful in the treatment of heat in the Stomach, especially when Stomach heat disturbs the Heart.

Basic herbal formula #1

Left Metal Pill *(zuo jin wan)* is a very commonly-used formula. The original prescription is as follows:

Rhizoma Coptidis *(huang lian)*..18g
Fructus Evodiae Rutaecarpae *(wu zhu yu)* 1-3g

Explanation of basic herbal formula #1

This formula was originally used in treating a pattern of Liver fire transversely attacking the Stomach. The main symptoms of this pattern are distending pain in the hyperchondriac, intercostal, and abdominal regions, regurgitation, indeterminate gnawing hunger, belching, vomiting, nausea, a red tongue with a yellow coating, and a wiry and rapid pulse. In this pattern, stagnant Liver qi has transformed into fire, and the Liver can no longer facilitate the free-flow of qi. This has also affected the upward- and downward-movement of the Spleen and Stomach qi, causing distention, fullness, and pain as well as the symptoms associated with the reversal of Stomach qi.

There are only two herbs in this formula. Rhizoma Coptidis *(huang lian)* is bitter in flavor and cold in nature; it promotes the downward-movement of qi. Fructus Evodiae Rutaecarpae *(wu zhu yu)* is acrid, bitter, and hot; it promotes the upward-movement of qi. These two herbs are completely opposite in character, but both are associated with the Liver and Stomach channels.

The dosage of Rhizoma Coptidis *(huang lian)* is quite large. Its purpose is to clear heat and remove fire, which it does especially well with respect to the middle burner and Stomach. It also clears heat from the Heart. This is a good choice for heat-disturbed Heart spirit. It serves here as a chief herb.

Fructus Evodiae Rutaecarpae *(wu zhu yu)* is very hot in nature and belongs to the category of herbs that warm the middle burner, remove the retention of cold, and alleviate pain. It is used in treating patterns of cold in the middle burner. In this case, however, there is a pattern of Stomach heat, and the dosage of this herb is therefore very small. Its acrid and dispersing actions are used to remove pathogenic heat and disperse pathogenic fire. It is especially suitable for treating patterns of stagnant heat. When combined with Rhizoma Coptidis *(huang lian)*, which is bitter and cold, its hot, dry qualities are ameliorated, though its pungency and ability to disperse are retained. Fructus Evodiae Rutaecarpae *(wu zhu yu)* is also bitter and can promote the downward-movement of qi. Here, combined with Rhizoma Coptidis *(huang lian)*, it promotes the downward-movement of Stomach qi, thereby correcting the reversal in the direction of Stomach qi.

In sum, this formula is used to clear Liver heat, drain fire, promote the downward-movement of qi in the middle burner, correct the reversal of qi, and relieve vomiting. It is not only useful in treating Liver fire transversely attacking the Stomach, but also pure Stomach fire, which is another problem of excess.

Basic herbal formula #2

Clear the Stomach Powder *(qing wei san)* is typically used for treating patterns of Stomach heat. The formula contains the following ingredients:

Radix Rehmanniae Glutinosae *(sheng di huang)* 12g
Radix Angelicae Sinensis *(dang gui)* 6g
Cortex Moutan Radicis *(mu dan pi)* 9g
Rhizoma Coptidis *(huang lian)* 5g
Gypsum *(shi gao)* 15g
Rhizoma Cimicifugae *(sheng ma)* 6g

Explanation of basic herbal formula #2

This formula is used for symptoms associated with Stomach heat like swelling, pain, and bleeding of the gums, swelling and pain in the cheeks and lips, foul-smelling breath, dryness of the mouth, yellow urine, dry stools, a red tongue with a yellow coating, and a slippery, rapid pulse. The pathogenesis of this pattern is that heat travels along the leg yang brightness channels and moves upward, where it affects the teeth, gums, lips, and cheeks. The heat also causes various symptoms associated with injury to the body fluids.

In this formula, Rhizoma Coptidis *(huang lian)* serves as a chief herb; it is bitter and cold, and is associated with the Stomach channel. It is used to clear heat and remove fire.

The heat in the Stomach here pertains to heat in the qi level. Gypsum *(shi gao)*, which is acrid and cold, is therefore selected, along with Rhizoma Coptidis *(huang lian)*, in order to clear the pathogenic heat from the qi level. However, the Stomach is a yang Organ, rich in qi and blood. Thus heat in the Stomach can very easily affect the blood, leading to heat in the blood. Radix Rehmanniae Glutinosae *(sheng di huang)*, which is sweet, bitter, and cold, is used with Cortex Moutan Radicis *(mu dan pi)*, which is acrid and slightly cold. Both of these herbs are associated with the Heart, Liver, and Kidney channels, and both serve to cool the blood. They do not directly clear the heat from the Stomach. Cooling the blood will assist Rhizoma Coptidis *(huang lian)* in clearing the Stomach heat. Radix Rehmanniae Glutinosae *(sheng di huang)* also nourishes the yin of the body, and can be used to treat the thirst, yellow urine, and dry stools caused by heat consuming the body fluids. This is why these three herbs all serve as deputies.

Rhizoma Cimicifugae *(sheng ma)* and Radix Angelicae Sinensis *(dang gui)* are the assistant herbs. Rhizoma Cimicifugae *(sheng ma)* is acrid, sweet, and slightly cold, and is associated with the Spleen, Stomach, and Large Intestine channels. Its characteristics of rising and dispersing are used to clear the heat and fire from the qi level. Radix Angelicae Sinensis *(dang gui)* is sweet, acrid, and warm, and is associated with the Heart, Liver, and Spleen channels; here it is used to dispel the heat and blood stasis from the blood system. As Rhizoma Cimicifugae *(sheng ma)* is associated with the yang brightness channels, it also functions as an envoy herb.

Modified herbal formulas

First prescription:

Rhizoma Coptidis *(huang lian)* 10g
Fructus Evodiae Rutaecarpae *(wu zhu yu)* 1g
Cortex Moutan Radicis *(mu dan pi)* 6g
Rhizoma Corydalis Yanhusuo *(yan hu suo)* 6g
Radix Glycyrrhizae Uralensis *(gan cao)* 6g

Second prescription:

Gypsum *(shi gao)* [pre-cook for 20 minutes] 30g
Rhizoma Coptidis *(huang lian)* 5g
Fructus Gardeniae Jasminoidis *(zhi zi)* 10g
Cortex Moutan Radicis *(mu dan pi)* 10g
Pericarpium Citri Reticulatae *(chen pi)* 10g
Os Sepiae seu Sepiellae *(hai piao xiao)* 15g
Concha Arcae *(wa leng zi)* [pre-cook for 20 minutes] 30g
Radix Paeoniae Lactiflorae *(bai shao)* 10g
Rhizoma Corydalis Yanhusuo *(yan hu suo)* 5g

Explanation of modified herbal formulas

The first prescription is a modification of Left Metal Pill *(zuo jin wan)* and the second is a modification of Clear the Stomach Powder *(qing wei san)*.

In this case there is excessive heat in the Stomach; the antipathogenic factors are not deficient. The two formulas are therefore used here to clear heat from the Stomach. Heat in the Stomach can very easily affect the blood, leading to heat in the blood. This patient suffers from restlessness and insomnia—the Heart spirit is affected by heat in the blood. Rhizoma Coptidis *(huang lian)* is the central herb in both formulas, as it can clear heat from both the Stomach and Heart.

First prescription

Compared with the original formula, the number of herbs associated with the blood system has been increased. The purpose is to more effectively clear heat from the Stomach, while also clearing heat from the Heart, and thereby calming the Heart spirit. This prescription is designed to clear Stomach heat. It is intended for treating acute epigastric pain, and can only be used for a short period of time.

Second prescription

For herbs associated with the qi level, Fructus Gardeniae Jasminoidis *(zhi zi)* replaces Rhizoma Cimicifugae *(sheng ma)* as it has a stronger action in clearing heat. Pericarpium Citri Reticulatae *(chen pi)* is added to regulate the qi, and to reinforce the combination of the first three herbs in clearing heat from constraint. For the herb associated with the blood system, Radix Paeoniae Lactiflorae *(bai shao)*) replaces Radix Rehmanniae Glutinosae *(sheng di huang)*. Although both herbs nourish the yin and blood, the latter's action is stronger in this respect, while the former is better suited for treating the acute disorder and for alleviating pain. Rhizoma Corydalis Yanhusuo *(yan hu suo)* replaces Radix Angelicae Sinensis *(dang gui)*. While Rhizoma Corydalis Yanhusuo *(yan hu suo)* does not nourish the blood, it is effective in dispelling blood stasis, regulating qi, and alleviating pain in this particular case. The combination of Os Sepiae seu Sepiellae *(hai piao xiao)* and Concha Arcae *(wa leng zi)* acts to reduce stomach acid. (These herbs are used for the treatment of the symptoms only.) As a whole, this prescription is bitter and cold, and is used mainly for the purpose of clearing heat, and regulating the qi and blood. The point is to improve the qi activity, remove the heat, and thereby alleviate the pain.

Follow-up

At the beginning of the first stage of treatment, acupuncture was used once a day for two weeks, at the end of which the frequency of pain had declined dramatically, as had the burning sensation in the epigastrium. The stifling sensation in the chest and the restlessness were also alleviated. The patient's sleep improved slightly, and he also calmed down considerably. Although this man is over fifty years of age, his interior heat is fairly strong.

Because the duration of his illness was rather long, herbal treatment was started at the beginning of the third week. One dose of the first prescription was administered daily; at the same time, the frequency of the acupuncture treatments was reduced to every other day. Because of its bitter and cold qualities, and its tendency to injure the Stomach yang if over-used, the first herbal prescription was used for only five days during the third week. The second prescription was used during the fourth and fifth weeks, during which no acupuncture was given. The epigastric pain became much more controlled, and the patient did not regurgitate or feel restless. The herbal treatment was accordingly terminated.

The patient continued to complain of slight discomfort in the epigastrium, and acupuncture was therefore resumed (same points) during the sixth week, at the end of which most of the symptoms had largely disappeared. However, because of the length of the illness, and the tendency of the patient to accumulate interior heat, the ingredients of the second prescription were made into pills, which the patient took during the ensuing two months (two 5g pills daily).

For about half a year thereafter the patient suffered from occasional mild attacks of epigastric pain. These were remedied each time by two to four acupuncture treatments. The following year treatment was terminated as the symptoms had virtually disappeared and the patient felt very well.

CASE 16: **Male, age 42**

Main complaint

Epigastric pain

History

Six years ago the patient began to have epigastric pain. He was sent to the hospital where he received an endoscopic exam and was diagnosed as having a duodenal ulcer. He experienced a recurrent stinging pain in the upper right part of the epigastrium. The attacks lasted varying lengths of time, sometimes short, sometimes long. The pain was alleviated when the patient had something to eat. When the pain was severe he took pain medication.

Over the past six years the patient complained of regurgitation, and had indeterminate gnawing hunger in the epigastrium. While he had no history of hematemesis (vomiting with blood), his stools have been bloody. An occult blood test done during this period was positive. Otherwise his general health has not been too bad.

At the moment the patient feels pain when his stomach is empty; sometimes it is severe, other times not. The site of the pain is fixed. It is burning and sharp, and increases with pressure. The patient's appetite has diminished. When he came to the clinic for treatment, the color of his stools was normal, and an occult blood test was negative.

Tongue

Dark red with a thin and slightly yellow coating

Pulse

Wiry and thin

Analysis of symptoms

1. Epigastric pain—obstruction of qi activity.
2. Stinging, fixed pain—blood stasis.
3. Burning sensation, regurgitation, and indeterminate gnawing hunger in the middle burner—internal disturbance of heat.
4. Relief of pain after eating—deficiency of antipathogenic factors.
5. Dark red tongue—poor circulation of blood.
6. Yellow tongue coating—heat pattern.

Basic theory of case

Blood stasis is commonly seen in the clinic. It may arise from poor circulation or from blood stasis inside the vessels, or blood from broken vessels accumulating inside the body. Examples would include subcutaneous hemorrhage, and blood accumulation from an internal visceral hemorrhage which stays inside the body.

Common causes of blood stasis are injury, cold invasion, qi stagnation, and qi deficiency. Trauma can directly injure the vessels and collaterals, leading to blood stasis. Cold, internal or external, can constrict the blood vessels, impeding the circulation of blood, which then leads to blood stasis. Qi is the force underlying the circulation of blood. When it becomes deficient or stagnates, the normal circulation of blood is impeded, and blood stasis ensues.

In Chinese medicine, prolonged disease can also cause blood stasis. In general, the basic pathological change is as follows: a chronic illness leads to injury of the yin, yang, qi, and blood or body fluids, leaving the blood vessels relatively empty; or it depletes the underlying power needed to circulate the blood. This is referred to as "prolonged disease entering the collaterals *(jiǔ bìng rù luò)*." Thus a patient with a long history of disease may possibly have blood stasis. Of course, an examination of the clinical symptoms is necessary to establish whether or not such a pattern exists. For example, if there is a sharp pain locally, together with a fixed mass or lump, this diagnosis would be appropriate.

Fig. 4-7

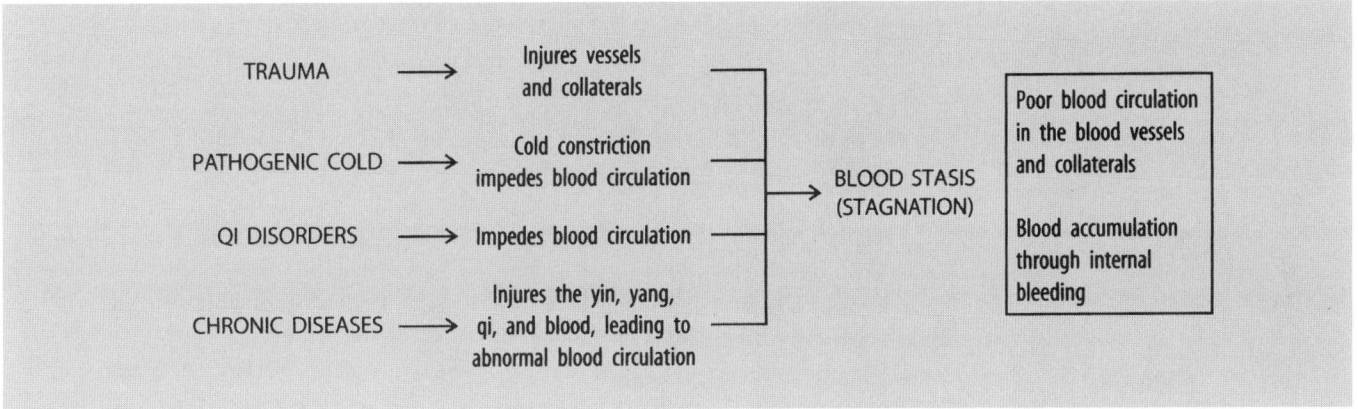

Cause of disease

Blood stasis

The patient feels a sharp pain at a fixed spot in the epigastrium. The pain worsens with pressure. This matches the characteristics of blood stasis.

Site of disease

Stomach

The site of the pain, the indeterminate gnawing hunger in the epigastrium, and the regurgitation identifies the site of disease as the Stomach.

Pathological change

Epigastric pain has various causes. Diagnosing the cause depends on the characteristics of the pain. This patient has chronic burning pain, indicating that the stasis obstructs the vessels in the Stomach. Blood stasis is a substantial pathogenic factor. Once it has occurred, the position of the blockage generally stays fixed, as does the pain. Pressure can increase the obstruction of qi and blood, and thus aggravate the epigastric pain.

The patient's appetite is slightly diminished, indicating a dysfunction in the middle burner. In clinical practice, if there is a pattern of excess, the pain in the Stomach usually worsens after eating. In this case, however, the pain is partially relieved after eating a little. This indicates that the chronic Stomach disorder has already injured the antipathogenic factors. Eating replenishes the qi in the middle burner, and the symptoms are thereby somewhat relieved. But compared with the general symptoms, the qi deficiency is not very obvious in this case.

Generally speaking, simple blood stasis does not lead to either heat or cold. In this instance, however, the presentation includes symptoms that point to Stomach heat. This indicates that the long history of blood stasis has led to poor circulation of qi, or stagnation of qi. Thus the yang qi of the body has become stagnant in this area for a long time, which has given rise to heat from constraint. The heat has disturbed the Stomach, resulting in burning pain. The Stomach qi rises up with the heat, and the patient regurgitates.

Fig. 4-8

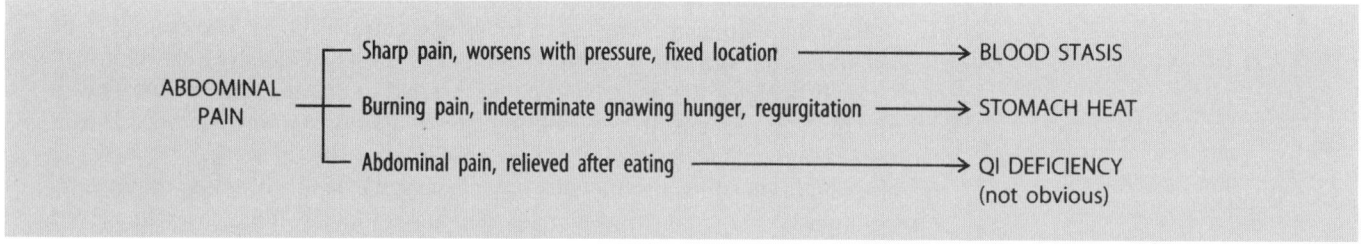

The dark red tongue indicates poor circulation of blood. The thin and slightly yellow tongue coating suggests the presence of internal heat from excess.

Pattern of disease

The sharp pain in the Stomach and the location of the disease in the blood vessels indicate an interior pattern.

The patient has a burning sensation in the epigastrium, indeterminate gnawing hunger, regurgitation, and a yellow tongue coating, all of which are evidence of heat.

The pain in the Stomach is aggravated with pressure, indicating a pattern of excess.

Although the antipathogenic factors have been injured, the symptoms are not very severe, and this is not considered significant at this time.

Additional notes

1. What caused the dark stools?

From a biomedical perspective, hematemesis and melena (dark stools) along with a positive test for occult blood are common symptoms of an ulcer in the digestive tract. The characteristics of this bleeding include coffee-colored or deep brown vomitus and tarry stools. In Chinese medicine, however, the bleeding is attributed to blood stasis. When the patient was examined, no hemorrhage in the digestive system was found. This aspect can therefore be ignored during treatment.

2. What does the wiry, thin pulse in this case indicate?

The wiry pulse indicates an obstruction of the qi activity, which is evidence of the pathological change in the Stomach. The thin pulse indicates that there is some deficiency of qi and blood, or the blood vessels have narrowed, or there is retention of dampness in the body. In this case the thin pulse is due to a slight deficiency of qi and blood.

3. What is the cause of the blood stasis in the Stomach?

As mentioned above, there are many causes of blood stasis. In this case, the long-term, chronic illness has affected the blood vessels. The patient here has more or less the same length of illness as the patient in the previous case, so is there any blood stasis in the channels and collaterals in the previous case? The diagnosis of blood stasis can be affected by a long history of chronic illness. However, there were no symptoms involving blood stasis in the previous case, so this diagnosis cannot be made. Here, on the other hand, not only is there a long history of illness, but there are also very definite symptoms indicating blood stasis. This is why the case differs from the previous one.

Conclusion

1. According to the eight principles:
   Interior, heat, excess.

2. According to etiology:
   Blood stasis.

3. According to Organ theory:
   Blood stasis obstructing the Stomach vessels.

Treatment principle

1. Dispel blood stasis.

2. Regulate the vessels and collaterals.

3. Clear heat from the Stomach and alleviate the pain.

Explanation of treatment principle

There is a saying in Chinese medicine that where there is obstruction, there will be pain. Blood stasis obstructs the vessels and channels, and the pain cannot be alleviated if the obstruction persists. Thus, the fundamental principle is to cure the blood stasis by promoting the circulation of blood and dispelling the stagnation from the vessels and collaterals.

Blood stasis can remain in other parts of the body, and can also appear as a different type of pattern, such as deficiency, excess, cold, or heat. Thus, there may be different methods of treatment, including the use of different acupuncture points on different channels, or Chinese herbs associated with different Organs. These methods may focus simply on removing the pathogenic factor, or they may also reinforce the antipathogenic factors. In addition, depending on the nature of the case, the cooling or warming method may be used. In this case there is excess and heat, so the cooling method is indicated. The focus of treatment is on the expulsion of the pathogenic factor and the removal of obstruction from the channels and collaterals.

In the relationship between qi and blood, qi provides the underlying energy for circulating the blood. That is why the qi must be regulated in order to strengthen the removal of the blood stasis from the vessels and collaterals.

Selection of points

CV-13 *(shang wan)*
SP-10 *(xue hai)*
PC-6 *(nei guan)*
ST-44 *(nei ting)*

Explanation of points

CV-13 *(shang wan)* is a meeting point of three channels: the conception vessel, leg yang brightness Stomach channel, and arm greater yang Small Intestine channel. This point harmonizes the functions of the middle burner, promotes the downward-movement in the qi activity, and clears heat. This is one of the most commonly used points in the treatment of peptic ulcers. It is used as a local point and is effective for alleviating pain in the upper abdominal region, whether on the right or left. It can also strengthen the functions of the Spleen and Stomach. In this case, the draining method is used at this point.

This point is only 1 unit above CV-12 *(zhong wan)*, which is one of the most commonly used points for abdominal problems. Both of these points are used to regulate qi, alleviate pain, and clear heat, but CV-13 *(shang wan)* is mainly used for patterns of excess, while CV-12 *(zhong wan)* can be used for either deficiency or excess, or a combination of the two. This is one of the reasons why the latter point is so commonly used in the clinic. In practice, however, these two points can be used separately or together.

SP-10 *(xue hai)*, meaning "sea of blood," is used in treating various blood disorders, hence the name. As a Spleen channel point, it can be used to clear heat from the middle burner. It also brings the blood back to the Spleen. In practice, it is used to regulate and cool the blood, and is suitable for patterns involving blood stasis or heat in the blood (as here). Because the point can clear heat from the blood throughout the body, it is helpful in removing heat from the Stomach.

PC-6 *(nei guan)* is a connecting point on the Pericardium channel. It is one of the eight confluent points, and serves as the "master" point in the pair of yin linking vessels. The yin linking vessels can be used for treating such conditions as pain in the pericardium, chest, abdomen, epigastrium, and hypochondrium. They are also helpful in treating distention in the upper abdominal region, abdominal masses, and rumbling in the abdomen. Thus, the yin linking vessels can be used to regulate the qi and blood throughout the body. As PC-6 *(nei guan)* is associated with these channels, it shares many of the same functions. It can be used for alleviating pain, relieving vomiting, and promoting the downward-moving action of the Stomach qi. It can also be used for regulating the blood, for example, when heat affects the blood and causes problems during menstruation, or dizziness after childbirth. In this particulate case, the point is used for regulating the blood and qi, and alleviating the pain in the middle burner.

ST-44 *(nei ting)* is a spring point among the transporting points, and is used for removing heat from the qi level. The Stomach is a yang Organ which is very rich in qi and blood. When there is blood stasis and heat, the heat must be removed not only from the blood level, but also from the qi; this point is used to clear the heat from the qi level and to alleviate pain. In this case it serves as a distant combination point.

Combination of points

SP-10 *(xue hai)* and ST-44 *(nei ting)*. The first point is associated with blood and clears heat from the blood, the second, a spring point, is associated with qi and clears heat from the qi level. In combination, these two points can clear heat and cool the blood. As SP-10 *(xue hai)* is on the Spleen channel and ST-44 *(nei ting)* is on the Stomach channel, the use of this combination draws on two channels. The yang brightness is associated with the yang Organs, which are rich in qi and blood.

CV-13 *(shang wan)* and CV-12 *(zhong wan)*, which are used in the follow-up (see below), are situated very close to one another: CV-13 *(shang wan)* is only 1 unit above CV-12 *(zhong wan)*. The object of using both points is to extend their influence locally over the affected area. This is a very commonly used combination for the treatment of epigastric pain. Both points alleviate pain, clear heat, and regulate qi. In Chinese the Stomach area is called *wǎn*. It is divided into upper, middle, and lower regions. There are three points on the conception vessel which correspond to these three regions, and which incorporate the term *wǎn* in their names: *shàng wǎn* (upper Stomach region), *zhōng wǎn* (middle Stomach region), and *xià wǎn* (lower Stomach region). The combination chosen here uses the upper and middle *wǎn* points for clearing heat and alleviating pain.

Basic herbal formula #1

Melia Toosendan Powder *(jin ling zi san)* is used in treating patterns associated with qi and blood stagnation or stasis. The formula includes the following ingredients:

Fructus Meliae Toosendan *(chuan lian zi)* 30g
Rhizoma Corydalis Yanhusuo *(yan hu suo)* 30g

Explanation of basic herbal formula #1

This formula was originally designed for treating a pattern of heat from constraint caused by stagnation of Liver qi. Symptoms include episodic pain in the precordial, epigastric, abdominal, intercostal, and hypochondrial regions. Other symptoms are a bitter taste in the mouth, a red tongue with a yellow coating, and a wiry and rapid pulse. The pathological change is Liver qi stagnation causing heat from constraint; the stagnant qi and poor circulation of blood gives rise to pain in various parts of the body, as well as symptoms of interior heat.

Fructus Meliae Toosendan *(chuan lian zi)* is bitter and cold, and is associated with the Liver and Stomach channels. It serves as the chief herb, and acts to promote the movement of qi, and to clear Liver fire. It is used in treating such symptoms as pain and distention in the intercostal, hypochondrial, epigastric, and abdominal regions, and heat symptoms associated with a pattern of Liver qi stagnation, or a pattern involving disharmony between the Liver and Stomach.

Rhizoma Corydalis Yanhusuo *(yan hu suo)* is acrid, bitter, and warm, and is associated with the Liver and Spleen channels. It is used in treating various patterns of blood stasis. It regulates the blood, dispels blood stasis, and is very effective in alleviating pain. It serves as a deputy herb, and is very commonly used in treating the pain associated with blood stasis. When combined with Fructus Meliae Toosendan *(chuan lian zi)*, the latter herb is directed at the qi, while Rhizoma Corydalis Yanhusuo *(yan hu suo)* is directed at the blood. In clinical practice this combination is used in treating a variety of patterns associated with qi and blood stagnation and stasis, rather than just the heat from constraint associated with Liver qi stagnation.

Basic herbal formula #2

Salvia Decoction *(dan shen yin)* is another formula that is commonly used in the treatment of qi and blood stagnation or stasis.

Radix Salviae Miltiorrhizae *(dan shen)* 30g
Lignum Santali Albi *(tan xiang)* 5g
Fructus Amomi *(sha ren)* 5g

Explanation of basic herbal formula #2

This formula is mainly used in treating blood stasis of a type characterized by a sharp, stabbing pain in the chest or epigastrium, accompanied by a dark tongue (with or without ecchymosis) and a sunken, choppy pulse.

Radix Salviae Miltiorrhizae *(dan shen)* is bitter and slightly cold, and is associated with the Heart and Liver channels. It can be used in treating various patterns of blood stasis, in that it regulates the blood and alleviates pain. Because of its cold nature, it cools the blood and removes the heat which has accumulated in the blood. This herb can also help buffer the heat from herbs that regulate the qi. It serves as the chief herb in this formula, and its dosage is relatively large.

Lignum Santali Albi *(tan xiang)* and Fructus Amomi *(sha ren)* are both acrid and warm in nature. They enter the Spleen and Stomach channels, and are very effective in warming the middle burner and regulating the qi. They serve as assistant herbs. Lignum Santali Albi *(tan xiang)* also expels cold and alleviates pain, and can therefore be used to treat cold and pain in the Stomach. Because of their acrid, warm, and drying characteristics, only a small amount (5g) of each is used in the prescription. In this formula, herbs associated with the qi are combined with those associated with the blood, but the primary function here is to remove the stasis of blood.

Modified herbal formula

Fructus Meliae Toosendan *(chuan lian zi)* 10g
Rhizoma Corydalis Yanhusuo *(yan hu suo)* 6g
Rhizoma Coptidis *(huang lian)* 10g
Concha Arcae *(wa leng zi)* [pre-cook for 20 minutes] 10g
Radix Salviae Miltiorrhizae *(dan shen)* 6g
Lignum Santali Albi *(tan xiang)* 2g
Radix Scutellariae Baicalensis *(huang qin)* 6g

Explanation of modified herbal formula

The cause of the epigastric pain in this case is blood stasis blocking the Stomach vessels and collaterals, and obstructing the qi and blood. Melia Toosendan Powder *(jin ling zi san)* and Salvia Decoction *(dan shen yin)* can both be used to treat abdominal and epigastric pain caused by qi and blood stagnation or stasis. However, because of the relatively small dosage of the herbs in those formulas, and their correspondingly mild actions, the two formulas were combined here, with the necessary modifications made for the patient's condition.

The essential function of this modified formula is to regulate the qi and dispel the blood stasis in order to improve the circulation of qi and blood and thereby alleviate the pain. Because of the presence of internal heat in this case, Fructus Amomi *(sha ren)*, which is acrid, warm, and associated with dry heat, is omitted to avoid adding to the existing heat. Rhizoma Coptidis *(huang lian)*, which is bitter and cold and clears heat from the middle burner (the Stomach in particular), has been added. Radix Scutellariae Baicalensis *(huang qin)*, which promotes the functions of the Spleen and insulates the antipathogenic factors from the pathogen-expelling actions of the other herbs in the formula, is combined with Concha Arcae *(wa leng zi)*, which alleviates the symptoms in this case.

Follow-up

Acupuncture and herbal treatment were used together here. For the first two weeks, acupuncture was administered three times a week, and the herbal formula was also administered. The formula was made in the following manner: Concha Arcae *(wa leng zi)* was pre-cooked for 10 minutes, then all the other herbs were boiled together for 30 minutes. The liquid was strained off using a sieve, and more water was added to the solids. This was then boiled gently for another 30 minutes. Finally, the liquid was strained off and combined with the first portion of liquid. Half of this amount was given to the patient in the morning, and the other half in the evening. The patient took the herbs every day for two weeks, during which the sharp, burning pain in the epigastrium gradually diminished, the regurgitation decreased, the appetite improved slightly, and the indeterminate gnawing hunger was sometimes better, sometimes worse.

After two weeks the amount of Concha Arcae *(wa leng zi)* was increased to 20 grams in order to control the acid, and CV-12 *(zhong wan)* was added to the acupuncture prescription. As discussed earlier, this point and CV-13 *(shang wan)* were used together. These modified treatments were continued for another three weeks. The abdominal pain decreased, and the patient occasionally complained of slight pain, though at other times he felt no pain at all. His energy level and alertness improved, and his bowel movements were normal.

After the additional three weeks the patient was treated for a second three-week period, during which the amount of Rhizoma Coptidis *(huang lian)* was reduced to 5 grams, Fructus Meliae Toosendan *(chuan lian zi)* to 8 grams, and the dosage was spread over two days, rather than one: one-half the first day, and the other half on the next, both taken in the evening. The reason for this was that the main symptoms had now subsided, and the bitter and cold herbs in the prescription had to be reduced in order to avoid injuring the Stomach. Acupuncture was continued during this period, but was reduced to twice weekly.

Over the next four months the patient's work schedule precluded regular treatment. He came to the clinic for acupuncture when he could, and usually took the herbs when acupuncture treatment was impractical. At the end of this period the symptoms had disappeared, and the treatment was terminated.

Three months later, after the patient ate a large meal and drank too much alcohol, the symptoms recurred for two days. However, compared with before, the symptoms this time were mild. Treatment was resumed along the lines described above for the initial two week period, then acupuncture was stopped and the herbal remedy continued for another two weeks. By this time the symptoms had lessened. The patient was advised to give up alcohol, avoid eating big meals, and refrain from eating hot, spicy foods. On follow-up eighteen months later, there had been no further attacks.

CASE 17: **Male, age 36**

Main complaint

Abdominal pain

History

Ten days ago, for no apparent reason, the patient began to feel pain in the upper middle and (especially) lower left parts of the abdomen. The pain was not very severe, and the duration of the attacks since then have not been very long. The location is not always fixed. When the patient experiences an onset of pain, he tends to have a bowel movement. The stools are not very loose. After the bowel movement the pain is often partially alleviated. The patient can also achieve some relief by passing gas, but he can't seem to pass enough. His appetite is very poor, and the abdominal distention becomes severe after eating. He does not belch, experience nausea, or feel particularly thirsty. His sleep and urination are both normal, and his complexion is slightly dark.

Tongue

Slightly red with a thick, greasy, and slightly yellow coating

Pulse

Wiry

Analysis of symptoms

1. Upper middle and lower left abdominal pain, not always fixed—qi stagnation in the Spleen and Stomach.

2. Relief of pain after passing gas or bowel movement—pattern of excess.

3. Poor appetite and increased abdominal distention after eating—Spleen's transportive and transformative functions impaired.

4. Thick, greasy tongue coating—retention of food in the Spleen and Stomach.

5. Dark complexion and wiry pulse—poor circulation of qi and blood.

Basic theory of case

To distinguish between abdominal pain of a deficient and an excessive nature, we must consider (1) the characteristics of the pain; and (2) the relationship among the pain, eating, and bowel movements.

The pain associated with excess is usually severe. In the worst cases the pain will seem unbearable, though it seldom lasts for more than a day. Although the disease itself may last for several months or even years, the duration of individual attacks will always be short. Pressure usually increases the pain.

Abdominal pain associated with deficiency is seldom severe, but the history of the complaint and the attacks themselves can be quite prolonged. Very often the pain is dull and continuous. Unlike the pain associated with excess, which comes and goes, the periods between pain and relief from pain are less marked, and there is always some background pain. In most cases, local pressure and massage will bring some relief. Such patients are often observed placing their hands on their abdomens.

Abdominal pain associated with excess is caused by retention of a pathogenic factor, which results from the obstruction of qi activity. Eating can aggravate the obstruction; thus, patients do not enjoy eating. Bowel movements can remove certain types of abdominal obstruction, and can, at least temporarily, relieve the obstruction of a pathogenic factor. This is why the pain may be reduced after a bowel movement.

Abdominal pain associated with deficiency is caused by insufficiency of the antipathogenic factors, or malnourishment of the Organs. The essence from food can reinforce the antipathogenic factors; thus, eating can relieve the pain. In general, bowel movements have no effect on abdominal pain associated with deficiency.

Fig. 4-9   Comparison of Abdominal Pain in Patterns of Deficiency and Excess

	EXCESS PATTERN	DEFICIENCY PATTERN
DURATION of PAIN	Short	Long
SEVERITY of PAIN	Severe	Dull
PAIN with PRESSURE	Increases	Decreases
CHANGE in PAIN AFTER EATING	Aggravated	Relieved
CHANGE in PAIN AFTER BOWEL MOVEMENT	Diminishes	No change or aggravated

In practice, the symptoms often change a great deal. In order to properly distinguish between deficiency and excess, besides noting the main symptoms, one should also consider such things as the general condition of the body, and the tongue and pulse.

Cause of disease

Qi stagnation

In this case, the pain is not fixed, eating can aggravate the abdominal distention, and the pain may be relieved after passing gas or a bowel movement. This suggests an obstruction caused by a pathogenic factor, but not a substantial pathogenic factor such as phlegm, dampness, or blood stasis. We may therefore conclude that the cause of the illness here is qi stagnation.

Site of disease

Spleen and Stomach

The pain is located in both the upper and lower abdominal regions. The symptoms associated with eating and bowel movements suggest that the site of the disorder is the Spleen and Stomach.

Pathological change

The Spleen and Stomach are the main Organs of the middle burner. Besides transforming and transporting food and fluids, these two Organs have a very important function in regulating qi activity, that is, regulating the upward and downward movement of qi in the middle burner. In this case, the dysfunction of the Spleen and Stomach results in obstruction in the middle burner, interfering with the normal qi activity. Stagnation occurs in some areas. This explains why the patient feels pain in only certain parts of the abdomen, specifically the upper middle and lower left. Although the pathway of qi is obstructed, the qi continues to circulate and move, albeit slowly. The obstruction itself can therefore be moved around by the qi activity, and this is one of the reasons why the pain does not remain fixed in the one spot.

The obstruction in the middle burner impairs the Spleen and Stomach's transportive and transformative functions. Food and water remain in the middle burner much longer than normal. The patient's appetite is thus reduced, and the abdominal distention worsens after eating.

In general, qi stagnation causes one to belch and pass gas excessively, but in this case the obstruction of qi activity appears to be more severe, especially in its upward and downward movements. Thus, the qi cannot easily move beyond the middle burner. This explains why the patient does not belch as much, or pass so much gas.

Bowel movements can help remove some of the waste from the Intestines, which in turn seems to relieve somewhat the qi stagnation in the middle burner. This is why the abdominal pain diminishes after a bowel movement. The stools are not loose, indicating that the digestive function of the Spleen and Stomach is still within its normal limits.

There is no thirst in this case, and the patient's sleep and urination are normal. This suggests that the disease remains localized, and has not yet affected the other Organs. However, we can see that the blood circulation has been affected somewhat, as the complexion is slightly dark.

A wiry pulse is commonly associated with obstruction of qi activity.

This case has many similarities with cases 13 and 14, such as the location of the pain in the epigastric and abdominal regions, a relationship between the pain on the one hand and eating and bowel movements on the other, and the fact that there is stagnation of qi in all three cases. However, although there is qi stagnation and a pattern of excess in case 13, there is also an invasion of pathogenic cold. External cold constricts the yang qi of the body, which contributed to the problem in that case. Here, there is no involvement of heat or cold, just qi stagnation. And with respect to case 14, this case and that one are actually opposites, in that one involves excess and the other deficiency.

Fig. 4-10

	CASE 13	CASE 17	CASE 14
CAUSE	Cold retention	Qi stagnation	Qi deficiency
SITE	Stomach	Spleen and Stomach	Spleen and Stomach
ABDOMINAL SYMPTOMS	Coldness and distention in epigastric region	Abdominal pain, not fixed	Dull abdominal pain
TONGUE COATING	Distention aggravated after overeating and relieved after belching	Distention aggravated after overeating and relieved after bowel movement	Pain relieved after eating, and pronounced after bowel movement
	Thin, white, and slightly greasy	Thick, slightly yellow, and greasy	Thin, mixture of yellow and white coating
PULSE	Slippery	Wiry	Wiry and slightly moderate
CONCLUSION	Cold retention and qi stagnation in middle burner	Qi stagnation in Spleen and Stomach	Qi deficiency and qi Stagnation in Spleen and Stomach
TREATMENT	Warm the Stomach and regulate the qi	Regulate the qi	Tonify and regulate the qi

Pattern of disease

This is an interior pattern. The illness is located in the middle burner (Spleen and Stomach).

The patient feels no thirst, and the stools are not loose or dry, therefore it is neither a hot nor a cold pattern.

The obstruction of the qi activity is consistent with a pattern of excess.

Additional notes

1. Is there any heat in this case?

From the symptoms, there is little evidence of heat, but the tongue coating is slightly yellow. We can therefore surmise that, even though stagnant qi has a tendency to generate heat, in this case it was mild.

2. What is the cause of the thick, greasy tongue coating?

It is well known that a thick, greasy tongue coating is a common manifestation of the retention of phlegm, dampness, or food. In this case there are no other symptoms indicating retention of phlegm or dampness. However, there is qi stagnation in the middle burner, and thus the transportive and transformative functions of the middle burner have been impaired. This means that the food is not being properly digested, but is accumulating in the middle burner; thus, the thick, greasy coating in this case.

3. Why does the patient experience abdominal pain before a bowel movement?

The most common reason for this disorder is disharmony between the Liver and Spleen. According to five-phase theory, the relationship between these two Organs is one of wood controlling earth. Thus, a disorder of the Liver or Spleen will often affect the other Organ, such as when Liver qi stagnation causes Spleen deficiency. If Liver qi stagnation becomes severe and overwhelms the Spleen and Stomach, it can impede the upward and downward movement of the qi in the middle burner. This will lead to qi stagnation in the middle burner, and thus abdominal pain preceding bowel movements and diarrhea. Defecation itself may reduce the stagnation, which in turn will bring relief from the pain. However, in this case the Liver qi stagnation is not very severe; it results in part from the qi stagnation in the Spleen and Stomach, and therefore the focus of treatment is still on the Spleen and Stomach.

Conclusion

1. According to the eight principles:
   Interior, neither cold nor heat, excess.

2. According to theory of qi, blood, and body fluids:
   Qi stagnation.

3. According to Organ theory:
   Qi stagnation in the Spleen and Stomach, combined with Liver qi transversely attacking the Spleen.

Treatment principle

1. Regulate the qi.

2. Remove the stagnation.

Explanation of treatment principle

Regulating the qi is the basic principle for treating patterns of qi stagnation. The idea is to promote the qi activity, and the actual method will vary from case to case. Here, apart from regulating the qi, it is important to reduce the retention of food that has affected the Spleen, Stomach, and Intestines. Although food is the source of nutrition for the body, if it remains in the Stomach too long, it can obstruct the qi activity and disturb the normal upward and downward movement of qi. Retained food can thus become pathogenic; it is important to remove this obstruction so that the qi activity can resume its normal movement. The functions of the middle burner will likewise recover.

In Chinese medicine this method is referred to as guiding out stagnation (*dǎo zhì*). This means promoting digestion and removing the accumulated food. It is a common method for dealing with disorders of the Spleen and Stomach, and is one of the methods for removing pathogens from the body. When guiding out stagnation is used in treating a pattern of deficiency, caution must be exercised to avoid injuring the antipathogenic factors.

Because the pathology in this case also involves Liver qi stagnation, adding small quantities of herbs that promote the Liver function of regulating the free-flow of qi will indirectly help regulate the qi in the middle burner.

Selection of points

ST-21 *(liang men)*
SP-14 *(fu jie)*
LI-10 *(shou san li)*
ST-37 *(shang ju xu)*

Explanation of points

ST-21 *(liang men)* is located 2 units lateral to CV-12 *(zhong wan)*. In classical Chinese medicine, *liáng* or *fú líang* refers to a palpable accumulation in the area below the heart, accompanied by irritability. It is attributed to stagnation, especially food stagnation. The word *mén* literally means door or gate. This point can be used to remove severe qi stagnation and epigastric pain, and to relieve stagnation and food accumulation below the Heart. It is very suitable for regulating qi. In this particular case, qi stagnation has occurred in the Spleen and Stomach, which makes this point a very good choice. It is located in the upper middle abdomen, which corresponds to one of the main areas of abdominal pain in this case. Use of this point will help regulate the qi, remove the qi stagnation, and alleviate the local pain.

SP-14 *(fu jie)*. The word *fù* means abdomen, and *jié* means knot or clump. Here "clump" means that the qi activity is stopped up in the abdomen. This point can be used for regulating both qi and blood, as well as the functions of the Intestines. It is located on the Spleen channel and is an important point for treating abdominal pain caused by qi stagnation in the middle burner. It is therefore quite suitable for this case.

One of the main symptoms is pain in the lower left abdominal region; SP-14 *(fu jie)* therefore serves as a local point. The reason for selecting the point bilaterally is that the side that is not affected by the disease (the right) is used in order to help the qi activity on the left. If the qi can circulate smoothly, the pain will be alleviated. This point needs to be punctured obliquely. The needle is angled from the Spleen channel toward the Stomach channel. In the neighborhood of the point, the two channels are only 2 units apart. The threading method is used, from the Spleen to the Stomach channel; this is called the "one point/two channel" puncturing method.

Nearby this point are two others on the Stomach channel: ST-26 *(wai ling)* and ST-27 *(da ju)*. The former regulates the Intestines and Stomach, and can alleviate pain. The latter tonifies the qi, calms the spirit, and controls seminal emissions. In other words, the actions of these two points are completely different. When puncturing obliquely at SP-14 *(fu jie)*, the needle should be angled toward ST-26 *(wai ling)*, as this is the relevant point in this case.

LI-10 *(shou san li)* is a distant point that regulates the Stomach and Intestines, and alleviates pain. The point is chosen here because the qi has stagnated in the Spleen and Stomach and caused abdominal pain.

ST-37 *(shang ju xu)* is the lower sea point of the Large Intestine. Although it is located on the Stomach channel, it is associated with the Large Intestine. This means that the point is closely related to both the arm and leg yang brightness channels. It is an effective distant point for clearing heat, regulating qi, and harmonizing the Stomach and Intestines. It is a very important point in clinical practice. The draining (reducing) method is used here in order to vigorously regulate the qi and thereby alleviate the pain. This point also regulates the functions of the yang brightness channels.

Combination of points

SP-14 *(fu jie)* and ST-37 *(shang ju xu)*. This is an important combination for the treatment of patterns of qi stagnation in the Spleen and Stomach, or qi stagnation in the Spleen and Stomach leading to accumulated heat, or slight damp-heat in the Spleen and Stomach. SP-14 *(fu jie)* is located on the Spleen channel, 2 units lateral to ST-25 *(tian shu)*. This point can be punctured perpendicularly or obliquely, angled toward the Stomach channel (the "one point/two channel" method). The idea is to reduce the number of needles. This point can also be used to regulate the functions of both the Spleen and Stomach. However, because it located on the Spleen channel, it is an especially good choice for patterns involving the Spleen. The point can regulate both qi and blood. It is used as a local point.

ST-37 *(shang ju xu)* regulates the functions of the arm and leg yang brightness channels; it is very good for regulating qi and clearing heat. It is an especially good choice for treating patterns in which qi stagnation, retention of dampness, or retention of food leads to heat. This point is 3 units below ST-36 *(zu san li)*, and is relatively more effective in treating patterns of excess. However, unlike ST-36 *(zu san li)*, it is not suitable for tonification. It does serve well as a distant point, and, when combined with the local point SP-14 *(fu jie)*, is very effective in treating symptoms in the middle and lower abdominal regions such as abdominal pain, distention, or discomfort.

ST-21 *(liang men)* and LI-10 *(shou san li)*. The first of these is an important point for regulating qi, and is very effective in removing stagnant qi. It is located in the upper middle abdomen. The second point is used in regulating the Intestines and Stomach, and is an important point in the regulation of qi. It is also mildly tonifying. It serves as a distant point in this combination. Together, these can be used for regulating the functions of the Stomach and Large Intestines, that is to say, the yang brightness channels and Organs. The draining (reducing) method of needle manipulation can be used at both points when treating a pattern of excess. For a combined pattern of deficiency and excess, even needle manipulation is often used at ST-21 *(liang men)*, and either tonifying or draining needle manipulation (depending on the type of pattern) at LI-10 *(shou san li)*. The combination of these points is very effective in relieving symptoms in the middle and upper abdominal regions such as abnormal appetite, nausea, vomiting, belching, anorexia, or an abnormal taste in the mouth.

Analyzing these point combinations, it is apparent that the four points can be divided into two pairs: one is used in treating the Stomach and Large Intestine for symptoms in the middle and upper abdomen, and the other pair is used for problems in the middle and lower abdomen. These two pairs can be used together or independently, and can also be joined with other combinations, depending on the case. This is a good example of a "[small] prescription within a [big] prescription *(fāng zhōng yǒu fāng)*."

Basic herbal formula	Bupleurum Powder to Spread the Liver *(chai hu shu gan san)* is frequently used to treat patterns of Liver qi stagnation. The formula includes the following ingredients:

Radix Bupleuri *(chai hu)* 6g

Rhizoma Cyperi Rotundi *(xiang fu)* 5g

Pericarpium Citri Reticulatae *(chen pi)* 5g

Radix Ligustici Chuanxiong *(chuan xiong)* 5g

Radix Paeoniae Lactiflorae *(bai shao)* 5g

Fructus Citri Aurantii *(zhi ke)* 5g

Radix Glycyrrhizae Uralensis *(gan cao)* 2g

Explanation of basic herbal formula	This formula is used in treating presentations with distention and pain in the intercostal and hypochondrial regions, alternating sensations of hot and cold, poor appetite, and abdominal distention. The pathological change in this pattern is impaired qi activity and poor circulation of qi and blood in the channels, collaterals,

and vessels which have affected the upward and downward movement of qi in the middle burner. This obstruction to the qi activity leads to disorders of the Liver and Spleen.

In the formula, Radix Bupleuri *(chai hu)* is bitter, acrid, and slightly cold, and is associated with the Liver and Gallbladder channels. It serves as the chief herb in this formula, and is used to relieve the stagnation of Liver qi. Rhizoma Cyperi Rotundi *(xiang fu)* is acrid and neutral, and is associated with the Liver channel. It regulates Liver qi and removes Liver qi stagnation, one of its most common uses. Fructus Citri Aurantii *(zhi ke)* is bitter, acrid, and slightly cold, and is associated with the Spleen, Stomach, and Large Intestine channels. Pericarpium Citri Reticulatae *(chen pi)* is acrid, bitter, and warm, and is associated with the Spleen channel. Together, these two herbs regulate and harmonize the Organs of the middle burner, resolve abdominal distention, and remove obstruction from the Spleen and Stomach. All of these herbs serve as deputies here.

Radix Ligustici Chuanxiong *(chuan xiong)* is acrid and warm, and is associated with the Liver and Gallbladder channels. It regulates qi and dispels blood stasis. Radix Paeoniae Lactiflorae *(bai shao)* is sour and cold, and is associated with the Liver and Spleen channels. It nourishes the blood, and relaxes and softens the Liver qi. These two herbs are used to regulate the circulation of Liver blood in order to facilitate the free-flow of Liver qi. They serve as assistants in this formula.

Radix Glycyrrhizae Uralensis *(gan cao)* strengthens the Spleen, harmonizes the Organs of the middle burner, and, with Radix Paeoniae Lactiflorae *(bai shao)*, alleviates pain. Radix Glycyrrhizae Uralensis *(gan cao)* thus serves as an envoy.

Modified herbal formula

Rhizoma Cyperi Rotundi *(xiang fu)* 6g

Pericarpium Citri Reticulatae *(chen pi)* 10g

Fructus Amomi *(sha ren)* [broken into pieces] 3g

Fructus Citri seu Ponciri Immaturus *(zhi shi)* 5g

Fructus Citri Sarcodactylis *(fo shou)* 6g

Flos Rosae Rugosae *(mei gui hua)* 4g

Massa Fermentata *(shen qu)* 6g

Explanation of modified herbal formula

In this case there is qi stagnation in the Spleen and Stomach as well as in the Liver, but the problem in the Spleen and Stomach is the main one. Here, Bupleurum Powder to Spread the Liver *(chai hu shu gan san)*, with certain modifications, is used to promote the functions of the middle burner and to remove both the qi stagnation and the retention of food.

Because stagnant Liver qi is not the main problem in this case, the number of herbs used to regulate the Liver qi has been reduced in this modified formula, while the number of herbs used to regulate the Spleen qi and promote digestion in order to remove the obstruction to the qi activity has been increased. Herbs that regulate both the Liver and Spleen qi have been added to harmonize the Liver and Spleen functions.

Follow-up

The patient was given acupuncture every day for three days, during which there was a marked decrease in the abdominal pain, which was reduced to short spasms. Passing gas afforded some additional relief, and the patient's appetite increased. The distention was significantly reduced.

After the first three days, two packets of the herbal formula were taken over four days: two quarter doses each day, one in the morning and one in the evening. During this time, acupuncture treatments were reduced to once every other day. By the end of the four days the patient's appetite was almost back to normal; there was no abdominal pain, but slight distention remained after eating. Bowel movements had become normal, and there was no longer any abdominal pain preceding a bowel movement.

At this point acupuncture was stopped, but two more packets of the herbal formula were taken over the next four days, as before. A week later all the symptoms were alleviated and the patient had fully recovered. Six months later the patient came back for a check-up, and was still symptom-free.

In this case, as the duration of the illness was short, priority was given to acupuncture, which always yields good results for such cases in which qi stagnation is the main problem. The herbs were used as a supplement; the dosage was accordingly quite small, but it was still necessary. This case serves as a good example of this type of treatment.

CASE 18: **Male, age 41**

Main complaint

Abdominal pain

History

The patient has experienced recurrent attacks of upper and middle abdominal pain for the last three years. The pain is accompanied by a distending sensation that can radiate to both hypochondria. When the pain becomes severe, the patient can experience nausea, excessively watery saliva, and a tendency to vomit. His appetite is very poor, and when he does eat, the abdominal distention becomes worse and he suffers from indigestion. He does not feel especially thirsty, but he can experience intense fatigue. His stools are watery and loose. He has two to three bowel movements daily. His urination is normal. He had an upper gastro-intestinal study with barium and was diagnosed as having a duodenal ulcer. He is very emaciated, and his lips are pale.

Tongue

Pale with a thick, white, and moist coating

Pulse

Wiry and thin

Analysis of symptoms

1. Pain with distention in the upper and middle abdominal region— qi stagnation in the Spleen and Stomach.
2. Pain radiating to both hypochondria—poor circulation of Liver qi.
3. Nausea and excessively watery saliva—reversal of Stomach qi.
4. Poor appetite, abdominal distention, and indigestion— Spleen's transportive and transformative functions impaired.
5. Fatigue, loose stools, and frequent bowel movements—Spleen deficiency.
6. Pale tongue and lips—inability of yang qi to circulate blood to the upper part of the body.
7. Thick, white, and moist tongue coating—retention of damp-cold.
8. Wiry pulse—Liver qi stagnation.
9. Thin pulse—deficiency.

Basic theory of case

There are two very common patterns associated with a disorder of the Liver and the Organs of the middle burner (Spleen and Stomach): disharmony between the Liver and Spleen, and between the Liver and Stomach. A brief review of the basic theory concerning the relationship among these Organs will be helpful here.

This relationship mainly revolves around the qi activity of the Liver, Spleen, and Stomach. The Liver governs the free-flow of qi, which regulates the qi activity of the entire body. The Spleen and Stomach are the Organs responsible for the transportation and transformation (metabolism) of food and water, as well as the upward and downward movement of the qi activity in the middle burner. In fact, these movements are also supported by the Liver's role in regulating the free-flow of qi. Apart from the Spleen and Stomach's function in producing food essence and clear qi, they also play an important role in replenishing the Liver blood and qi. In clinical practice, any change in these relationships can very easily cause disharmony between the Liver and Spleen or Liver and Stomach. These patterns are called, respectively, "no regulation between the Liver and Spleen *(gān pí bù tiǎo)*" and "disharmony between the Liver and Stomach *(gān wèi bù hé)*."

According to five-phase theory, each of these disorders is viewed separately. In the first, "wood becomes exuberant and overwhelms earth *(mù wàng chéng tǔ)*," and in the second, "earth becomes deficient [such that] wood overwhelms it *(tǔ xū mù chéng)*."

An explanation of the first pattern is as follows. The Liver is associated with wood. Just as wood keeps earth in check, so too does the Liver keep the Spleen and Stomach in check; this is a controlling relationship. However, if the Liver qi becomes overactive ("exuberant"), it can injure the Spleen and Stomach.

The second pattern occurs when there is initially no problem with the Liver, but the Spleen and Stomach have been injured for some unrelated reason. Although the Liver qi is still normal, it is out of balance relative to the diminished qi of the Spleen and Stomach. Thus, the now-greater Liver qi over-controls or overwhelms the depleted qi of the Spleen and Stomach.

Despite the fact that these two patterns have different causes, the manifestations are the same: the Liver is too strong relative to the Spleen and Stomach, and so overwhelms them. The clinical presentations of these two patterns likewise have much in common.

Fig. 4-11

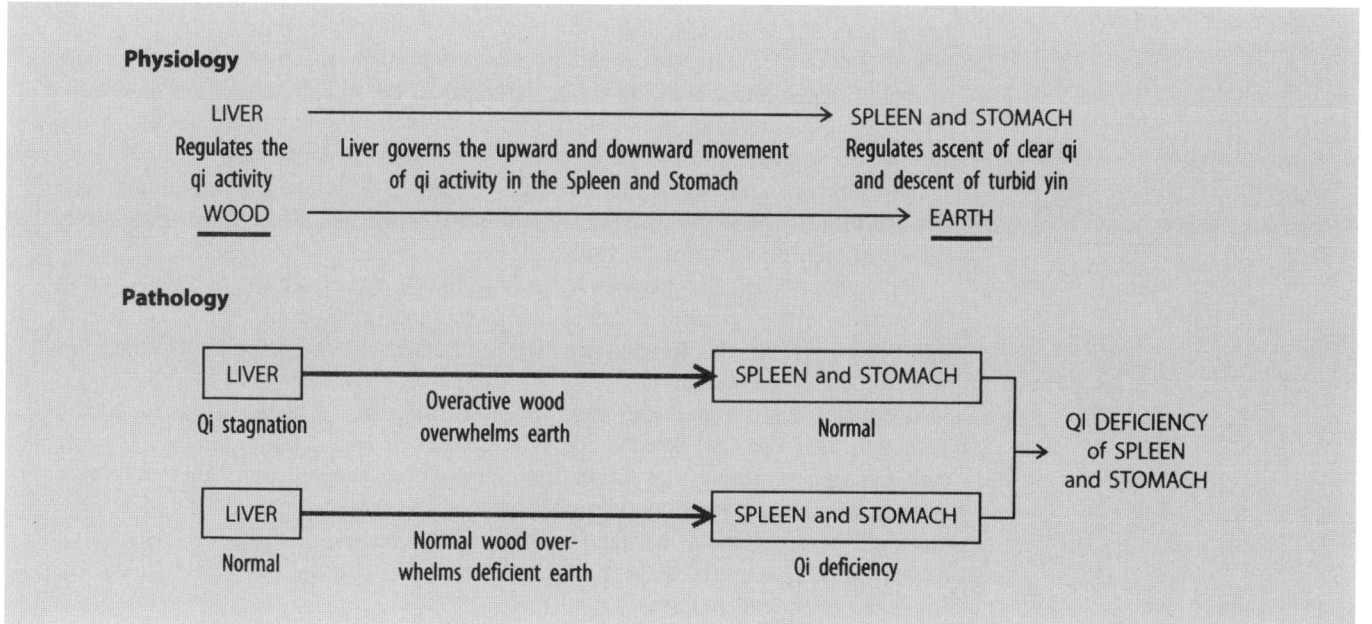

Physiology

LIVER ──────────────────────────────→ SPLEEN and STOMACH
Regulates the   Liver governs the upward and downward movement   Regulates ascent of clear qi
qi activity   of qi activity in the Spleen and Stomach   and descent of turbid yin
WOOD ──────────────────────────────→ EARTH

Pathology

LIVER ──────────→ SPLEEN and STOMACH
Qi stagnation   Overactive wood   Normal   QI DEFICIENCY
                  overwhelms earth   of SPLEEN
                                                              and STOMACH
LIVER ──────────→ SPLEEN and STOMACH
Normal   Normal wood over-   Qi deficiency
           whelms deficient earth

Cause of disease	Qi stagnation and retention of damp-cold
	The patient experiences pain and distention, which is evidence of qi stagnation. When the pain worsens, there is also nausea, excessively watery saliva, and watery, loose stools. The tongue coating is white and moist. All of these signs and symptoms indicate the retention of damp-cold in the body. We may therefore conclude that the problem is one of qi stagnation and retention of damp-cold.
Site of disease	Spleen, Stomach, Liver
	There is pain in the middle and upper abdomen, which, when it worsens, leads to nausea and excessively watery saliva. Thus, the site of disease is the Stomach.

The patient has a poor appetite, abdominal distention, and loose stools, indicating a disorder of the Spleen.

The abdominal pain that radiates to the hypochondria, and the wiry pulse, are evidence of Liver involvement.

Pathological change

Qi stagnation in the middle burner may be caused by a disorder of the Spleen and Stomach. It may also be caused by the Liver qi transversely attacking the Spleen and Stomach. Clinically, one can distinguish between the two mainly by the appearance of Liver symptoms, such as those involving the hypochondrial and intercostal regions, or emotional changes. In this case, the qi stagnation in the middle burner is caused by the Liver disorder.

The Stomach is located in the upper middle part of the abdomen. When qi stagnation occurred in the Stomach, the patient experienced pain and distention in this area of the body. The Liver channel passes around both hypochondria. When the Liver qi stagnates, it will cause pain and distention in the hypochondrial and intercostal regions. Stagnant Liver qi is also unable to regulate the free-flow of qi, which may in turn affect the upward and downward movement of the Spleen and Stomach's qi activity. If the Stomach qi is unable to descend, a reversal in the movement of the Stomach qi may occur, manifested as nausea and excessively watery saliva. As the condition becomes more severe, there can also be vomiting.

Conversely, if the Spleen qi is unable to ascend, impeding its functions of transporting and transforming food and water, food can accumulate in the middle burner, reducing the appetite and interfering with digestion; under these circumstances, eating may aggravate the distention. Because the Spleen controls the flesh and limbs, Spleen deficiency may lead to malnourishment. This accounts for the patient's fatigue and weight loss. Similarly, when the Spleen's function of metabolizing water is impaired, water and dampness will accumulate in the body, and the dampness can drain into the Large Intestine, resulting in loose stools.

The pale lips and tongue are evidence of yang qi deficiency, which reduces the upward-movement of blood. This is manifested in the lack of luster in the various tissues of the upper part of the body.

The white, thick, and greasy tongue coating indicates retention of damp-cold in the body. The wiry pulse indicates Liver qi stagnation and constraint of qi, and its thin quality reflects the deficiency of the antipathogenic factors, and also the malnourishment of the vessels.

Both this and the previous case involved disharmony between the Liver and Spleen or the Liver and Stomach *(Fig. 4-12)*. However, the patient in the previous case experienced abdominal pain before his bowel movements, and his stools were normal, because the main pathological change was the qi stagnation in the Spleen. Here, on the other hand, the main problem is Spleen yang deficiency. There is no relationship between the abdominal symptoms and the bowel movements, and the stools are loose and watery.

Pattern of disease

This is an interior pattern because there is no evidence of an invasion by a pathogenic factor, and also because the site of disease is in the Organs.

There is an absence of thirst, the stools are loose, and the tongue coating is white, all of which is evidence of cold.

There is a combination of excess and deficiency in this case. The pain and distention in the abdomen and hypochondrial regions is indicative of excess. Yet the patient also has Spleen deficiency, fatigue, and emaciation, which reflect the deficiency of the antipathogenic factors.

Additional notes

1. Is there qi or yang deficiency in the Spleen?

Patterns of both Spleen qi and Spleen yang deficiency can be associated with digestive disorders, with such symptoms as poor appetite and loose stools. The

Fig. 4-12

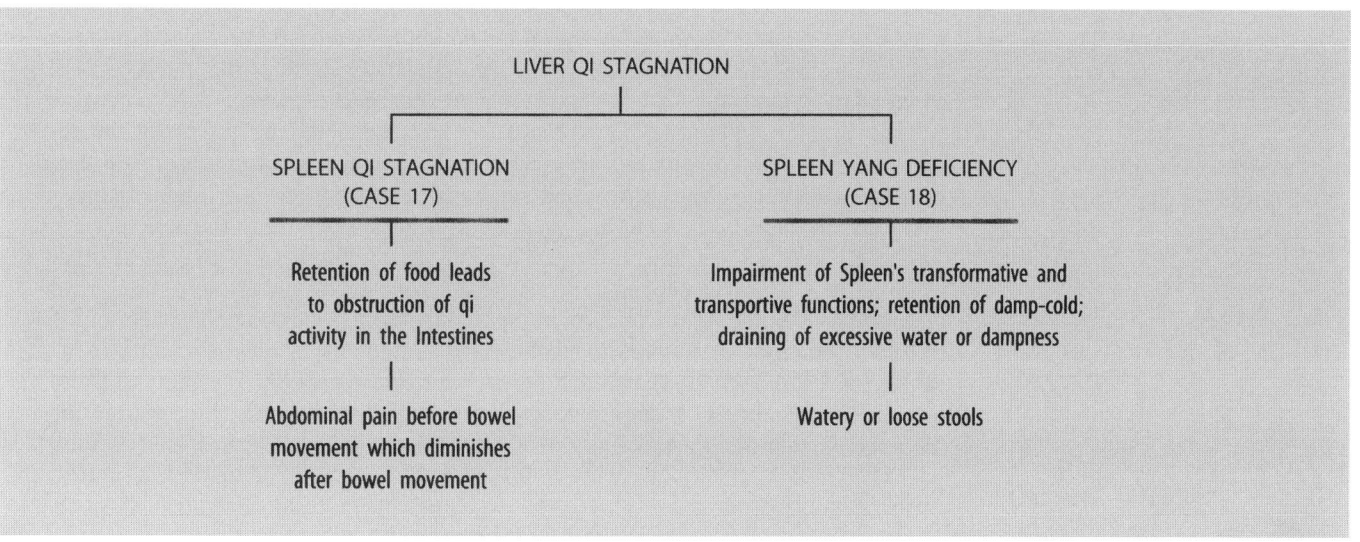

main distinguishing point is whether there are any symptoms of cold. Yang deficiency will present with cold symptoms, while qi deficiency will not. The relationship between yang deficiency and qi deficiency was previously discussed. Yang deficiency may be a progression of qi deficiency.

In this case there are very obvious symptoms of qi deficiency. The patient is showing early symptoms of yang deficiency, such as absence of thirst, clear, watery and loose stools, and a white, thick, moist tongue coating. This is evidence of mild cold, which indicates that the Spleen yang has been injured to a certain degree.

2. In terms of five-phase theory, is this an example of "wood becomes exuberant and overwhelms earth" or "earth becomes deficient [such that] wood overwhelms it"?

These two patterns are both associated with problems of deficiency and excess. In the first, qi stagnation is a pattern of excess, which leads to qi deficiency, a pattern of deficiency. But in the second, it is just the opposite—meaning that the pattern of deficiency leads to the qi stagnation, a pattern of excess. In this case, there is qi stagnation as well as qi deficiency in the Spleen and Stomach, but the symptoms of qi stagnation are obvious and are combined with the general symptoms in the body. Thus, we may say that the pattern of excess is the primary one: "wood becomes exuberant and overwhelms earth" is the underlying pattern in this case.

Conclusion

1. According to the eight principles:
   Interior, cold, and a combination of deficiency and excess (deficiency within excess).

2. According to etiology:
   Qi stagnation and retention of damp-cold.

3. According to Organ theory:
   Disharmony between the Liver and Stomach, together with Spleen yang deficiency.

Treatment principle

1. Regulate the qi and promote the Liver function of governing the free-flow of qi.

2. Warm the middle burner and strengthen the functions of the Spleen.

Explanation of treatment principle

Regulating Liver qi is a very important principle for treating patterns of disharmony between the Liver and Spleen or the Liver and Stomach. The Liver is responsible for regulating the general qi activity of the entire body, including the upward and downward movement of the Spleen and Stomach qi. If the Liver qi activity is well regulated ("smooth"), the qi activity of the entire body will improve, including the Spleen and Stomach qi, thus alleviating the underlying cause of the illness as well as the main symptoms.

The retention of damp-cold in this patient has obstructed the qi activity, impeding the upward and downward movement of the Spleen and Stomach qi, and thus interfering with their transportive and transformative functions. Treatment methods that warm and tonify the middle burner are indicated. Because of the deficiency in this case, caution must be exercized when regulating the qi so as to avoid further injuring the already weakened antipathogenic factors. The retention of damp-cold is caused by the deficiency of yang in the middle burner and the impairment of the Spleen's functions of transporting and transforming (metabolising) water. If the Spleen and Stomach functions are normalized, the retention of damp-cold will resolve spontaneously. In other words, it is not always necessary to address the treatment of damp-cold directly.

Selection of points

Prescription #1:

PC-6 *(nei guan)*
CV-12 *(zhong wan)*
ST-36 *(zu san li)*
SP-4 *(gong sun)* [right side]
LR-3 *(tai chong)* [left side]

Prescription #2:

BL-18 *(gan shu)*
BL-20 *(pi shu)*
BL-21 *(wei shu)*
SP-6 *(san yin jiao)*

Explanation of points

Prescription #1:

PC-6 *(nei guan)* is the connecting point on the arm terminal yin Pericardium channel. It is also one of the eight confluent points, serving as the master point on the yin linking vessel. It regulates the qi and blood, and relieves such symptoms as pain, fullness, and distention in the chest and abdomen. This point is very effective in regulating qi, especially in the regions of the chest, epigastrium, and abdomen. In this case, it is used to alleviate the fullness and pain in the epigastric region. As this point is on the arm terminal yin Pericardium channel, which is related, through its qi, to the leg terminal yin Liver channel and is thereby associated with the Liver, the point can also be used to dispel stagnation of Liver qi. This relationship is referred to as "those of the same qi can rescue each other *(tóng qì xiāng qiú),*" which means that, although the channels are associated with different Organs and have different pathways in the body, they share the same quality of qi and can thus be accessed to treat each other's disorders.

CV-12 *(zhong wan)* is the alarm point of the Stomach channel, and is also one of the eight meeting points of the yang Organs. This point regulates the functions of the middle burner, removes qi stagnation, regulates qi and blood, reduces the retention of food, and promotes digestion. Here it serves as a local point. Because there is both deficiency and excess in this case, even needle manipulation is indicated. This will serve to regulate the qi and alleviate the pain while preventing injury to the antipathogenic factors. The moxa box is also used at this point for twenty minutes during each treatment.

ST-36 *(zu san li)* is one of the most commonly used points in the clinic. It serves as a general tonifier, regulates the Stomach and Spleen, and removes obstruction from the channels and collaterals. The needling method depends on the pattern to be treated. In this case, because the point is used to tonify the middle burner for treating the Spleen yang deficiency and Stomach disorder, the tonification (reinforcement) method of needle manipulation is used.

SP-4 *(gong sun)* is the connecting point of the Spleen channel, and is thus associated with both the Spleen and Stomach channels. As one of the eight confluent points, it is also associated with the penetrating vessel. It regulates the functions of the Spleen, harmonizes the Organs of the middle burner, and regulates the functions of the Intestines. It promotes the upward and downward movement of the middle burner qi, and can alleviate pain.

LR-3 *(tai chong)* is the source point of the Liver channel. It regulates Liver qi and removes qi stagnation. Here, the draining (reducing) method is used to regulate the qi and alleviate pain. It directly relieves the pain in the hypochondria, and the distention in the abdomen.

Prescription #2:

BL-18 *(gan shu)* is a back associated point of the Liver. It promotes the functions of the Liver, regulates the Liver qi, and removes Liver qi stagnation. It is very effective in alleviating symptoms associated with obstruction of the Liver qi. The draining method is used for this purpose.

BL-20 *(pi shu)* is the back associated point of the Spleen. It strengthens the Spleen, harmonizes the functions of the Stomach, and resolves dampness.

BL-21 *(wei shu)* is the back associated point of the Stomach. It tonifies the middle burner, harmonizes the Spleen and Stomach, and promotes the downward movement of Stomach qi, thus correcting its upward reversal. This point and BL-20 *(pi shu)* are used in this case to treat the deficiency in the middle burner; the tonification method is therefore utilized. Moxa sticks are also held over the points for ten minutes during each treatment.

SP-6 *(san yin jiao)* regulates and harmonizes the functions of the Spleen and Stomach. The tonification method is used here in treating the Spleen and Stomach deficiency.

Combination of points

PC-6 *(nei guan)*, SP-4 *(gong sun)*, LR-3 *(tai chong)*. The first two are connecting points, and the third is the source point of the Liver channel. PC-6 *(nei guan)* is punctured bilaterally, whereas SP-4 *(gong sun)* and LR-3 *(tai chong)* are needled on only one side. This combination regulates the qi, removes qi stagnation from the Liver and middle burner, and alleviates pain. In clinical practice this combination is often used for pain in the abdominal and hypochondrial regions, or for abdominal and epigastric pain radiating to the hypochondrial region. Four needles are inserted at the three points, one on each of the three channels. This is an example of engaging more channels with fewer needles. In addition, PC-6 *(nei guan)* and SP-4 *(gong sun)* are both confluent points; they form a combination of points from the eight extraordinary channels. They are very effective in treating qi stagnation in the chest and epigastrium, and can be used for the associated pain and other symptoms in this area.

CV-12 *(zhong wan)* and ST-36 *(zu san li)* is one of the most commonly used combinations in the clinic. It is used especially for patterns of deficiency, for abdominal and epigastric pain, and for poor digestion leading to such symptoms as abdominal pain and distention, as well as diarrhea. This combination can also be used for general tonification of the body.

BL-18 *(gan shu)*, BL-20 *(pi shu)*, and BL-21 *(wei shu)* are all back associated points, associated with the Liver, Spleen, and Stomach respectively. They are used for disorders involving the Liver and middle burner, especially in patterns associated with the Liver overwhelming the Spleen or Stomach. They can also be used for patterns of Spleen deficiency resulting in the hyperfunction of the Liver. The most commonly used methods of needling are the draining (reducing) at BL-18 *(gan shu)* and reinforcing (tonifying) at BL-20 *(pi shu)* and BL-21 *(wei shu)*. This combination can also be used in treating deficiency of qi and blood, but in that case, the reinforcing method is indicated at all three points.

Basic herbal formula #1

Galangal and Cyperus Pill *(liang fu wan)* is typically prescribed in treating patterns of cold caused by Liver qi stagnation transversely attacking the Stomach. The formula consists of only two herbs:

Rhizoma Alpiniae Officinari *(gao liang jiang)* 5g
Rhizoma Cyperi Rotundi *(xiang fu)* 5g

Explanation of basic herbal formula #1

The primary symptoms associated with this pattern are a feeling of cold, fullness and pain in the epigastric region (which is often partially relieved by warmth); pain, and a feeling of distention radiating from the epigastrium to the chest and hypochondrial region; vomiting (clear and watery vomitus), poor appetite, a white, greasy tongue coating, and a wiry and tight pulse. The pathological change in this pattern is either impairment of the Liver's function in governing the free-flow of qi, or pathogenic cold invading the Stomach, which interferes with the upward and downward movement of middle burner qi, and reversal of the downward movement of Stomach qi.

In this formula, Rhizoma Alpiniae Officinari *(gao liang jiang)* is acrid, hot, and enters the Spleen and Stomach channels. It is used especially for warming the Spleen and Stomach, expelling pathogenic cold, and alleviating the vomiting and epigastric pain. Rhizoma Cyperi Rotundi *(xiang fu)* is acrid, bitter, and neutral, and enters the Liver channel. The focus of this herb is on regulating Liver qi and promoting the Liver's function in governing the free-flow of qi. It is very effective in alleviating pain. Together, these two herbs can be used in treating Liver and Stomach disorders. In clinical practice, the dosage of the chief herb, which can be either of the two in the formula, can be modified in accordance with the main problem in the case. Thus, if the primary pattern is one of cold in the Stomach, Rhizoma Alpiniae Officinari *(gao liang jiang)* serves as the chief herb, and its dosage can be increased accordingly; if Liver qi stagnation is the main problem, Rhizoma Cyperi Rotundi *(xiang fu)* will serve as the chief herb, and its dosage increased.

Basic herbal formula #2

Four-Gentlemen Decoction *(si jun zi tang)* is another basic formula used in tonifying the qi. It contains the following ingredients:

Radix Ginseng *(ren shen)* 10g
Rhizoma Atractylodis Macrocephalae *(bai zhu)* 9g
Pericarpium Citri Reticulatae *(chen pi)* 9g
Radix Glycyrrhizae Uralensis *(gan cao)* 6g

Explanation of basic herbal formula #2

This formula can be used in treating various types of qi deficiency, especially of the Spleen and Stomach. Symptoms include fatigue, weakness in the limbs, weak voice, poor appetite, loose stools, pale tongue, and a thin, forceless pulse. The basic pathological change here is that the body has become malnourished owing to general qi deficiency.

In this formula, Radix Ginseng *(ren shen)* serves as the chief herb. It is sweet and warm, and is very effective in tonifying the source qi of the body; it can also promote the Spleen and Lung qi. Rhizoma Atractylodis Macrocephalae *(bai zhu)* is the deputy herb. It is bitter, sweet, and warm, and tonifies the Spleen qi. It can assist the chief herb in strengthening the body qi, and can dry dampness and relieve the disorder in water metabolism caused by the deficiency. Pericarpium Citri Reticulatae *(chen pi)* is sweet and bland, and can strengthen the Spleen and promote the metabolism of water, thereby draining dampness. It assists the deputy herb, Rhizoma Atractylodis Macrocephalae *(bai zhu)*, in tonifying Spleen qi and removing dampness, and serves here as an assistant herb. Radix Glycyrrhizae Uralensis *(gan cao)* is an envoy. It is sweet, neutral, and regulates the function of the middle burner.

Modified herbal formula

Rhizoma Alpiniae Officinari *(gao liang jiang)* 6g
Rhizoma Cyperi Rotundi *(xiang fu)* 10g
Fructus Meliae Toosendan *(chuan lian zi)* 6g
Radix Ginseng *(ren shen)* 12g
Pericarpium Citri Reticulatae *(chen pi)* 12g
Radix Scutellariae Baicalensis *(huang qin)* 10g
Fructus Citri Medicae seu Wilsonii *(xiang yuan)* 6g
Pericarpium Citri Reticulatae *(chen pi)* 6g

One packet per day, divided into two doses, one taken in the morning, the other in the evening.

Explanation of modified herbal formula

In this case, wood (Liver) overwhelms earth (Spleen) and there is retention of damp-cold. The combination of Galangal and Cyperus Pill *(liang fu wan)* and Four-Gentlemen Decoction *(si jun zi tang)* is therefore used, with modifications, in order to expel the pathogenic factors and reinforce the antipathogenic factors.

In light of the patient's presentation, the quantity of Rhizoma Cyperi Rotundi *(xiang fu)* is greater than that of Rhizoma Alpiniae Officinari *(gao liang jiang)*, compared with their respective dosage in Galangal and Cyperus Pill *(liang fu wan)*, where they are equal. Also, Rhizoma Cyperi Rotundi *(xiang fu)* is combined with Fructus Meliae Toosendan *(chuan lian zi)* and Fructus Citri Medicae seu Wilsonii *(xiang yuan)*. Thus, the primary purpose of this formula is to regulate the qi; warming the Stomach is a secondary purpose. Fructus Meliae Toosendan *(chuan lian zi)* is bitter and cold, and regulates the Liver qi, but the dosage must be limited here. Four-Gentlemen Decoction *(si jun zi tang)* is used to warm and tonify the Stomach and Spleen qi, as well as to warm and resolve damp-cold. However, because tonifying the qi can aggravate the qi stagnation, Radix Glycyrrhizae Uralensis *(gan cao)* is omitted, and Pericarpium Citri Reticulatae *(chen pi)* is added to promote the qi activity and thereby indirectly remove the qi stagnation. In general, the action of this formula in expelling pathogenic factors is stronger than its action in strengthening the antipathogenic factors.

Follow-up

Two acupuncture prescriptions were used in this case. The first was used when the pain became severe and the symptoms were very obvious. Whenever the pain diminished, the second prescription was utilized. The two prescriptions were therefore administered alternately, depending on the patient's condition.

Acupuncture was administered once a day for the first two weeks, six times a week in all. After two weeks, treatment was given every other day, that is, three times a week. The patient was treated for six weeks, though treatment was interrupted for about a week when he caught a very mild cold. After six weeks the patient's appetite was much improved, the abdominal and epigastric pain had diminished, and the nausea was alleviated. Although the stools remained fairly loose, the frequency of bowel movements declined to once or twice a day. There was also an improvement in the hypochondrial distention and pain, but these symptoms persisted. Nevertheless, the patient was very satisfied with the results up to that time.

Because of the necessity of returning home (he lived far from the clinic), the patient was unable to stay longer for acupuncture treatment. The herbal therapy was therefore introduced. The hebs were combined with acupuncture for a week, during which the symptoms improved even more, and the patient felt that his physical energy was returning. After the week of combined treatment, the herbs were used alone during the following month, at the end of which the symptoms had all but disappeared. Although the pain and distention were more or less alleviated, the patient still suffered from some of the symptoms of Spleen deficiency. Therefore, those herbs that were prescribed for regulating qi were reduced, and the remaining herbs were used primarily for tonifying the Spleen. Treatment was concluded after one month, and the patient was able to resume his normal life and work.

During the following year the patient occasionally suffered from abdominal pain, but as soon as he took the herbs, the symptoms were alleviated. One year later he underwent another upper GI study with barium, and no ulcer was found.

Diagnostic Principles for Abdominal and Epigastric Pain

The epigastrium and abdomen encompass the entire abdominal cavity, which contains many organs. In this chapter we have focussed on abdominal and epigastric pain associated with Spleen and Stomach disorders.

Causes and pathological change

Pathogenic factors from the environment can cause abdominal and epigastric pain, as can diet and dysfunction of the internal Organs:

- Invasion of cold: Of the six external pathogenic factors, an invasion of cold can manifest in two different ways. It can directly affect the Spleen and Stomach, without leaving an exterior pattern in its wake. Or it can invade by means of overeating cold and raw food. Both can directly injure the yang qi in the Spleen and Stomach, cause stagnation of the qi activity in the middle burner, and lead to disorders in the Stomach and Spleen.
- Retention of heat: If one often overindulges in hot and spicy foods, heat can accumulate in the middle burner. This may disturb the circulation of qi and blood in the middle burner, causing pain.
- Qi stagnation in the middle burner: Spleen and Stomach qi stagnation, or stagnant Liver qi, can impair the upward and downward movement of the Spleen and Stomach qi, leading to stagnation of the qi activity in the middle burner.
- Blood stasis: Qi stagnation can lead to blood stasis, and chronic illness can gradually affect the circulation of blood. In a long-term illness the antipathogenic factors can be injured, eventually leading to poor blood circulation. Chronic illness of the Spleen and Stomach can obstruct the qi and blood.
- Retention of food: Overeating, as well as impairment of the transportive and transformative functions of the Spleen, can both cause food to accumulate in the middle burner, which then becomes pathogenic.
- Deficiency of Spleen and Stomach: Qi or yang deficiency in connection with this disorder is frequently seen in the clinic. Qi deficiency can impede the transportation and transformation of food, while yang qi deficiency can lead to

Fig. 4-13

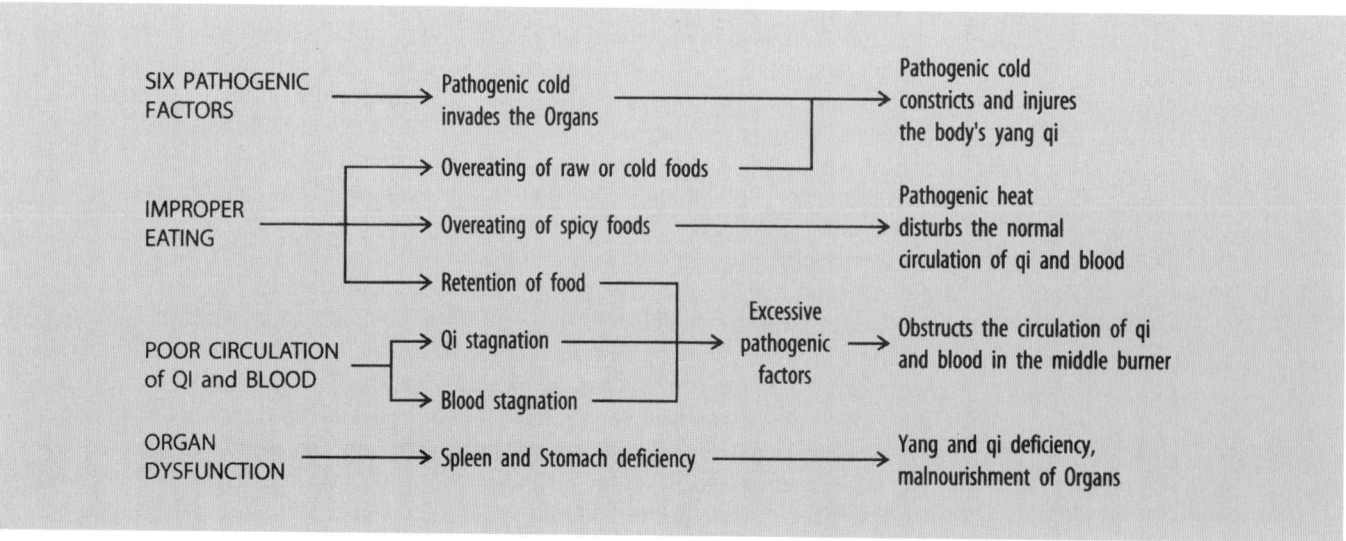

internal cold, compromising the warmth in the middle burner. Both conditions can lead to abdominal pain.

Symptoms and distinguishing criteria   When a patient is diagnosed with pain in the epigastrium and abdomen, two major aspects should be noted: the characteristics of the pain, and common symptoms.

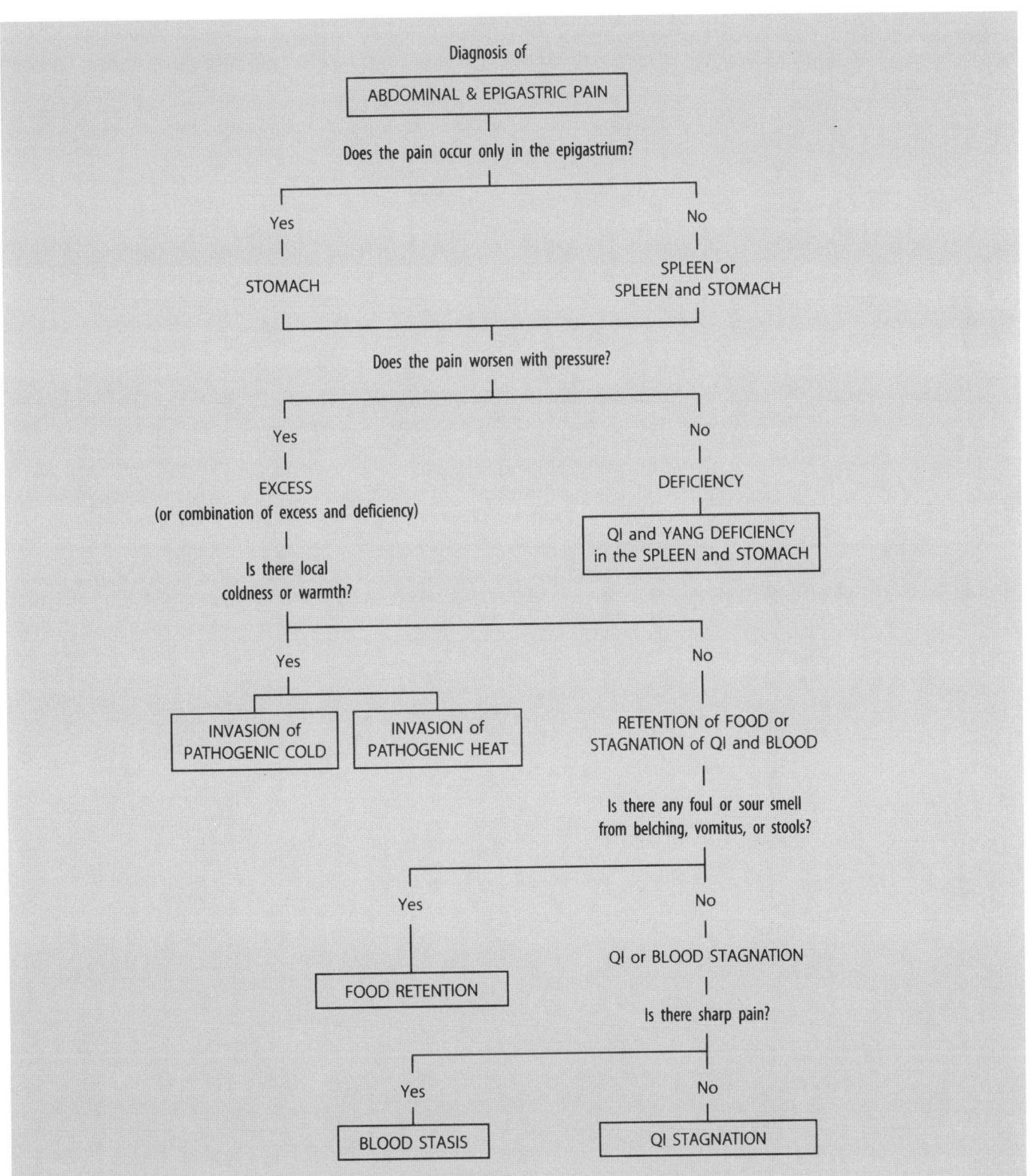

Abnormal Bowel Movements

CASE 19: **Female, age 74**

Main complaint

Diarrhea

History

This patient has long had a very weak digestive system and often suffers from diarrhea after eating improper foods. Two days ago she ate some corn on the cob, after which she felt pain and distention in her upper abdomen, but without nausea or vomiting. That evening she began to have diarrhea, which has continued to the present. She has bowel movements four or five times a day, and her stools, which are clear and watery, contain obvious traces of undigested food. She feels cold in the abdomen, especially below the umbilicus. She has no fever or aversion to cold, but her hands and feet are cold. Her appetite is poor and she has little desire to eat; when she does eat, even though it may be only a very little, her intestines rumble loudly and her upper abdomen becomes very distended. There is no excessive belching, and she does not drink much. She feels very tired. Even a little activity will bring shortness of breath and palpitations. She wakes easily at night.

Tongue

Very dark with a thin, yellow coating

Pulse

Thin and slightly slippery, forceless under deep pressure

Analysis of symptoms

1. Long history of diarrhea after eating improper foods—Spleen deficiency.

2. Poor appetite, disinterested in food, upper abdominal distention, and stools containing undigested food—impairment of Spleen's transportive and transformative functions.

3. Diarrhea four to five times a day, clear and watery stools—retention of damp-cold.

4. Cold feeling in the abdomen, especially below the umbilicus, cold hands and feet, and little inclination to drink—Spleen yang deficiency.

5. Fatigue, lassitude, and shortness of breath after any physical activity—qi deficiency.

6. Palpitations, easily wakes, and unsound sleep—disturbance of Heart spirit.

7. Dark tongue, thin pulse, forceless under deep pressure—qi deficiency.

8. Slightly slippery pulse—retention of dampness.

Basic theory of case

In Chinese medicine the Stomach and Spleen provide the necessary warmth for breaking down, transforming, and transporting food and water. The Spleen is responsible for the transformation and transportation of ingested liquids, their transformation into body fluids, and the transportation of these fluids to various parts of the body. The Spleen is also responsible for expelling excessive fluids from the body.

When water enters the body it is warmed to the correct temperature, and then nutrition is extracted to form the body fluids. This is then mixed with food essence and transported to the Lung. From there it is distributed to the rest of the body where it performs various physiological functions such as providing moisture for the skin, muscles, and sensory organs, and supplying nourishment to the blood, brain, marrow, Organs, and tissues. Excess water, which has not been used to make body fluids, is passed along through the Small and Large Intestines, from which it will be expelled. In addition, the waste liquids from metabolism are discharged from the body through the Triple Burner and Bladder.

Because most of the water taken into the body is transformed into body fluids, the amount that enters the Small and Large Intestines is limited. There it serves to soften the feces, which explains why normal feces have a recognizable form, and contain a certain amount of moisture. They are neither too dry nor too watery. If for some reason there is excessive liquid in the Intestines, the feces will become too soft and often lose their form completely, and the patient will have symptoms such as diarrhea.

Fig. 5-1

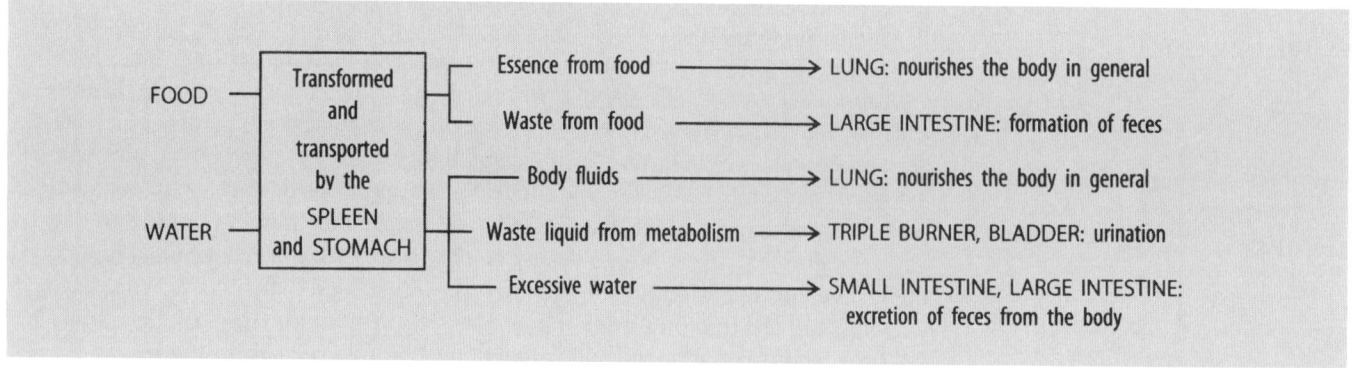

Cause of disease

Pathogenic dampness

The patient has diarrhea which is watery, loose, and unformed. She has bowel movements four to five times a day. Her intestines rumble, and her pulse is slippery, indicating the presence of excessive water in the body. Thus, the condition is caused by water and dampness.

Site of disease

Spleen

The patient's diarrhea has been caused by eating improper foods, her appetite is poor, and she suffers from general lassitude and coldness in the abdominal region. Her stools contain particles of undigested food. All of this is evidence of a Spleen disorder.

Pathological change

If the Spleen yang is deficient, digestion will become very weak, and the metabolism of water will be impaired. Thus, when liquids are ingested, they are not properly transformed into body fluids which can nourish the body. Instead, water remains in the Spleen, where it becomes harmful or transforms into dampness, both of which are pathogenic. This is referred to as "Spleen deficiency generating dampness *(pí xū shēng shī)*." This is a variety of internal dampness.

In this particular case the patient has a history of recurrent diarrhea caused by eating improper foods. The digestion is thus very weak, and any change in diet can very easily overload the Spleen's ability to transform and transport food and water. When this occurs, symptoms of Spleen dysfunction begin to appear. As the Spleen's transportive and transformative functions become impaired, the food, instead of being transformed into essence that will nourish the body, remains in the Spleen and Stomach. Here it obstructs the normal upward and downward movement of the qi activity in the middle burner, and the patient thus experiences fullness and distention in the epigastric region, and has a poor appetite.

The Spleen governs the limbs. When there is Spleen yang deficiency, the limbs are deprived of warmth, and the arms and legs feel cold. Spleen deficiency also interferes with the transportation and transformation of water. Excessive water thus accumulates in the middle burner and drains into the Large Intestine, causing the patient to have diarrhea with loose and watery stools.

Spleen deficiency also affects the transportation and transformation of food. It cannot be properly digested or expelled from the body, which explains why undigested food may appear in the feces. Because eating aggravates the already overloaded Spleen and Stomach, as well as the Intestines, there is rumbling in the lower abdomen. This also reflects the retention of excessive water in the Intestines.

The Spleen and Stomach are the source for production of qi for the entire body. When the Spleen's ability to transport and transform food and water is impaired, the production of qi will decline and the patient will suffer from general lassitude, fatigue, and shortness of breath after any kind of physical activity.

Qi provides energy for the circulation of blood. This energy is reduced where there is qi deficiency. In addition, yang deficiency will cause internal cold that can constrict the vessels. Blood circulation thereupon slows down, and the tongue becomes dark. The thin, forceless pulse in this case indicates yang deficiency, and its slippery quality reflects the retention of dampness.

Fig. 5-2

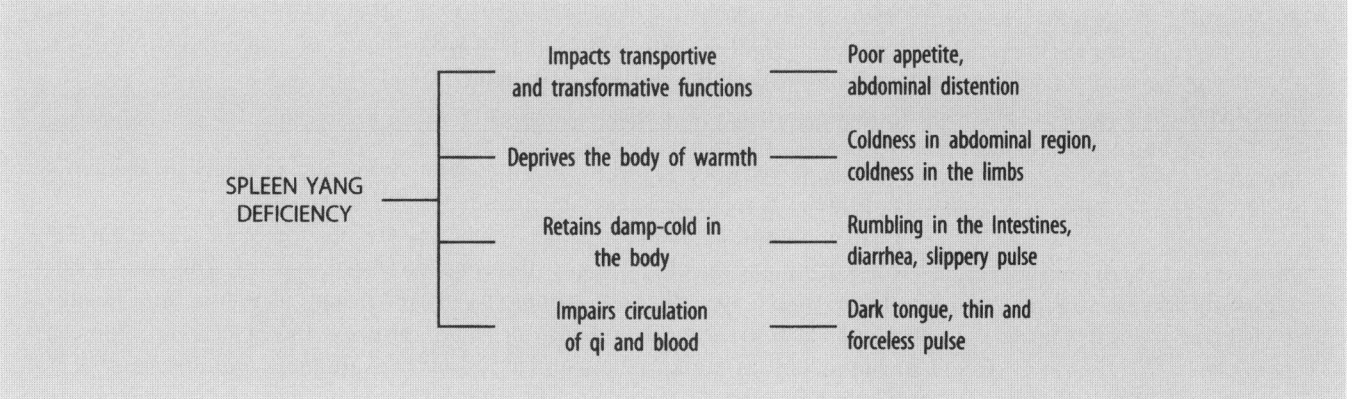

SPLEEN YANG DEFICIENCY	Impacts transportive and transformative functions	Poor appetite, abdominal distention
	Deprives the body of warmth	Coldness in abdominal region, coldness in the limbs
	Retains damp-cold in the body	Rumbling in the Intestines, diarrhea, slippery pulse
	Impairs circulation of qi and blood	Dark tongue, thin and forceless pulse

Pattern of disease

There is no history of invasion by an external pathogenic factor, and the site of the disease is the middle burner (Spleen and Stomach). Accordingly, this is an interior pattern.

Because of the yang deficiency, there is a feeling of cold in the abdomen and limbs, the stools are loose and watery, and the patient has little inclination to drink. These symptoms are indicative of cold.

The deficiency of Spleen yang has impeded the transportation and transformation of food, thus the patient's appetite is poor, and she suffers from fatigue and general lassitude. Her pulse is thin and forceless. All of these symptoms reflect a pattern of deficiency.

Additional notes

1. Is there any retention of food in this case?

While pathogenic dampness has been established as the cause of disease in this case, we also know that the patient's current crisis began after eating corn on the cob. Thus, one may wonder if retention of food isn't the cause of this illness.

According to the history, the patient has diarrhea, a poor appetite, epigastric and abdominal distention, and lassitude; these symptoms are associated with Spleen deficiency. There are no symptoms like belching, bad breath from regurgitating food, or vomiting of undigested food. There is undigested food in the feces, which are loose and watery, but not sticky or greasy. These are characteristics of a deficiency pattern, and the eating of the corn was only the precipitating episode for the onset of this illness. Thus, retention of food can be ruled out in this case.

2. Is there a pattern of excess?

Spleen yang and Spleen qi insufficiency pertain to a deficiency pattern; retention of dampness pertains to a pattern of excess. In this instance, the cause of disease is dampness, but it is dampness due to deficiency. Dampness here is only a secondary pathogenic factor resulting from the Spleen deficiency, which impaired its function of transporting and transforming water. Furthermore, the dampness itself has not caused any severe symptoms. At the moment, then, there is neither a pattern of excess nor a combination of deficiency and excess.

3. What is the cause of the yellow tongue coating?

From the history we can see that all the symptoms indicate a cold pattern, so why is there a yellow coating on the tongue? A detailed analysis must be given in order to understand this coating.

The tongue coating here is not the thick, dry, yellow coating produced by heat, but a thin layer of a moist and slightly yellow coating, which is normally associated with retention of dampness in the middle burner. As dampness is a turbid pathogenic factor, when it mixes with turbid qi from the Stomach, the dampness and turbid qi "steam" upward and quite often form this particular type of coating on the tongue. To summarize, this coating is characteristic of dampness in the Stomach, and is completely different from the coating produced by heat.

4. Is there any Heart qi deficiency?

According to the history, the patient has palpitations and is easily awakened at night. Should Heart qi deficiency be included in the diagnosis?

First, it should be said that these symptoms are not the main reason for the patient's coming to the clinic, nor are these symptoms very severe. This patient suffers from general qi deficiency, symptoms of which may include a mild insufficiency of Heart qi and a disturbance of Heart spirit. As the Spleen and Stomach functions return to normal, the palpitations and wakefullness will disappear. It is therefore inappropriate to include Heart qi deficiency as part of the diagnosis in this case.

Conclusion

1. According to the eight principles:
   Interior, cold, deficiency.

2. According to etiology:
   Retention of damp-cold.

3. According to Organ theory:
   Spleen yang deficiency.

Treatment principle

1. Warm and tonify the Spleen yang.
2. Dry dampness.

Explanation of treatment principle

Both qi and yang pertain to the yang aspect of the body. The difference in treating yang deficiency and qi deficiency is that yang deficiency, which is part of a cold pattern, is treated by warming the yang to dispel cold, and tonifying the qi. Qi deficiency has no symptoms associated with cold, and therefore treatment only requires tonifying the qi.

In this case there is Spleen yang deficiency and retention of damp-cold, so it is necessary to use the warming method to warm and strengthen the Spleen yang. This will also help remove the damp-cold. Thus, warming the yang and tonifying the qi are the main methods used to restore the yang qi of the Spleen and Stomach. We should also use, to a lesser extent, the method of drying dampness to help expel the pathogenic factors from the Spleen and Stomach.

Selection of points

CV-12 *(zhong wan)*
GV-20 *(bai hui)*
ST-25 *(tian shu)*
ST-36 *(zu san li)*
LR-13 *(zhang men)*
SP-9 *(yin ling quan)*

Explanation of points

CV-12 *(zhong wan)* is the alarm point of the Stomach, and the influential point of the yang Organs. It regulates the qi of the middle burner, dispels blood stasis, eliminates retention of food, and stops the vomiting and diarrhea. It serves as the main point in this case, as the patient suffers from retention of dampness. This point will improve the transportive and transformative functions of the middle burner. The primary focus of the point is on improving Stomach function. It is located in the epigastric region, and is a local point in this prescription. Moxibustion is used in this instance because of the deficiency of Spleen yang, and the pattern of interior cold.

ST-25 *(tian shu)* is the alarm point of the Large Intestine. It regulates the functions of the Stomach and Large Intestine, and removes qi stagnation. This is one of the most common points used in treating diarrhea and constipation. It has a bi-directional action for the Intestines and Stomach. For diarrhea caused by Spleen yang deficiency, the tonification (reinforcement) method of needle manipulation, or tonification with moxibustion, can be used at this point. In this case, strong moxibustion is recommended.

LR-13 *(zhang men)* is the alarm point of the Spleen, and the influential point of the yin Organs. It regulates the Liver functions, strengthens the Spleen, regulates the qi, and dispels blood stasis. It is located in the hypochondrial region, and is a very important point for promoting the proper functioning of the Spleen. As it is selected here primarily to strengthen the Spleen, the tonification method is used.

GV-20 *(bai hui)*. The name of this point, which is located in the middle of the top of head, means "a hundred meetings," which refers to the head as the meeting place of many channels, especially those of the yang. This point is used to recapture the yang and strengthen prolapse in the body, as well as treating diarrhea, especially chronic diarrhea, caused by the sinking of qi. In this case, because the patient is quite elderly, readily developed diarrhea after eating improper food, and has been suffering from yang and qi deficiency in the middle burner, this point is used as a secondary point to assist in raising the yang qi and stopping the diarrhea.

ST-36 *(zu san li)* is the sea point on the Stomach channel. It regulates and strengthens the Spleen and Stomach and removes obstructions from the channels and collaterals. Here it is used to tonify the Spleen and harmonize the Spleen and Stomach. The focus is on improving the transportive and transformative functions of these Organs. The tonification method is used in order to strengthen the yang qi of the middle burner, remove dampness, and stop the diarrhea. Only the right side is needled in this case.

SP-9 *(yin ling quan)* is the sea point of the leg greater yin Spleen channel. It tonifies the Spleen qi and also improves water metabolism and the functions of the Triple Burner. It is an assistant point to ST-36 *(zu san li)*, helping to remove dampness, improve water metabolism, and stop diarrhea. Even needle manipulation is used, and only the left-hand side is punctured. Owing to the patient's age, these two points are needled unilaterally in order to limit the number of points that are needled.

Methods of needling and moxibustion

Only moxibustion is used at CV-12 *(zhong wan)* and ST-25 *(tian shu)*. Two moxa boxes are placed on the abdominal region. One 3-inch stick is used at CV-12 *(zhong wan)*. The second box, containing two sticks on each side, is placed in the area of the umbilicus, with the sticks—which are replenished twice during each treatment—positioned over the ST-25 *(tian shu)* points.

Needling is used at GV-20 *(bai hui)*, LR-13 *(zhang men)*, ST-36 *(zu san li)*, and SP-9 *(yin ling quan)*. Thus, a total of five needles is used at four points (one bilaterally).

Combination of points

CV-12 *(zhong wan)*, ST-25 *(tian shu)*, and LR-13 *(zhang men)*. This is a combination of the alarm points of the Stomach, Large Intestine, and Spleen. They are used to regulate the functions and qi of these three Organs. Moxibustion is used at the first two of these points, and needling at the third. The purpose is to strongly tonify the yang qi of the middle burner, dispel the qi stagnation and pain, strengthen the functions of the Spleen, harmonize the middle burner Organs, and stop the diarrhea.

ST-36 *(zu san li)* and SP-9 *(yin ling quan)*. These two points are a very commonly used combination for strengthening the functions of the Spleen and Stomach, and improving the metabolism of water. They serve to tonify the middle burner yang and remove qi stagnation. They can be punctured bilaterally or unilaterally. In this instance, ST-36 *(zu san li)* is needled on the right side and SP-9 *(yin ling quan)* on the left in order to regulate the Spleen and Stomach, remove the dampness, and stop the diarrhea.

Follow-up

Acupuncture and moxibustion was administered once daily for three days, after which the diarrhea stopped. The patient had one bowel movement each day, though the stools were still fairly loose. The cold feeling in the abdomen, which was still distended, was greatly alleviated, but her appetite was still poor. Treatment was continued, once every other day (three times a week), for another two weeks. The patient's appetite was gradually restored, the abdominal distention alleviated, and the bowel movements continued as before; her stools were still slightly loose on occasion. The patient's physical and mental energy was also restored, and treatment was accordingly terminated.

The patient was advised to use the prepared Chinese medicine Regulate the Middle Pill *(li zhong wan)*, which consists of Radix Ginseng *(ren shen)*, Radix Scutellariae Baicalensis *(huang qin)*, Rhizoma Zingiberis Officinalis *(gan jiang)*, and Radix Glycyrrhizae Uralensis *(gan cao)*. She took two pills each day, one in the morning and one in the evening, for another two months, and was told to return to the clinic if there was any recurrence of the symptoms. By the time she had finished her pills, she had no further trouble.

Because this patient is elderly and her condition has both acute and chronic aspects, caution and patience are needed during treatment, which must not be overdone, as the antipathogenic factors must not be injured. Very strong moxibustion is used, but few acupuncture needles; the purpose is to treat the root of the illness by tonifying the yang and strengthening the qi of the body. The prepared herbal pills were prescribed for a period of two months to treat the chronic deficiency of the Spleen.

CASE 20: **Male, age 48**

Main complaint

Diarrhea

History

The patient's illness began in the summer. One week before coming to the clinic he went on a business trip. On the first day the weather was extremely hot, and he soon became very tired and thirsty. He drank a large quantity of cold beverages and ate only melons and other cold fruit. That night he developed severe abdominal and epigastric pain. He experienced nausea, vomited a quantity of watery liquid, and had an attack of diarrhea. He had ten bowel movements during the night, and passed loose, watery stools containing particles of undigested food. He was rushed to the hospital where he was diagnosed with acute gastroenteritis. He was given antibiotics, antispasmodics, and a digestive tonic. The following day he did not vomit but the diarrhea continued. The abdominal pain diminished, but his appetite was extremely poor. He was advised to continue this course of conventional medication for the rest of the week but it yielded little change. He therefore came to the clinic.

One week after the initial attack he still has diarrhea, with four to six bowel movements a day. The feces are very loose and foamy. The patient feels cold all over and experiences a cold sensation in the abdominal region. He often feels pain in the abdomen, and has distention in the central abdomen and epigastrium. His appetite is still poor. He is not inclined to drink much, and can only tolerate a little warm water. He looks tired and feels fatigued. His complexion is pale. His urine is yellowish, and the quantity is reduced.

Tongue

Pale, slightly swollen, with a thick, white, and moist coating

Pulse

Slow and forceful under deep pressure

Analysis of symptoms

1. Consumption of cold food and beverages leading up to complaint—invasion of pathogenic damp-cold.
2. Vomiting, abdominal pain, diarrhea, and watery stools—damp-cold in the middle burner.
3. Reduced appetite, distention, and fullness in the epigastric and abdominal regions—impairment of Spleen's transportive and transformative functions.
4. General feeling of cold, and inability to drink anything other than warm water—yang injured by pathogenic cold.
5. Fatigue, general lassitude, and pale complexion—qi deficiency.
6. Reduced volume of yellow urine—injury to body fluids.
7. Pale, slightly swollen tongue with a thick, white, and moist coating, and a slow pulse—cold pattern.

Basic theory of case

In Chinese medicine there are two patterns of damp-cold in the Spleen, each of which has a different pathogenesis. The first, described in case 19, is Spleen deficiency producing dampness *(pí xū shēng shī)*. As the name suggests, this is a pattern of deficiency. The second, damp-cold encumbering the Spleen *(hán shī kùn pí)*, is a pattern of excess caused by an invasion of pathogenic damp-cold from the environment.

It is this second pattern which pertains to this case. When the invasion is too strong, the resistance of the antipathogenic factors is overcome, and it affects the

Stomach and Spleen. The yang qi of the middle burner becomes obstructed, impeding the transportive and transformative functions. In this particular case, still in its early stage, there was little evidence of a pathological change involving Spleen qi or yang deficiency, but if the illness had lasted a little longer, the cold could have obstructed the Spleen yang and led to Spleen yang deficiency. This pattern could therefore have changed into one of deficiency, or a combination of deficiency and excess.

Characteristic symptoms of patterns shared in common by the two Spleen patterns include abdominal and epigastric distention, poor appetite, and loose stools. These are symptoms associated with a disorder of the digestive system.

It is important, however, that one be able to distinguish between these two patterns. Although there are certain similarities between them, the pattern associated with deficiency of the Spleen leading to retention of dampness is usually of long duration; the symptoms come and go, and there are recurrent attacks. There may also be accompanying symptoms such as very poor appetite, fatigue, and emaciation. This type of pattern often occurs in patients with weak constitutions. On the other hand, the pattern of damp-cold invasion of the Spleen is associated with acute attacks, and the symptoms—including severe epigastric and abdominal pain, very severe nausea, vomiting, and diarrhea—indicate that the pathogenic factors are very strong. This pattern can affect people who have previously been very healthy. Again, it is important that one distinguish between these two patterns of deficiency and excess.

Fig. 5-3

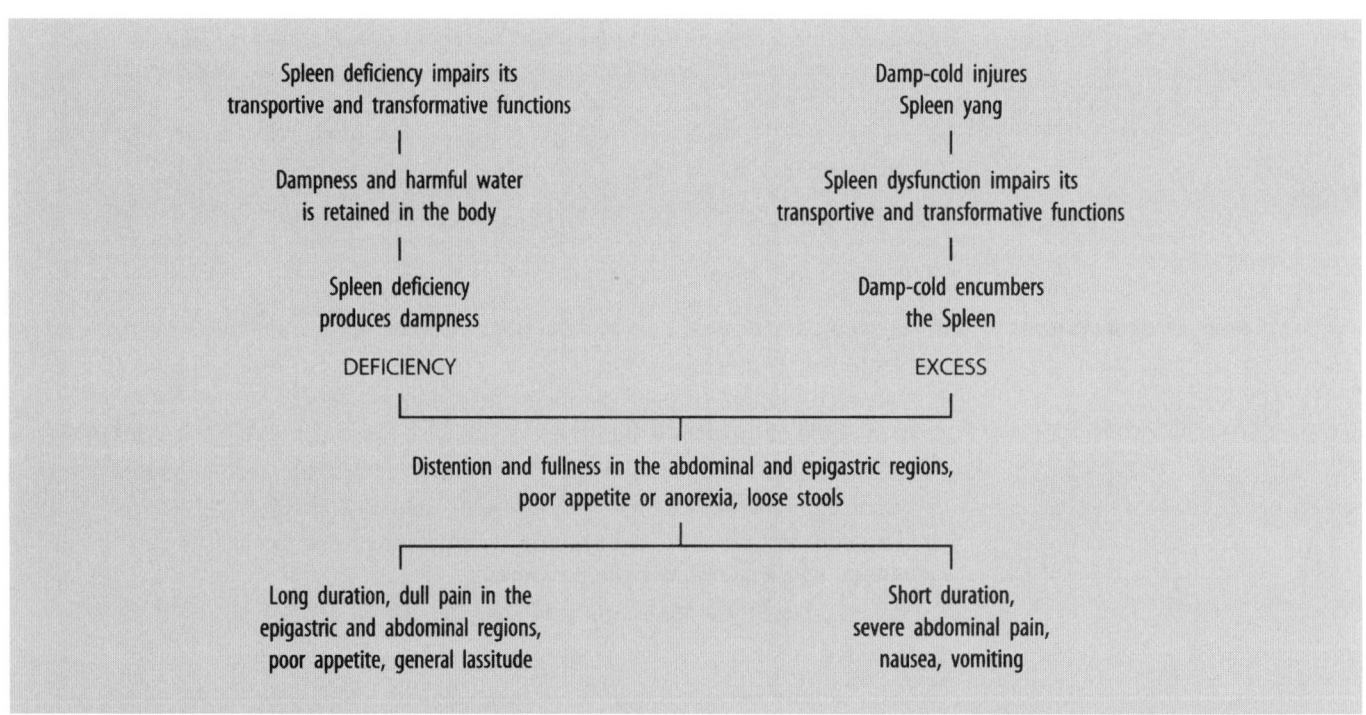

Spleen deficiency impairs its transportive and transformative functions	Damp-cold injures Spleen yang
Dampness and harmful water is retained in the body	Spleen dysfunction impairs its transportive and transformative functions
Spleen deficiency produces dampness	Damp-cold encumbers the Spleen
DEFICIENCY	EXCESS

Distention and fullness in the abdominal and epigastric regions, poor appetite or anorexia, loose stools

| Long duration, dull pain in the epigastric and abdominal regions, poor appetite, general lassitude | Short duration, severe abdominal pain, nausea, vomiting |

Cause of disease   Damp-cold

Before the onset of this illness the patient consumed too much cold food and drink. He then developed diarrhea, loose and watery stools, and severe vomiting. His tongue coating is white and moist. All of these signs and symptoms are evidence of damp-cold, a yin pathogenic factor; when it causes illness, the symptoms are of a clear, cold, and watery nature.

Site of disease   Spleen and Stomach

The patient has epigastric pain, nausea, and vomiting, indicating that the illness has affected the Stomach.

The abdominal pain, diarrhea, and reduced appetite are evidence of a Spleen disorder.

Pathological change

Pathogenic cold and dampness can cause disease in different ways, the most common of which include the following:

1. Pathogenic cold and dampness from the external environment invade the body through the skin, channels, and collaterals, causing exterior patterns or pain in the lower back or legs.

2. Yang deficiency leads to cold inside the body, which, if allowed to persist, leads to internal damp-cold problems such as retention of dampness and edema.

3. Eating improper foods, such as cold or raw fruit or vegetables, causes symptoms in the digestive system. That is to say, the Organs are directly affected by cold and dampness through the digestive system. That is what happened in this particular case.

Damp-cold can obstruct the yang qi of the Spleen and Stomach, causing blood stasis, qi stagnation, and poor circulation; the patient will experience severe abdominal and epigastric pain. When the upward and downward movement of qi in the middle burner is impaired, the Stomach qi may not descend properly, but instead reverses upward, causing nausea and vomiting. When the transportive and transformative functions of the Spleen become disrupted, the clear yang will fail to rise properly; thus, instead of being transformed into essence and transported throughout the body to provide nourishment, the food and water simply drain into the Large Intestine, causing frequent bowel movements and loose, watery stools containing particles of undigested food.

In this case, after one week the patient still had abdominal pain and diarrhea, and felt cold all over. This indicates that the damp-cold was not expelled, and that the yang qi of the body had already been injured. Since there is yang deficiency and a feeling of cold inside the body, the patient prefers to drink warm water in order to relieve the coldness in the Spleen and Stomach. As the yang deficiency has reduced the patient's energy level, he experiences symptoms such as lassitude and fatigue. And because of the qi stagnation in the middle burner, there is also abdominal and epigastric distention.

The pale tongue and complexion reflect yang qi deficiency and poor circulation of blood. The swollen tongue with its thick, white, and moist coating points to retention of damp-cold inside the body. The slow pulse suggests a pattern of cold, and its forceful quality under deep pressure means that the injury to the antipathogenic factors is not very severe *(Fig. 5-4).*

Pattern of disease

In this case, damp-cold has injured the Spleen and Stomach. It is therefore an interior pattern.

The patient feels cold all over, experiences pain with a cold sensation in the epigastric and abdominal regions, diarrhea, watery stools containing undigested food, a pale tongue with a thick, white, and moist coating, and a slow pulse. All of this is evidence of cold.

The damp-cold pathogenic factor is very strong. The illness has lasted for only one week, it has blocked the qi activity in the middle burner, and the abdominal pain is severe. It is thus a pattern of excess.

However, the patient also suffers from general lassitude, feels cold all over, and shows some symptoms associated with deficiency of yang qi. This is therefore a combination of deficiency and excess. As the main problem is excess, and the deficiency is not too pronounced, the pattern may be characterized as one of deficiency within excess.

Fig. 5-4

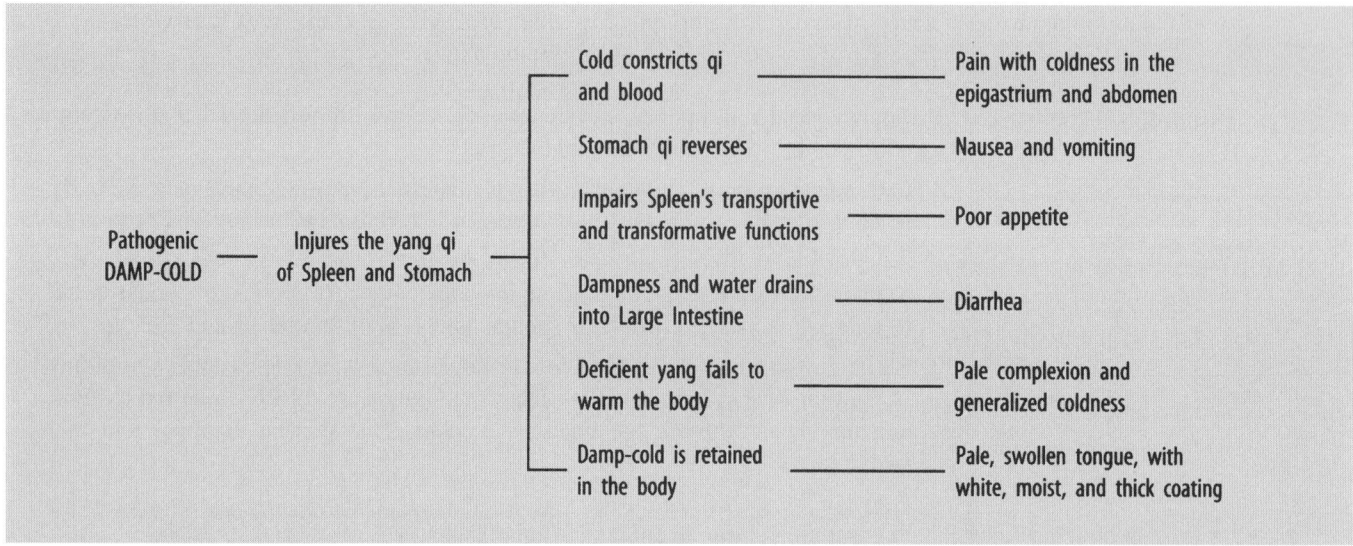

Additional notes

1. The abdominal pain in the early stage of this illness had different characteristics from that in the later stage. What is the significance of this?

In the early stage of the illness the abdominal pain was very severe, which is typical of pain associated with pure excess. The pathological change at that stage was that the pathogenic factors were blocking the qi activity in the middle burner, and cold was constricting the vessels; this explains why the pain was so severe.

In the later stage of the illness the pathogenic factors were not as strong as at the beginning, and therefore the abdominal pain decreased. However, the symptoms associated with yang deficiency became more apparent, and thus the pain acquired the characteristics of deficiency, that is, intermittent and with a feeling of cold. Because the qi stagnation in the middle burner persisted, the patient continued to experience abdominal distention. Thus, this later stage in the illness suggests a combination of excess and deficiency.

2. What is the cause of the smaller quantity of yellow urine?

The patient had diarrhea continuously for a week, and was not inclined to drink, so there was an obvious loss of body fluids. Because of the yang deficiency, water accumulated in the middle burner; rather than being transformed into normal body fluids, it became a pathogenic factor. This pathological change is part of the illness, and accounts for the smaller quantity of urine. Because the urine is concentrated, it becomes yellow in color. In this instance the change in the urine was not been caused by heat.

3. Is there any involvement of the external pathogenic factors of summer-heat and dampness?

Summer-heat and dampness are very common pathogenic factors encountered during the summer. They often combine and invade the body. Since the illness in this case occurred in mid-summer, it is appropriate to ask whether there was any summer-heat or dampness. The answer depends on the characteristics of the pathogenic factors. Summer-heat and dampness pertain to heat, yet everything in this case suggests that the pathological change involved cold. There is simply no evidence of summer-heat and dampness in this case.

Conclusion

1. According to the eight principles:
Interior, cold, combination of deficiency and excess (deficiency within excess).

2. According to etiology:
   Invasion of damp-cold.

3. According to Organ theory:
   Retention of damp-cold in the Spleen, and yang deficiency in the middle burner.

Treatment principle

1. Remove the pathogenic damp-cold by warming the yang of the body.

2. Regulate the qi and strengthen the Spleen.

Explanation of treatment principle

Because the basic problem in this case is the disturbance of the Spleen by damp-cold, the main treatment principle is to expel the pathogenic factors. The warming method is used to remove the cold and dampness.

Because there is qi stagnation in the middle burner, regulating the qi in this area is very useful in facilitating the metabolism of water; it can also assist in restoring the transportive and transformative functions of the Spleen and Stomach. Thus, regulating the qi and strengthening the Spleen are both used. These two methods can strengthen the yang qi of the Spleen and Stomach, thereby helping to remove dampness from the body.

Selection of points

GV-9 *(zhi yang)*
CV-10 *(xia wan)*
ST-37 *(shang ju xu)*
PC-6 *(nei guan)*
SP-4 *(gong sun)*

Explanation of points

GV-9 *(zhi yang)*. The literal translation of this point's name is "reaching the yang." This can be explained by its location at the spinal process of the seventh thoracic vertebra, and the fact that seven, according to tradition, is a yang number. This point strengthens the Spleen and regulates the functions of the middle burner and the Spleen and Stomach qi. This is one of the main points in this prescription, since the damp-cold, which is yin in nature, obstructs the functioning of the Spleen and injures the yang qi of the middle burner. Acupuncture and moxibustion (that is, the warm needle method) are both used at this point in order to warm the yang of the body, remove the dampness and cold, regulate the qi, and alleviate pain. A 2-unit needle is used. The point is punctured perpendicularly to a depth of about 25mm. The warm needle method is utilized, and the moxa sticks are replaced three times during treatment.

CV-10 *(xia wan)* is the meeting point of the conception and leg greater yin Spleen channels. It is used for harmonizing the Organs of the middle burner, regulating the qi, and removing the retention of food. It is a suitable choice in the treatment of such symptoms as abdominal pain, rumbling in the intestines, poor digestion and appetite, vomiting, and regurgitation. It can also be used for deficiency of the Spleen and Stomach. It is another of the main points in this prescription. In addition, this point can be used for treating patterns of excess involving digestive disorders and pain, for strengthening the functions of the Spleen, and for middle burner yang or qi deficiency. It is therefore an appropriate choice for treating the combination of deficiency and excess found in this case. Moxibustion and acupuncture—the warm needle method—are also used at this point (three moxa sticks).

ST-37 *(shang ju xu)* is the lower uniting point of the Large Intestine. It regulates the functions of the middle burner, harmonizes the Stomach and Large Intestine, and removes obstruction from the channels and collaterals. It is a very important point for promoting transportation through the Large Intestine. When a patient has a disorder of the Large Intestine and Stomach, the tenderness felt around the area of the point can be used as an indication for the diagnosis. In this case, the point is chosen for its effectiveness in regulating the qi in order to treat the abdominal pain, distention, and diarrhea. Because the patient must lie on his side, the point is punctured on the left side only.

PC-6 *(nei guan)* is the connecting point of the Pericardium channel. It regulates the qi, alleviates pain, treats disorders of the Heart, and calms Heart spirit. It is especially useful for treating pain in the areas of the chest, Heart, and Stomach that is associated with a pattern of qi stagnation. Combined with SP-4 *(gong sun)*, it is often used in treating abdominal disorders such as abdominal pain, distention, and poor digestion, as PC-6 *(nei guan)* is very effective in regulating the qi and removing obstruction.

SP-4 *(gong sun)* is a connecting point on the Spleen channel that can be used to regulate the Spleen, harmonize the functions of the Spleen and Stomach, and promote the functions of the Large Intestine. There is a very strong needling sensation elicited at this point. It is an important point for removing stagnation and alleviating pain when treating diarrhea. In this case, the point is combined with PC-6 *(nei guan)* in order to strengthen the functions of the Spleen, regulate the qi, and remove obstruction; thus, the pathogenic factors can be expelled, and the abdominal distention and diarrhea resolved.

Combination of points

GV-9 *(zhi yang)* and CV-10 *(xia wan)*. This is a combination of points on the governing and conception vessels, one on the back of the body, the other on the front. In clinical practice there are few opportunities to use a combination of points on both the front and back of the body, but when, as here, a suitable opportunity arises, it should be taken. Together, these two points remove stagnation and retention, and regulate the qi. GV-9 *(zhi yang)* tends to be more effective in tonifying the Spleen, while CV-10 *(xia wan)* is more effective in regulating the qi and removing problems of excess (stagnation, retention), although it also serves to strengthen the Spleen functions to a certain degree. Thus the two points, drawing upon both the yin and yang aspects of the body, can regulate the functions of the middle burner. Both needling and moxibustion are used at these points to increase their effectiveness in removing pathogenic dampness and cold associated with the the abdominal pain and diarrhea. The severity of the cold in the abdomen in this case indicates that the pathogenic dampness and cold have invaded fairly deeply into the body; this is why strong moxibustion is indicated.

ST-37 *(shang ju xu)*, PC-6 *(nei guan)*, and SP-4 *(gong sun)*. The second and third points in this combination are both confluent points, which are suitable for the treatment of qi stagnation and abdominal disorders. As they are also connecting points, they are very effective in regulating the qi. Moreover, PC-6 *(nei guan)* is associated with the yin linking vessel and SP-4 *(gong sun)* with the penetrating vessel; together, they regulate the blood, dispel blood stasis, and promote the circulation of blood to a certain degree. ST-37 *(shang ju xu)* is the lower uniting point of the Large Intestine. Combining this point with the other two strengthens their ability to regulate the functions of the Stomach and Intestines in the treatment of such abdominal disorders as pain, distention, and diarrhea. This combination is often used in clinical practice.

Follow-up

After the first treatment the abdominal cold and pain were largely alleviated, and the frequency of diarrhea was reduced. Thereafter, the patient received acupuncture and moxibustion once a day for four more days, during which the symptoms were relieved. His appetite returned to nearly normal, and his physical energy was much improved. Treatment was therefore terminated. The patient was advised to eat easily digested food for one week. A month later he was in good health, with no sign of digestive disorder.

CASE 21: **Male, age 22**

Main complaint

Fever and diarrhea

History

Two days ago the patient developed abdominal pain, diarrhea, aversion to cold, fever, and (at first) watery stools, which now contain blood, pus, and a considerable amount of greasy discharge. The patient has as many as twenty bowel movements a day. He experiences a burning sensation around the anus when he defecates, as well as a straining sensation in the same area. At the present time he has no aversion to cold, but feels very hot all over. He has a headache, lacks energy, and feels quite fatigued. He is nauseous, has a very poor appetite, and feels thirsty, but has little inclination to drink. The pain in the abdomen, especially in the lower region, is aggravated by pressure of any kind. The quantity of urine is diminished, and is yellow in color.

The conventional medical diagnosis is acute bacterial dysentery. His temperature is 38.7°C. The results of a blood test were WBC 16,000/(mm)^3, (N 76%, L 24%), and the feces showed RBC ++, WBC +++, with a large quantity of mucus.

Tongue

Red, with a yellow, greasy coating

Pulse

Sunken, rapid, and forceful

Analysis of symptoms

1. Diarrhea with stools containing blood and pus—severe retention of damp-heat in the Large Intestine.
2. Burning sensation around the anus during bowel movements—pathogenic heat draining down to the lower burner.
3. Straining sensation around the anus—qi stagnation in the Large Intestine.
4. Abdominal pain, especially in the lower abdomen, which is aggravated with pressure—obstruction of qi activity.
5. Headache, fatigue, and physical weariness—failure of clear yang to rise.
6. Nausea and very poor appetite—upward and downward movement of Spleen and Stomach qi is impaired.
7. Hot sensation all over the body, thirst, and diminished quantity of yellow urine—body fluids injured by pathogenic heat.
8. Red tongue and rapid pulse—heat.
9. Yellow, greasy tongue coating—pathogenic damp-heat.
10. Sunken pulse—interior pattern.

Basic theory of case

Dysenteric disorder *(lì jí)* in Chinese medicine has symptoms that are very similar to those of bacterial dysentery in conventional medicine. In Chinese medicine, dysenteric disorder is caused either by an invasion of damp-heat, epidemic toxic factors, or consumption of cold and raw foods, which can injure the Spleen, Stomach, and Large Intestine in such a way as to cause this disorder. The main symptoms include abdominal pain, tenesmus (ineffectual and painful straining at stool), and diarrhea with stools containing blood and a white, pus-like discharge.

There are a number of possible pathological mechanisms. The most common are summer-heat and dampness, damp-heat, or epidemic toxic factors invading the digestive system through the surface of the body, or directly injuring the Stomach and Intestines. Sometimes the disorder is due to ingesting unclean food, which injures the Spleen and Stomach qi. All these factors can lead to stagnation of qi, blood stasis, and qi obstruction in the yang Organs. The pathogenic damp-heat accumulates and "steams" in the Large Intestine, injuring the vessels, poisoning the Large Intestine itself, and decomposing the soft tissue. This is the cause of the pus and blood in the stools and other related symptoms.

Because dampness and heat have very different characteristics, a predominance of dampness or heat (relative to the other) has a clear effect on the pattern, as does the patient's individual constitution. For example, some patients may have a yang-excessive constitution, which means that the body tends to produce heat, whereas other patients may already have a certain degree of damp-heat in the Spleen and Stomach. Yet again, patients may have a yang-deficient constitution, especially yang deficiency of the middle burner. Thus, the symptoms will vary in each type of patient when they are invaded by these pathogenic factors.

Clinically, if the stools contain bright red-purple blood and pus, the heat pathogenic factor is strong. This condition is known as damp-heat or toxic dysenteric disorder, since the pathogenic heat has already deeply invaded the blood system. When there is not much blood in the stools, but there is a white, pus-like discharge along with other symptoms linked to retention of dampness, the condition is known as damp-cold dysenteric disorder, as the pathogenic factors accumulate mainly in the qi level.

Fig. 5-5

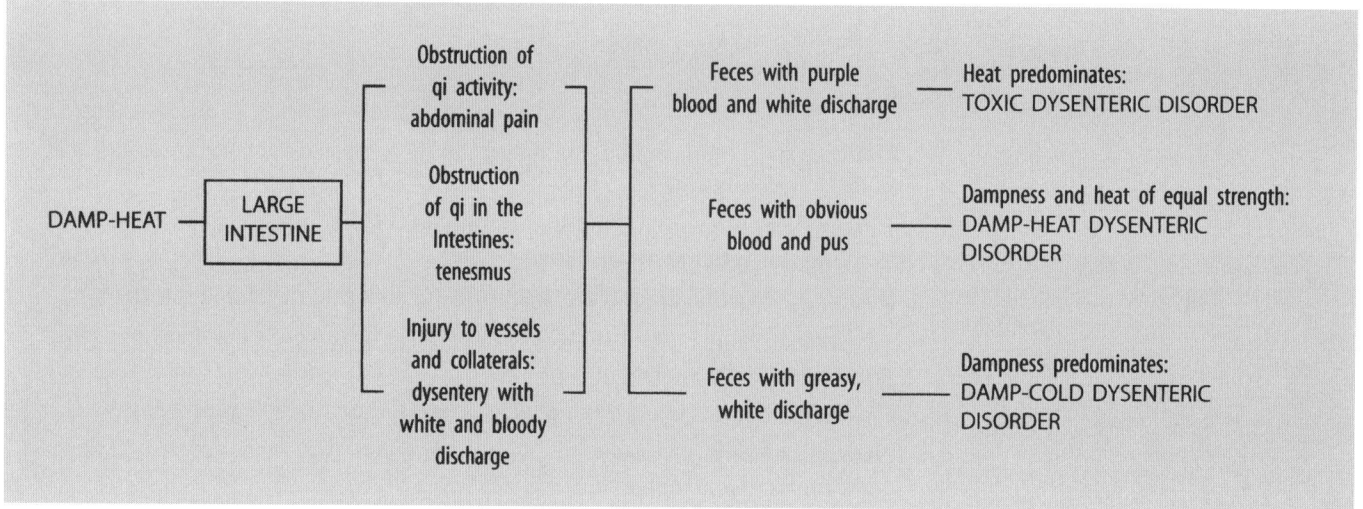

Cause of disease	Pathogenic damp-heat

The patient's fever, the sensation of heat felt all over the body, diarrhea, stools containing blood, pus, and a greasy discharge, frequent bowel movements, burning and straining sensation around the anus, diminished quantity of yellow urine, red tongue and greasy coating are all evidence of damp-heat. The pathogenic dampness has caused qi stagnation; heat has injured the vessels inside the Intestines, stimulated the blood into moving recklessly, and injured the body fluids. These are all characteristics of an invasion by pathogenic damp-heat.

Site of disease   Large Intestine

The main symptoms in this case are diarrhea, abdominal pain (especially in the lower abdomen), and discomfort around the anus during bowel movements. These symptoms point to the Large Intestine as the site of disease.

Pathological change   Dampness as a substantial pathogenic factor, and is characteristically greasy, sticky, turbid, and heavy. It can easily accumulate in the middle and lower burners where it obstructs qi activity and leads to various symptoms involving the digestive system.

In this case, dampness has accumulated in the Large Intestine; thus, the activity of the yang Organs is obstructed, and there is relatively intense pain in the abdomen (especially in the lower region). When pressure aggravates the pain, it indicates the accumulation of an excessive pathogenic factor. The impairment of the Large Intestine's transportive function, together with the injury to the vessels and the decomposition of the qi and blood in the Large Intestine caused by pathogenic heat, has led to the presence of pus, greasy mucus, and blood in the stools. The severity of the qi stagnation in the Large Intestine makes it very difficult for the patient to pass stool completely, which accounts for the frequency of bowel movements and the straining sensation around the anus. The patient experiences a burning sensation in this area when he defecates, because the feces remove some of the pathogenic damp-heat as they pass out of the body.

The qi stagnation in the Large Intestine has affected not only that Organ, but also the qi activity in the middle burner; thus, the Spleen's transportive and transformative functions have also been impaired. Also, the clear yang cannot properly rise, and the patient suffers from headaches and fatigue, and has a poor appetite. Since the Stomach qi cannot properly descend, the patient feels nauseous. Pathogenic heat injures the body fluids, causing the patient to feel thirsty, and his urine to be yellow and diminished in quantity. Because of the retention of dampness, he is not inclined to drink anything, despite his thirst.

The red tongue and rapid pulse indicate strong internal heat, which is over-stimulating the circulation of qi and blood. The greasy, yellow tongue coating suggests damp-heat, and the sunken pulse, an interior pattern. The pulse's forceful quality indicates that the antipathogenic factors have not been significantly weakened.

The cause of dysenteric disorder is usually damp-heat, but either the dampness or heat may predominate in a particular case. Here, however, the dampness and heat are of equal severity. Evidence of this is reflected in the stools, which contain pus, excessive mucus, and blood. This means that the patient's disorder is both in the qi and blood levels.

Fig. 5-6

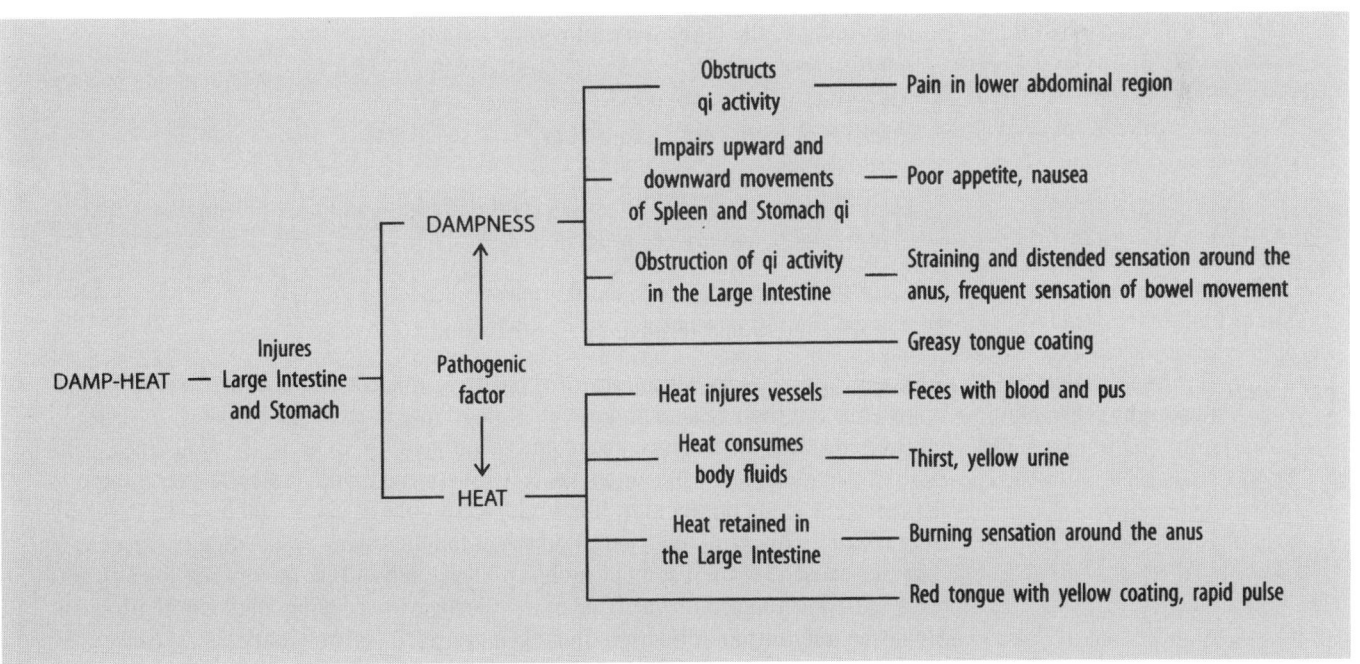

Pattern of disease   There is an interior pattern in this case, as the patient has diarrhea, abdominal pain, and fever, but no aversion to cold.

The fever, thirst, diminished quantity of urine (yellow in color), the burning sensation around the anus during bowel movements, the red tongue with a yellow coating, and the rapid pulse are symptoms of heat.

There is also excess in this case, relected in the abdominal pain—which is aggravated by pressure, and has lasted for only two days—and in the sunken and forceful pulse.

Additional notes

1. What is the source of the pathogenic damp-heat?

There are two primary sources of damp-heat for patients suffering from dysenteric disorder: the pathogenic factor can invade the digestive system (Large Intestine and Stomach) through the surface of the body, or the Spleen and Stomach can be directly affected by the consumption of unclean food.

The onset of this patient's symptoms began with abdominal pain, diarrhea, fever, and an obvious aversion to cold, which suggests that the source of the pathogenic factor is the external environment. The damp-heat and epidemic toxic factor entered the body and injured the protective qi, which explains why the patient has symptoms like fever and an aversion to cold. However, the exterior pattern lasted for only a short period of time, after which the pathogenic factor quickly penetrated further into the body, injuring the Stomach and Large Intestine. The patient then developed a fever without any aversion to cold. By this point, the exterior pattern had given way to an interior pattern.

2. Is there any deficiency here?

The patient suffers from lassitude, obvious fatigue, and has no appetite—symptoms associated with Spleen qi deficiency. Because the qi of the yang Organs is severely obstructed in this case, impairing the upward and downward movement of the qi in the middle burner, the clear yang cannot rise, which accounts for these symptoms. In view of the short duration of this disorder, and the sunken, forceful nature of the pulse, we may conclude that the antipathogenic factors have not been significantly injured; there is only a pattern of excess.

Conclusion

1. According to the eight principles:
   Interior, heat, excess.

2. According to etiology:
   Invasion of pathogenic damp-heat.

3. According to Organ theory:
   Damp-heat in the Large Intestine, with dampness and heat of equal severity (damp-heat dysenteric disorder).

Treatment principle

1. Clear the heat and resolve the dampness.

2. Regulate the qi and remove the obstruction.

Explanation of treatment principle

Although the primary symptom of dysenteric disorder is diarrhea, stopping the diarrhea is not the focus of treatment. Rather, one must regulate the qi in order to remove (relieve) the retained feces and the stagnation of qi in the Intestines. This is a very gentle method of purgation. In Chinese medicine, this treatment principle is known as "using unblocking [methods] for problems due to unblocking *(tōng yīn tōng yòng).*" This principle is applied when the treatment of diarrhea or dysenteric disorder caused by food stagnation or an invasion by toxic factors involves purgatives. At first glance, the treatment of diarrhea by purging may seem illogical. However, on further reflection it makes sense: if severe diarrhea is caused by damp-heat stagnating in the Intestines, where it impedes the transportive function of the Intestines, one can expel the pathogenic factors by removing the stagnation and regulating the qi. As soon as the pathogenic factor is expelled from the Large Intestine its function will be restored; the qi will then properly descend, and the diarrhea will stop. However, if the diarrhea is simply stopped, the pathogenic damp-heat will remain in the Intestines where it will continue to injure the qi and blood, and the problem will actually increase in severity.

Because the pathogenic damp-heat has already severely affected the blood system, the normal circulation of blood has been disrupted. Thus, besides using the main treatment principles discussed above, it is also necessary to cool the blood.

Basic herbal formula

Peony Decoction *(shao yao tang)* is commonly used in the treatment of dysenteric disorder. The formula contains the following ingredients:

Radix Paeoniae Lactiflorae *(bai shao)* 15g
Radix Angelicae Sinensis *(dang gui)* 9g
Rhizoma Coptidis *(huang lian)* 10g
Radix Scutellariae Baicalensis *(huang qin)* 9g
Semen Arecae Catechu *(bing lang)* 5g
Radix Aucklandiae Lappae *(mu xiang)* 5g
Radix et Rhizoma Rhei *(da huang)* 9g
Radix Glycyrrhizae Uralensis *(gan cao)* 5g
Cortex Cinnamomi Cassiae *(rou gui)* 2g

Explanation of basic herbal formula

This formula is suitable for the treatment of dysenteric disorder attributable to a variety of factors, but especially that which is caused by the invasion of damp-heat. This is true whether the dampness and heat are of equal severity, or if the heat is more severe than the dampness. The main symptoms include fever, thirst without desire to drink, abdominal pain, diarrhea, stools containing pus and blood or a discharge from the Large Intestine mixed with purple-red blood, burning sensation around the anus, tenesmus, diminished quantity of yellow urine, red tongue with a yellow, greasy coating, and a slippery, rapid pulse. The basic pathological change is damp-heat accumulating in the Large Intestine where it causes severe qi stagnation and consequently abdominal pain and tenesmus. Because the heat injures the blood in the Large Intestine, diarrhea and stools containing a white and bloody discharge will result, as well as a burning sensation around the anus.

There are two chief herbs in this formula: Radix Paeoniae Lactiflorae *(bai shao)*, which is bitter, sour, and cold, and regulates the nutritive qi and blood, and Rhizoma Coptidis *(huang lian)*, which is bitter, cold, clears heat, dries dampness, and relieves toxicity. As the former focusses on the blood and the latter on the qi, both serve as chief herbs.

The deputy herbs in this formula include Radix Angelicae Sinensis *(dang gui)*, which is sweet, acrid, and warm, dispels blood stasis, nourishes the blood, and assists Radix Paeoniae Lactiflorae *(bai shao)* in regulating the blood; Radix Scutellariae Baicalensis *(huang qin)*, which is bitter and cold, removes heat, and dries dampness; and Radix Aucklandiae Lappae *(mu xiang)*, which is acrid, bitter, and warm, and regulates the qi. The latter two herbs help Rhizoma Coptidis *(huang lian)* clear the heat from the qi level, since they are associated with the Large Intestine; in combination, they are very effective in regulating qi and removing heat.

The assistant herbs include Semen Arecae Catechu *(bing lang)*, Radix et Rhizoma Rhei *(da huang)*, and Cortex Cinnamomi Cassiae *(rou gui)*. In this formula the three herbs are divided into two groups, the first of which is comprised of Semen Arecae Catechu *(bing lang)*, which is acrid, bitter, and warm, is associated with the Stomach and Large Intestine channels, regulates qi, and removes food stagnation, and Radix et Rhizoma Rhei *(da huang)*, which is bitter and cold, is associated with the Spleen, Stomach, and Large Intestine channels, clears heat, and acts as a strong purgative. These two herbs serve to remove damp-heat from the Large Intestine and are used in the treatment of diarrhea by purgation. The second group is comprised of just Cortex Cinnamomi Cassiae *(rou gui)*, which is acrid, hot, and very effective in supporting the yang activities of the body. Here, however, it is used as a corrective assistant herb: its dosage is very small (2g), and it serves to counteract the bitter, cold qualities of the other herbs and thereby prevent injury to the antipathogenic factors. Its warmth also counteracts the cold characteristics of the other herbs, which can aggravate the retention of dampness, itself a yin pathogenic factor.

The envoy herb in this formula is Radix Glycyrrhizae Uralensis *(gan cao)*. It protects the antipathogenic factors in the Spleen and Stomach, assists Radix Paeoniae Lactiflorae *(bai shao)* in alleviating the acute pain, and harmonizes the actions of the other herbs in the formula.

Modified herbal formula

Radix Paeoniae Lactiflorae *(bai shao))* 10g

Rhizoma Coptidis *(huang lian)* 10g

Radix Aucklandiae Lappae *(mu xiang)* 6g

Fructus Citri seu Ponciri Immaturus *(zhi shi)* 5g

Cortex Moutan Radicis *(mu dan pi)* 8g

Radix et Rhizoma Rhei *(da huang)* 5g

Radix Glycyrrhizae Uralensis *(gan cao)* 5g

Explanation of modified herbal formula

This case involves a pattern of damp-heat. Because the dampness and heat are of equal severity, Peony Decoction *(shao yao tang)* is used, with only a few modifications. Cortex Cinnamomi Cassiae *(rou gui)*, which is acrid and hot, has been omitted in the modified formula because of the presence of pus and blood in the stools. Cortex Moutan Radicis *(mu dan pi)* is substituted for Radix Angelicae Sinensis *(dang gui)* as it is better able to remove heat from the blood, and to cool the blood. Although Fructus Citri seu Ponciri Immaturus *(zhi shi)* does not possess a strong purgative action, it is nonetheless better able to regulate the qi than Semen Arecae Catechu *(bing lang)*, for which it is substituted.

Follow-up

The patient was given one packet of the herbal formula per day, divided into three doses. After the first day his body temperature returned to normal, and the frequency of bowel movements declined significantly. The formula was continued for another two days, after which the abdominal pain diminished, and the frequency of bowel movements declined to just one to three times per day. Although the stools were still very loose, there was no more blood. Moreover, the discomfort which the patient experienced around the anus while defecating had disappeared.

The herbal formula was continued for another two days, but now the daily packet was taken in two half-doses. The body temperature remained constant, the bowel movements returned to their normal frequency, and the patient's appetite was restored. The herbal therapy was terminated to avoid injury to the Stomach from the bitter and cold herbs in the formula. The patient was advised to eat easily-digested foods for a period of a week. Thereafter, he was given three routine checkups for his blood and stools, which revealed that all was normal. The patient then returned to work.

Although acute bacterial dysentery can be treated successfully with conventional medicine, some patients may have a severe allergic reaction to antibiotics, or otherwise have a very sensitive constitution which is easily affected by biochemical treatment. Others simply dislike pharmaceuticals. An herbal remedy is appropriate for such patients as it is natural, has no side effects, and is generally effective.

CASE 22: **Male, age 54**

Main complaint

Recurrent diarrhea

History

The patient has been suffering from recurrent diarrhea for the past eight years. Each onset lasts from a few days to a few weeks. During these bouts he has a bowel movement immediately after getting up in the morning, and about ten minutes after eating a meal. When the diarrhea is severe, the stools are loose and there is some mucus, but no pus or blood. He does not experience a burning sensation around the anus, but he does feel a straining sensation in the area, and has a slight prolapse of the rectum. To treat the diarrhea he has taken antibiotics, digestants (such as *Saccharomycitis*), and simple herbal remedies, but the results are never satisfactory. He sometimes has abdominal pain, but it is never very severe and is relieved after a bowel movement. In general, the patient always feels cold, lacks energy, has a poor appetite, experiences abdominal distention after meals, and has no inclination to drink. His sleep and urination are both normal.

Tongue	Red tip and a thin, white, moist coating
Pulse	Sunken, thin, and wiry

Analysis of symptoms

1. Recurrent diarrhea—injury to the yang qi.
2. Diarrhea after waking and eating—deficiency of Spleen and Kidney yang.
3. Loose stools with no pus or blood, and no burning sensation around the anus—pathogenic cold.
4. Straining sensation around the anus, and mild prolapse of the rectum—sinking of Spleen qi.
5. Mild abdominal pain, which comes and goes—deficiency.
6. Cold sensation, lack of energy, and disinclination to drink—deficiency of yang qi.
7. Poor appetite, abdominal distention after eating—Spleen's transportive and transformative functions impaired.
8. Thin, white, and moist tongue coating—cold from deficiency.
9. Sunken, thin pulse—interior deficiency.

Basic theory of case

In Chinese medicine the Spleen is responsible for facilitating the rise of clear yang (including to the face and head), and also for transporting food essence throughout the body. Physiologically speaking, the clear yang is the energy that keeps the mind clear and alert, maintains the position of the internal Organs, and provides nourishment for the tissues and Organs in the body to enable them to perform their various functions. When affected by disease, the Spleen's ability to keep the clear yang rising may become impaired; the Spleen qi thereupon sinks, and the patient consequently suffers from such associated symptoms as dizziness, prolapse of the internal Organs, and malnourishment of the body.

Clinically, the sinking of Spleen qi can also cause recurrent diarrhea. The body can become over-sensitive to changes in the patient's environment or life-style, such as changes in the diet (for example, from hot to cold foods), weather, or sleeping patterns, all of which can induce a bout of diarrhea. Besides a poor appetite, lack of energy, and lassitude—which are symptoms of Spleen qi deficiency—patients usually do not experience the general symptoms associated with a strong attack by pathogenic factors, such as severe abdominal pain, fever, or nausea and vomiting. Some will complain of chronic, continuous diarrhea. When it has persisted, for a long time, the antipathogenic factors will become exhausted, and patients will often present with general symptoms associated with a pattern of deficiency.

The pathological change pertaining to diarrhea caused by Spleen qi sinking is that the Spleen's transportive and transformative functions are impaired, and because the essence is not completely extracted from the food, it becomes mixed in with the waste. The clear yang, that is, the food essence and qi, fails to be transported upward; instead, it sinks with the turbid yin and waste, which enters the

Fig. 5-7

Large Intestine and causes diarrhea. The stools are loose (unformed) and often contain particles of undigested food. Unlike the symptoms of damp-heat in the Large Intestine, this pattern shows no symptoms of excessive pathogenic heat, such as pus or blood in the stools, or a burning sensation around the anus.

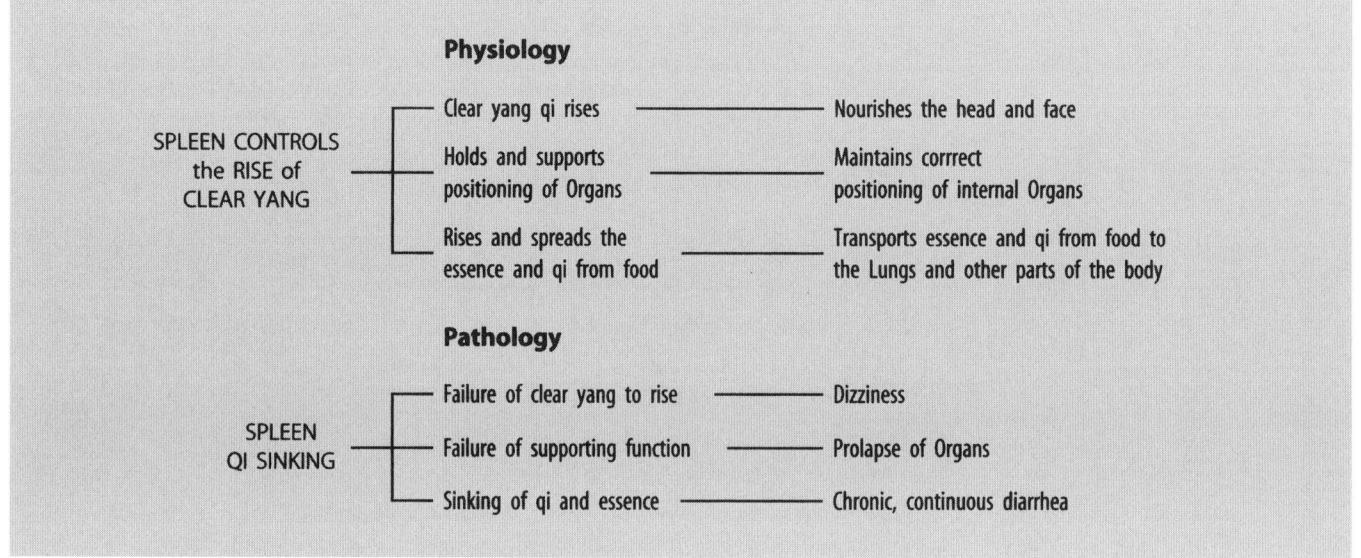

Physiology

SPLEEN CONTROLS the RISE of CLEAR YANG

- Clear yang qi rises ——————— Nourishes the head and face
- Holds and supports positioning of Organs ——————— Maintains corrrect positioning of internal Organs
- Rises and spreads the essence and qi from food ——————— Transports essence and qi from food to the Lungs and other parts of the body

Pathology

SPLEEN QI SINKING

- Failure of clear yang to rise ——————— Dizziness
- Failure of supporting function ——————— Prolapse of Organs
- Sinking of qi and essence ——————— Chronic, continuous diarrhea

Cause of disease	Qi deficiency

There is no evidence of invasion by pathogenic factors. The diarrhea is chronic and recurrent, the stools are loose and unformed. The patient therefore has a type of diarrhea caused by the sinking of qi, which has resulted from qi deficiency.

Site of disease   Spleen and Kidney

The recurrent diarrhea, loose or unformed stools, straining sensation around the anus, slight prolapse of the rectum, poor appetite, and abdominal distention after eating all suggest that the Spleen is the site of disease.

   The chronic diarrhea, especially first thing in the morning, indicates a dysfunction of the Kidney.

Pathological change   Normally, food, after it enters the Stomach and is warmed and softened by the Stomach yang, is later transformed by the Spleen yang into food essence, which can be absorbed by the body. The essence from food is transported upward into the Lung, and from there is dispersed throughout the body. After being digested, the waste from food is transported to the Large Intestine where it becomes feces, which are expelled from the body.

   In this case, the patient suffers diarrhea immediately after eating. The food stays for only a very short time in the middle burner, as the Spleen qi is deficient, and the middle burner functions of receiving, transporting, and transforming food are weakened. After the patient eats, the food essence and waste, which cannot be properly separated and are therefore mixed together, drain into the Large Intestine, causing loose stools and an onset of diarrhea. Because the Spleen qi sinks, the patient experiences a straining sensation around the anus and a slight prolapse of the rectum.

   Both the diarrhea and malnutrition caused by Spleen qi deficiency injure the yang qi of the middle burner, and after a long period of time, the yang of the lower burner will also be affected. Kidney yang contributes to the functions of defecation and urination, and secures and binds the Large Intestine; thus, Kidney yang deficiency can affect the functions of the Large Intestine. In the early morning, just before dawn, the yang of the environment is at its weakest. This is also the time when Kidney yang function is at its weakest, especially in relation to the Large Intestine. This is the mechanism underlying daybreak diarrhea *(wǔ gēng xiè),* which is characteristic of Kidney yang deficiency. Apart from this symptom, the patient in this case has no other symptoms of Kidney yang deficiency, such as coldness and pain in the lower back and knees, or coldness in the limbs. We may therefore conclude that Spleen yang deficiency is the main problem, and that the Kidney yang deficiency is not too severe yet.

Fig. 5-8

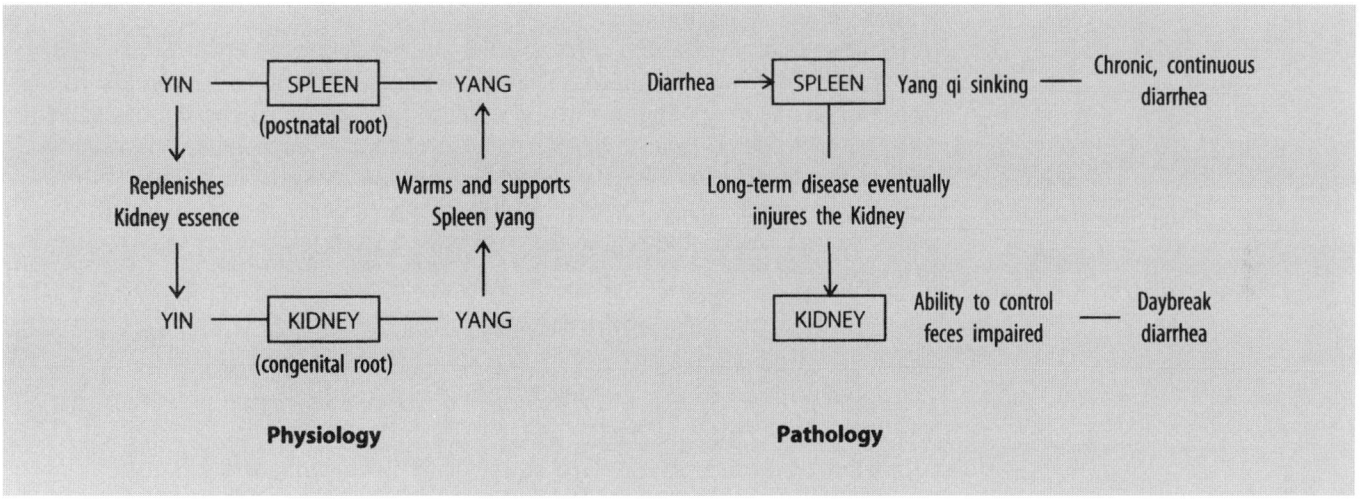

Physiology   **Pathology**

The poor digestion here is due to impairment of the Spleen's transportive and transformative functions. The patient's appetite is poor, and he suffers from abdominal distention after eating. His weak physical energy can be attributed to malnourishment owing to yang deficiency and the impairment of qi and blood production. Yang deficiency causes the body to become cold, which is why the patient feels cold and not thirsty.

The thin tongue coating indicates that the pathogenic factor is not very severe. Its moist, white characteristics suggest retention of cold. The sunken pulse is evidence of an interior pattern, while its thin quality points to deficiency of qi and blood and a diminishment in the vessels' normal fullness.

Because of the long duration of this disorder, it is very difficult to determine the initial cause of the Spleen deficiency. In any event, it is irrelevant to the present treatment.

Pattern of disease

The injury to the Spleen and Kidney caused by chronic diarrhea, and the eight-year history of the disorder, confirm the presence of an interior pattern.

Cold is evidenced by the patient's feeling cold but not thirsty, the loose stools, and the white, moist tongue coating.

The poor appetite and weak energy, caused by injury to the antipathogenic factors, are evidence of deficiency.

Additional notes

1. What is the cause of the abdominal pain prior to bowel movements, and why is the pain partially relieved afterwards?

Abdominal pain just prior to an onset of diarrhea is evidence that a pathogenic factor has been retained inside the body, where it is obstructing the qi activity, and thus causing pain. After diarrhea, the qi activity in the body improves somewhat and the pain is relieved. However, one must still determine which type of pathogenic factor is present.

The impairment in the Spleen's transportive and transformative functions indicates a pattern of Spleen qi deficiency. Also, the patient complains of abdominal distention after eating. Retention of food in the Stomach and Large Intestine is most likely the cause of the pain, but it is not very severe, and has not yet reached the level where the pattern itself can be said to be one of excess. If the functions of the Spleen and Stomach are restored to normal, the retention of food will disappear.

2. Is there a pattern of heat in this case?

All the general symptoms in this case are of a cold nature, and the pulse fails to reflect the presence of heat; yet the tip of the patient's tongue is red. Is it possible that this singular symptom could reveal a pattern of heat?

The answer is no. We may infer that the yin aspects of the body, after such a long illness, will tend to be injured. The singular heat sign found on the tongue has occurred because the body has lost too much fluids due to the chronic diarrhea, which has not been adequately replenished. We cannot diagnose a heat pattern based on this one sign, although it should be taken into consideration when warming and tonifying the body. Caution must be exercised during treatment, for if too much warmth is added, the heat of the body can be increased and the injury to the yin aggravated.

3. What is the significance of the wiry pulse?

In general, a wiry pulse indicates a disorder of the Liver. In this case, however, the site of disease is the Spleen and Kidney and there are no symptoms involving the Liver. What, then, accounts for the wiry pulse?

In Chinese medicine the Spleen is associated with earth, and the Liver with wood. The relationship between the physiological functions of these two Organs can be expressed in terms of wood controlling earth. At present the patient is suffering from Spleen qi deficiency, which means that wood is relatively stronger than earth, which in its weakened state can be easily controlled. Thus, the wiry pulse indicates that the Liver qi is strong relative to that of the Spleen. In order to prevent the Liver qi from overcontrolling the Spleen, we should supply a certain amount of tension by controlling wood (Liver) a little and supporting earth (Spleen) more.

Conclusion

1. According to the eight principles:
   Interior, cold, deficient.
2. According to Organ theory:
   Spleen and Kidney yang deficiency; the Spleen deficiency predominates.

Treatment principle

1. Strengthen the Spleen and warm the Kidney.
2. Raise the yang, bind the Intestines, and stop the diarrhea.

Explanation of treatment principle

The treatment principle for diarrhea caused by Spleen and Kidney yang deficiency is to control the diarrhea by binding the Intestines with astringents, while simultaneously warming and tonifying the Organs. The purpose of tonifying and warming is to get at the root of the disorder; controlling the diarrhea prevents further injury to the antipathogenic factors. Nevertheless, one must be cautious, as the use of astringent agents for stopping diarrhea can only be used in treating patterns of deficiency. The reason for this is that, if there is retention of a pathogenic factor within the body, the astringent method will aggravate the condition and interfere with its expulsion. The pathogenic factor will thus remain in the body and continue to injure the antipathogenic factors.

In this case the diarrhea is chronic. Besides the problem of deficiency, the patient also has a certain amount of food retention caused by Spleen deficiency, the overcontrol of wood (Liver) in response to the deficiency of earth (Spleen), and a slight tendency toward heat from deficiency due to the chronic diarrhea. Thus, when the binding method is used, these three minor problems should be kept in mind.

Basic herbal formula

Four-Miracle Pill *(si shen wan)* is typical of the formulas containing astringent herbs that are used to bind the Large Intestine and treat prolapse of the rectum. The formula contains the following ingredients:

Semen Myristicae Fragrantis *(rou dou kou)* 6g

Fructus Psoraleae Corylifoliae *(bu gu zhi)* 12g

Fructus Schisandrae Chinensis *(wu wei zi))* 6g

Fructus Evodiae Rutaecarpae *(wu zhu yu)* 3g

Rhizoma Zingiberis Officinalis Recens *(sheng jiang)* 8g

Fructus Zizyphi Jujubae *(da zao)* 5g

Explanation of basic herbal formula

Spleen and Kidney yang deficiency, which may be attributed to a variety of causes including long-term diarrhea, will impair the Large Intestine's ability to control the feces. The symptoms include recurrent or daybreak diarrhea, poor appetite, anorexia, coldness and pain in the abdomen, epigastric region, lower back and knees, weak energy, general lassitude, mental fatigue, coldness in the limbs, a pale, soft, and swollen tongue with a white, moist coating, and a sunken and forceless pulse.

In the basic formula, Fructus Psoraleae Corylifoliae *(bu gu zhi)* is bitter, acrid, and very hot. It is associated with the Kidney and Spleen channels, and has a very strong ability to fortify the body's yang. It also tonifies, warms, and strengthens the Spleen and Kidney, and effectively controls the diarrhea. It is commonly used to treat this type of diarrhea, and serves as the chief herb in this formula.

There are two deputy herbs. Semen Myristicae Fragrantis *(rou dou kou)* is acrid and warm, and is associated with the Spleen, Stomach, and Large Intestine channels. It warms the middle burner, and, as an astringent herb, binds the Large Intestine. Fructus Evodiae Rutaecarpae *(wu zhu yu)* is acrid, bitter, and hot, and is associated with the Liver, Spleen, and Stomach channels. It warms the middle burner, expels the cold from within the body, and is very effective in treating the retention of damp-cold caused by yang deficiency.

There are three assistant herbs. Fructus Schisandrae Chinensis *(wu wei zi)* is sour and warm, and is associated with the Heart and Kidney channels. It is astringent, and controls the diarrhea. Rhizoma Zingiberis Officinalis Recens *(sheng jiang)* is acrid and warm, and is associated with the Spleen channel. It warms the middle burner and expels coldness. Fructus Zizyphi Jujubae *(da zao)* is sweet and warm, and is associated with the Spleen and Stomach channels. It tonifies the middle burner and strengthens the qi of the body. Each of these three herbs supports the chief and deputy herbs in different ways.

In general, this formula is warm and astringent, and is used for tonification. None of the herbs expels pathogenic factors; this formula is used in treating pure deficiency with no retention of pathogenic factors.

Modified herbal formula

Rhizoma Zingiberis Officinalis *(gan jiang)* 3g

Fructus Psoraleae Corylifoliae *(bu gu zhi)* 12g

Charred Fructus Pruni Mume *(wu mei tan)* 6g

Radix Astragali Membranacei *(huang qi)* 15g

Charred Rhizoma Cimicifugae *(sheng ma tan)* 6g

Cortex Magnoliae Officinalis *(hou po)* 5g

Burnt Semen Arecae Catechu *(jiao bing lang)* 8g

Semen Myristicae Fragrantis *(rou dou kou)* 8g

Fructus Schisandrae Chinensis *(wu wei zi)*) 6g

Radix Paeoniae Lactiflorae *(bai shao)*) 10g

Radix Scutellariae Baicalensis *(huang qin)* 4g

Explanation of modified herbal formula

As this case involves chronic diarrhea in a pattern of deficiency, Four-Miracle Pill *(si shen wan)* has been selected as the basic herbal formula. The purpose here is to warm the body's yang qi and bind the Intestines so as to stop the diarrhea.

In the modified formula used in this case, Fructus Evodiae Rutaecarpae *(wu zhu yu)* and Rhizoma Zingiberis Officinalis Recens *(sheng jiang)* are replaced by Rhizoma Zingiberis Officinalis *(gan jiang)*, which, although similar in nature to the other two herbs, is very effective in warming the middle burner and promoting the functions of the Spleen and Stomach. The number of herbs that tonify the qi and nourish the blood is increased in this formula, as tonifying the qi strengthens the formula's action in promoting the rising of the qi to offset the sinking of the Spleen qi, and nourishing the blood harmonizes the functions of the Liver and thereby curbs the tendency of Liver-wood to overcontrol on Spleen-earth, owing to the deficiency of Spleen qi. Herbs that promote the digestive functions are used to strengthen the Spleen's transportive and transformative functions. The whole formula tends to be acrid and hot, characteristics that may aggravate the injury to the yin. A small amount of a bitter and cold herb has been added to act as a corrective assistant, preventing further injury to the yin and body fluids.

This formula contains two herbs treated with extreme heat: Charred Fructus Pruni Mume *(wu mei tan)* and Burnt Semen Arecae Catechu *(jiao bing lang)*. Many of the Chinese materia medica are specially treated before being used to treat certain types of problems. Often this preparation (known as *pào zhì)* is used to buffer or accentuate the properties of the basic substance, or to change its properties (cold or hot), or reduce its side effects. Here, the charring and burning (carbonization) of these two herbs increases their astringent properties and thereby augments their ability to stop the diarrhea.

Follow-up

The patient was given one packet of the herbal formula each day, divided into two doses. He continued to visit the clinic once a week. After four weeks the bowel movements had declined to two or three times a day. Because the patient felt that he had completely recovered, he stopped taking the herbs and did not return to the clinic. Not surprisingly, the symptoms returned and the bowel movements increased to four or five times a day. The patient came back for further treatment and resumed taking the above formula.

After two weeks the bowel movements were back to normal (two to three times a day). However, the stools were still unformed, although better than before. If the patient overate slightly, he felt very uncomfortable and the upper abdomen became distended. He also complained of palpitations, restlessness, and, at times, insomnia. A checkup revealed that his tongue had become quite red, with a thin, yellow coating, which was peeling slightly. The pulse was thin. This indicated that the yang qi of the body had gradually recovered, but the deficiency of yin and body fluids had become more apparent.

Because the original formula was predominantly acrid and warm, it was now modified for the purpose of not only tonifying the Spleen and Kidney, but also nourishing the yin. The newly-modified formula consisted of the following ingredients:

Honey-toasted Radix Astragali Membranacei *(zhi huang qi)* 15g

Semen Myristicae Fragrantis *(rou dou kou)* 6g

Burnt Rhizoma Atractylodis Macrocephalae *(jiao bai zhu)* 10g

Radix Paeoniae Lactiflorae *(bai shao)* 6g

Semen Dolichoris Lablab *(bian dou)* 6g

Radix Dioscoreae Oppositae *(shan yao)* 15g

Radix Rehmanniae Glutinosae Conquitae *(shu di huang)* 30g

Tuber Ophiopogonis Japonici *(mai men dong)* 6g

Fructus Schisandrae Chinensis *(wu wei zi)* 6g

The patient took this prescription for three months and visited the clinic once every two weeks. During this period his appetite improved and his tongue returned to normal. When the three months were over, there was an interval of one month during which no herbs were administered, and there was no recurrent diarrhea. Thereafter, the patient was given a small dosage of herbs for an additional three months to consolidate the result of the treatment. At the end of this period the treatment was terminated.

Over the ensuing two years the patient had very few attacks. When they occurred, he always used the Chinese herbal remedy, which yielded excellent results. For severe attacks the herbal remedy was based on the first formula. If the recurrence was not so severe, the prepared remedy Four-Miracle Pill with Nutmeg *(rou guo si shen wan)* was taken. None of the recurrent attacks lasted for longer than a week. His appetite, bowel movements, and sleep were normal, and he regained his normal body weight. All in all, he was very satisfied with the treatment.

Like the patient in this case, many patients who have experienced a long, chronic illness and have visited many doctors and received a variety of treatments gain a considerable amount of personal experience with the medical profession. They therefore develop their own ideas about medications, dosage, and how their illnesses are dealt with by practitioners. There is a Chinese expression, "A long-term illness makes a patient half a doctor." Also, many patients like to read about their illnesses. When an over-confident patient of this kind feels as if they know more than a young and relatively inexperienced practitioner or specialist who may be unsure about how to handle them, the patient may lose confidence in the treatment and resort to various means to disrupt it, just as the patient in this case stopped taking the herbs. All of this is understandable, and so practitioners should counsel their patients. The progress of the illness and treatment should be explained, as successful treatment is not solely the work of the practitioner, but is also the result of cooperation between the practitioner and patient. In addition, the practitioner can gain valuable experience by learning from his or her patients.

CASE 23: **Male, age 68**

Main complaint

Constipation

History

This patient previously had a very strong constitution and always enjoyed good health. Strong and muscular, he was seldom sick. However, he often suffered from constipation due to intensive work, lack of rest, and, because he is a highly emotional person, his propensity to argue with others. During the past two weeks the constipation recurred, and he now has only one bowel movement every two to three days. The stools are very dry and difficult to pass, and are accompanied by bleeding and pain around the anus. On his head, the area around the glabella is tense and painful. He feels restless, can be very irritable, and has "butterflies" and a hot sensation in the chest. His sleep is unsound and dream-disturbed. His gums are swollen and painful, his mouth is dry, and he constantly wants to drink. His appetite is normal.

Tongue

Red with a thick, dry, and yellow coating that covers the entire surface of the tongue

Pulse	Thin and slippery
Analysis of symptoms	1. Occurrence of symptoms after stressful work or strong emotional upset, like quarreling—rising of internal fire.
	2. Constipation with bowel movement every two to three days, dry stools which are difficult to pass, and bleeding and pain around the anus—injury of body fluids.
	3. Tension and pain around the glabella—internal heat and fire rising and disturbing the head.
	4. "Butterflies" and hot sensation in the chest, restlessness, irritability and dream-disturbed sleep—disturbance of Heart spirit by heat.
	5. Swollen and painful gums, dry mouth and desire to drink a lot of liquids—retention of Stomach heat.
	6. Red tongue with a thick, dry, and yellow coating—injury of body fluids by heat.
	7. Slippery pulse—excessive heat.

Basic theory of case

Constipation is a manifestation of abnormal bowel function, indicating that the frequency of bowel movements has decreased. The stools become dry and difficult to pass. There are various causes and accompanying symptoms. While some people require clinical attention, most who have no other symptoms apart from the constipation do not need to see a health practitioner.

The most common causes of constipation include the following:

1. Pathogenic heat in the interior

This can be associated with pathogenic factors from the external environment, where, for example, a pathogenic factor invades the body and is transformed into heat. Another source is heat in the Organs, which accumulates and injures the body fluids, causing constipation. This type of constipation usually has an acute onset, after which very obvious symptoms emerge.

2. Deficiency of body fluids

Deficiency of blood or yin can result in diminished body fluids, which can be a direct cause of constipation. Patients with this condition usually have a chronic history. Besides constipation, there may be no accompanying symptoms, or a few.

3. Qi deficiency

Qi is the energy of each of the Organs, and is essential for normal functioning. The main function of qi in the Large Intestine is to transport the feces and remove them from the body. Qi deficiency in the Large Intestine—or in the Spleen and Stomach, which may eventually lead to deficiency of the Large Intestine—can cause constipation. In such cases there can be accompanying symptoms of qi deficiency.

4. Yang deficiency in the lower burner

Yang deficiency can result in an accumulation of cold in the interior and deficiency of yang in the lower burner, which can directly affect the Large Intestine. The cold contracts the qi of the Large Intestine and affects the body fluids, causing the feces to remain too long in the Large Intestine; this leads to constipation. Besides the general symptoms associated with yang deficiency, patients will present with constipation, although the feces are usually not dry, but loose.

Cause of disease

Excessive pathogenic fire

This patient has a very short history of illness. The stools have become very dry and difficult to pass, which causes bleeding from and pain around the anus. The patient shows general heat symptoms: "butterflies" and a hot sensation in the chest, anxiety, dry mouth, thirst, and a red tongue with a yellow coating. This is evidence that the cause of the disorder is retention of pathogenic heat and fire, which has injured the body fluids.

Site of disease

Stomach and Large Intestine

The patient feels thirsty, has swollen and painful gums, suffers from constipation with dry stools that are difficult to pass, has pain around the anus, and bleeding. This indicates involvement of the Organs associated with the yang brightness channels, that is, the Stomach and Large Intestine.

Pathological change

Fire in the Heart, Liver, and Stomach can result in constipation symptoms associated with excessive heat. In this case, Stomach fire is the direct cause of the constipation. As the Stomach and Intestines are closely related, Stomach fire readily consumes body fluids in the Large Intestine. The stools then become dry and difficult to pass, owing to the diminished quantity of fluids. The dry, rough feces can break the surface of the anus, which causes severe pain and bleeding. Characteristic of heat and fire, the fire in the Organ can travel upward through the channels and collaterals. The Stomach channels ascend to the gums, thus the fire in this case moved upward and disturbed the gums, causing pain and swelling. The fire also affected the face and head, disturbing the qi activity. The circulation of qi and blood was thereby upset, causing the patient to feel tension and pain in the area around the glabella, which is associated with the yang brightness channels.

    The heat which has accumulated in the middle burner can also affect the neighboring upper burner, disturbing the Heart spirit. This accounts for the restlessness, "butterflies" and hot sensation in the chest, irritability, and dream-disturbed sleep. In other words, the Heart spirit in this case is not affected by heat in the Heart itself. This heat also consumed the body fluids, causing the patient's dry mouth and thirst. The red tongue with its dry, yellow coating are manifestations of pathogenic heat. The fact that the coating is thick and covers the entire surface of the tongue suggests that the pathogenic factor in the Stomach is one of excess.

Fig. 5-9

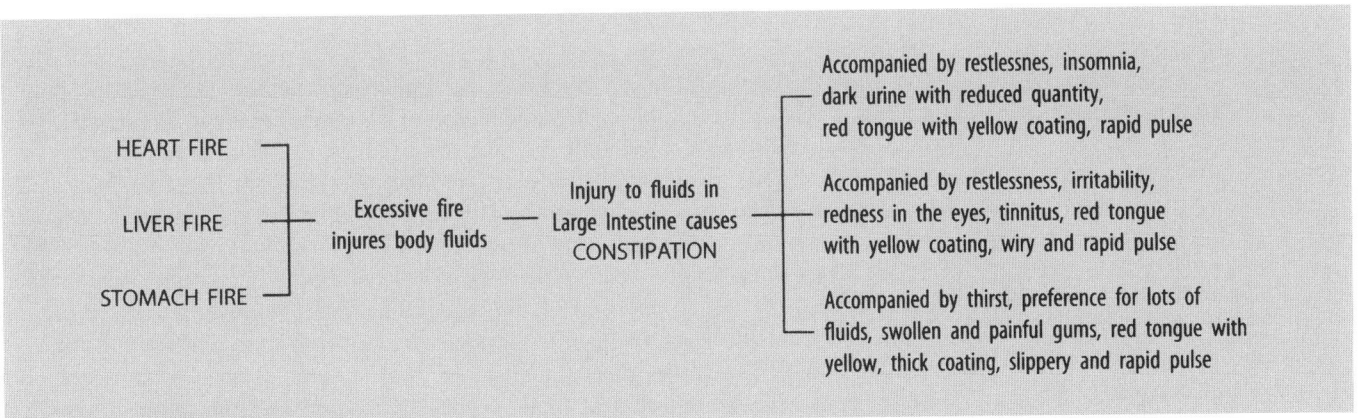

Pattern of disease

As the site of disease is the Stomach and Large Intestine, and there is no evidence of invasion by a pathogenic factor, this is an interior pattern.

    Retention of fire in the interior which is consuming the body fluids suggests a pattern of heat.

    The lack of injury to the antipathogenic factors indicates a pattern of excess.

Additional notes

1. Is there any evidence of Liver fire rising?

The patient's stressful work, lack of rest, and strong emotions are direct precipitating factors of this condition. In this episode the patient experiences tension and pain in the region of the glabella. Doesn't this evidence suggest retention of Liver fire?

We know from his history that the patient is a highly emotional person, and that his constitution could be linked to Liver fire; but there are no symptoms indicative of a Liver disorder, and the emotional change is not very obvious. The swollen and painful gums is a characteristic symptom of Stomach heat or fire. Thus, the diagnosis favors retention of Stomach fire, and not Liver fire rising.

2. What does the thin and slippery pulse mean?

In pulse diagnosis a thin pulse can be evidence of either deficiency or retention of dampness. A slippery pulse generally suggests retention of dampness or of substantial pathogenic factors. In this case, however, the pulse is both thin and slippery. Does this mean that there is dampness?

In this pattern there is no evidence to support a diagnosis of dampness; nor are there any signs of deficiency. The thin pulse here is caused by fire from excess injuring the body fluids. And although they have been injured, it is only a short-term injury that was not severe enought to cause deficiency. The slippery pulse can be indicative of heat from excess, which is precisely the case here. The pathogenic heat has accelerated the circulation of blood, and this is reflected in the slippery pulse.

Conclusion	1. According to the eight principles: Interior, heat, excess. 2. According to etiology: Pathogenic heat from excess. 3. According to Organ theory: Retention of fire in the yang Organs associated with the yang brightness channels (Stomach and Large Intestine).
Treatment principle	1. Clear the heat and reduce the fire. 2. Administer purgatives to remove the fire retained in the yang brightness Organs.

Explanation of treatment principle

Many different methods are suitable for the treatment of symptoms associated with patterns of heat or fire. In this case the retention of Stomach fire is the direct cause of the constipation, so just reducing the heat will not be sufficient. Purgatives must also be administered as the dry, hard stools are blocking the Large Intestine, where they are causing severe qi stagnation. This is also why the qi activity in the Stomach has been obstructed.

The reason that simply clearing the heat is not enough is because it does not enable the hard stools to pass out of the body, nor does it remove the severe qi obstruction from the yang Organs. If the feces are not removed, neither will the retention of fire. Purgatives must therefore be used to unblock the Stomach and Large Intestine, allowing the qi activity—especially the descending turbid qi—to recover; the heat and fire in the Stomach will then clear up on their own.

Basic herbal formula

In *Discussion of Cold-induced Disorders (Shang han lun)*, the most important Chinese classic on herbal treatment, there are three formulas listed for the treatment of constipation caused by retention of heat or fire: Major Order the Qi Decoction *(da cheng qi tang)*, Minor Order the Qi Decoction *(xiao cheng qi tang)*, and Regulate the Stomach and Order the Qi Decoction *(tiao wei cheng qi tang)*. All three of these formulas are very strong purgatives. However, compared with the other two, Regulate the Stomach and Order the Qi Decoction *(tiao wei cheng qi tang)* is relatively gentle. Included in this simple formula are the following herbs:

Radix et Rhizoma Rhei *(da huang)* 12g

Mirabilitum *(mang xiao)* 12g

Radix Glycyrrhizae Uralensis *(gan cao)* 6g

Explanation of basic herbal formula

The indications of this formula are constipation, fullness and distention in the abdomen, a hot sensation over the entire body, restlessness, thirst, swollen and painful gums and throat, red tongue with a dry, yellow coating, and a slippery and rapid pulse. The basic pathological change associated with this pattern is that, during the course of a febrile disease, external pathogenic factors enter the body, where they transform into heat. This pathogenic heat, which is very strong, injures the body fluids and causes the waste from food and feces in the yang brightness Organs (Stomach and Large Intestine) to become dry and hard. They therefore cannot be moved properly, but instead obstruct the qi in these Organs.

In clinical practice this formula, with minor modifications, can be used to treat this kind of constipation due to heat from excess, or a similar pattern caused by any type of heat, which need not necessarily come from outside the body.

In this prescription, Radix et Rhizoma Rhei *(da huang)* is the chief herb. It is bitter and cold, and is associated with the Spleen, Stomach, and Large Intestine channels. It is a strong purgative and very effective in clearing heat.

Mirabilitum *(mang xiao)*, which serves as the deputy, is salty, bitter, and cold, and is associated with the Stomach and Large Intestine channels. It too is a strong purgative. It reduces heat and removes waste from the Large Intestine. It also softens hard, dry feces to facilitate their removal from the Large Intestine.

Radix Glycyrrhizae Uralensis *(gan cao)* is the envoy herb. It harmonizes the functions in the middle burner and promotes the functions of the Stomach. It prevents the other two herbs, which are very strong, from injuring the antipathogenic factors.

Modified herbal formula

Radix et Rhizoma Rhei *(da huang)* 10g

Mirabilitum *(mang xiao)* 10g

Rhizoma Coptidis *(huang lian)* 8g

Radix Rehmanniae Glutinosae *(sheng di huang)* 8g

Radix Glycyrrhizae Uralensis *(gan cao)* 6g

Explanation of modified herbal formula

Because this case involves constipation due to retention of heat and fire from excess in the Stomach and Large Intestine, our modified formula is based on Regulate the Stomach and Order the Qi Decoction *(tiao wei cheng qi tang)*, which is a strong purgative that is able to remove the dry feces and reduce the heat and fire. The only modification is that the dosage of Radix et Rhizoma Rhei *(da huang)* and Mirabilitum *(mang xiao)* have both been reduced by 2 grams. Because there are accompanying symptoms associated with heat disturbing the Heart spirit and injuring the yin and blood, Rhizoma Coptidis *(huang lian)* and Radix Rehmanniae Glutinosae *(sheng di huang)* were added to strengthen the formula's ability to clear the heat and cool the blood. The latter herb also nourishes the yin and blood in order to compensate for the injury to the body fluids caused by pathogenic heat.

Follow-up

The patient was given one packet of the formula daily, divided into two doses. After two days the bowel movements were smooth, so Mirabilitum *(mang xiao)* was removed from the formula, and the dosage of Radix et Rhizoma Rhei *(da huang)* was reduced to 5 grams. After another two days, all of the symptoms had disappeared and treatment was therefore terminated.

Because the patient had a very strong yang constitution and a tendency towards heat, he was advised to eat certain foods at different times of the year. In part this advice was based on the traditional Chinese belief that the best vegetables are those which grow locally in the season during which they are consumed. This particular patient had a prepoderance of yang. People with this type of constitution often follow the changes in the yang qi of nature throughout the seasons. It is accordingly very helpful for people like him to use diet as an adjunct to treatment.

Below are the dietary recommendations that were made to this patient, who lives in Northern China. Depending on where you live, the specific foods that would be useful to your patients will of course vary.

In the spring he was asked to make a porridge consisting of half a lily leaf and 50 grams of polished nonglutinous rice, which was enough to last for two days. He would be free to eat this from time to time, whenever he liked. Lily leaves are thought to very gently clear heat. They also have a dispersing action, and are thus compatible with the characteristics of yang qi during the spring (gradually rising). Nonglutinous rice is used to protect the stomach qi.

In the summer he was advised to eat bitter melon, either stir-fried or made into a soup. Bitter melon is effective at clearing heat, and is very useful in the summer when the yang qi in nature becomes excessive.

When autumn comes around everything changes quickly, and strong heat-clearing substances are no longer appropriate. During this time, winter melon (*dōng guā*, also known as wax gourd) made into a soup was recommended. Winter melon gently clears heat, in a manner similar to lily leaves, but has no dispersing action, which would be inappropriate during the fall.

During the winter, a soup should be made from white radishes. These do not clear heat, but are effective in removing qi stagnation and promoting the movement of qi. They also improve digestion and facilitate the removal of waste through the bowels.

The purpose of these dietary changes was to reduce the heat in the body and adjust the patient's constitution, so that he would suffer no further episodes of this disorder. He was also advised to reduce his intake of food or beverages of a "hot" nature, such as lamb, ginger, chili, spices, and alcohol.

Each person has his or her own constitutional tendencies, for example, toward yin or yang, deficiency or excess. One is then more easily affected by a precipitating factor whose nature is similar to that of their constitution. For example, people with a qi stagnation constitution are more susceptible to Liver disorders, those with a hot or fire constitution are more susceptible to Heart disorders, and those with cold constitutions are predisposed toward problems of deficiency. This does not mean that they will necessarily have this kind of illness, only that they have a greater tendency to do so. Diet can be used to adjust these constitutional tendencies, and is a very safe and effective method. In this case the patient readily accumulated heat in his body, and the recommended foods were chosen to adjust this tendency. It is important to remember that sensible people prevent disease by keeping healthy, rather than always relying on treatment.

According to our records, this patient had no significant recurrence of constipation.

CASE 24: **Female, age 28**

Main complaint

Constipation

History

Two months ago after a trouble-free labor, this young woman gave birth to a baby girl. She did not breast-feed the baby. Until now she has had no bloody discharge from the vagina. She has been suffering from constipation since the birth of the baby, with one bowel movement every four to six days. The stools are very dry and extremely difficult to pass. She requires an enema of soapy water or glycerin to move the stools and alleviate the pain during bowel movements. Her appetite is slightly reduced, and she has constant bad breath. She reports slight abdominal distention, but no fever or aversion to cold. Although her mouth is dry, she neither feels thirsty nor drinks much. Her sleep is normal, her urine is yellow, and there are no abnormal symptoms when she urinates. Her bowel movements were normal before labor.

Tongue

Pale tongue body with a thin, yellow coating

Pulse

Thin

Analysis of symptoms

1. Disorder following labor—injury to the blood.
2. Constipation, very dry stools that are difficult to pass, and bowel movements every four to six days—lack of moisture in the Large Intestine.
3. Bad breath and abdominal distention—dysfunction of turbid qi in the Stomach.
4. Dry mouth and yellow urine—deficiency of body fluids.
5. Thin, yellow tongue coating—heat.
6. Pale tongue and thin pulse—blood deficiency.

Basic theory of case

Constipation caused by a deficiency of body fluids or dryness in the Large Intestine is very frequently seen in the clinic. Common causes of this disorder include the following:

1. Yin deficiency

The body fluids pertain to the yin aspect of the body. If there is a tendency toward yin deficiency and a preponderance of yang, or if a patient is suffering from the later stages of a febrile disease or a chronic illness that has injured the body's yin, or if an elderly person suffers from yin deficiency, then an insufficiency of body fluids will result, manifested as a lack of moisture in the Large Intestine, and thus constipation. This type of pattern may involve chronic, long-term constipation, with bowel movements once every few days. The stools are usually very dry and hard. The patient may experience a hot sensation, low-grade fever or tidal heat, night sweats, restlessness, insomnia, dry mouth, bad breath, and have yellow urine, a red tongue with a thin, yellow coating, or very little coating. The pulse is often thin and rapid.

2. Blood deficiency

Constipation is not necessarily one of the symptoms typically associated with a pattern of blood deficiency, but if a large quantity of blood is lost in a short time, due to labor or trauma for example, constipation can result. This is also commonly seen in practice. The loss of blood causes a reduction in body fluids, which results in a lack of moisture in the Large Intestine. This is why, apart from passing dry, hard stools every few days, such patients can present with symptoms of blood deficiency: pale complexion and lips, dizziness, palpitations, pale tongue with a white coating, thin pulse. Female patients may have menstrual disorders.

3. Depletion of body fluids

This can be caused by deficiency in the production of body fluids, or by the loss of or injury to the body fluids, such as a failure to drink enough liquids, or severe diarrhea, vomiting, or sweating. Both of these conditions can injure the body fluids, which leads to a lack of moisture in the Large Intestine. Besides constipation, patients can also have a dry mouth, throat, nose, and skin, and dry and cracked lips. Such patients feel thirsty and drink a lot of liquids, but their urine is yellow and the quantity is reduced. The tongue is slightly red, with a dry coating, and the pulse is thin.

In addition, one also sees patients with habitual constipation due to depletion of body fluids. The stools are dry and hard, and there is no regularity to the bowel movements. This type of patient has no general symptoms or abdominal discomfort. A common cause of habitual constipation is deficiency of fluids in the Large Intestine.

Cause of disease

Deficiency of body fluids after labor

Before labor the patient was very healthy and her bowel movements were regular. As the constipation only began after labor, we may infer that it was caused by a loss of blood, resulting in deficiency of body fluids and a lack of moisture in the Large Intestine.

Site of disease

Large Intestine

The patient's main complaint is constipation. Besides the very mild symptoms associated with the digestive system, there are few other symptoms of a general nature. We may therefore conclude that the site of the disease is the Large Intestine.

Pathological change

In Chinese medicine both the body fluids and blood have a common source. Both pertain to the yin aspect of the body and are derived from food essence. Physiologically speaking, apart from nourishing and moistening the skin, sensory organs, tissues, and internal Organs, the body fluids flow continuously into the vessels, replenishing the liquid constituent of the blood. When there is a deficiency of blood and a demand for more fluids to replenish this deficiency, an insufficiency of body fluids can result. This is how symptoms involving the lack of normal moisture and nourishment can develop.

Fig. 5-10

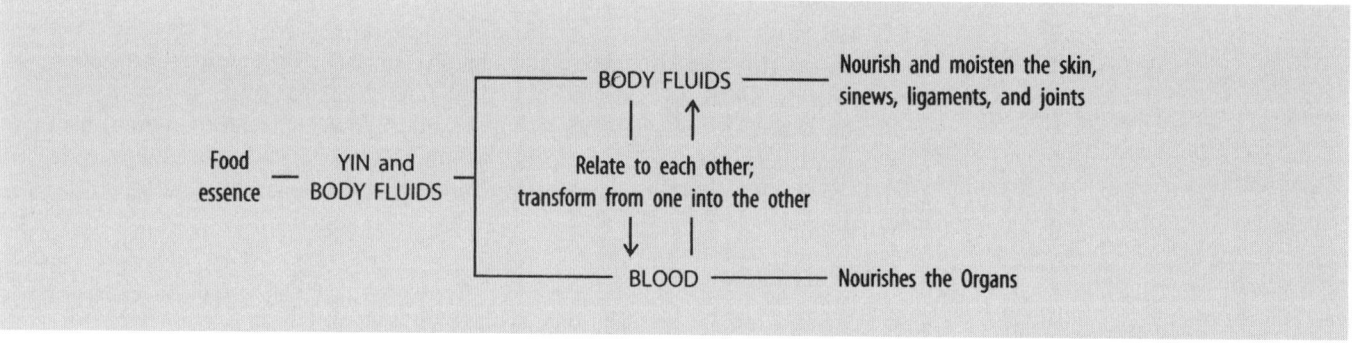

This patient's constipation is due to the loss of a large quantity of blood after labor, and the resulting insufficiency of body fluids. This has led to a lack of moisture in the Large Intestine, which prevents the feces from moving.

This condition has caused an obstruction of qi in the yang Organs, hence the abdominal distention. Since the Stomach is closely related to the Intestines, the turbid qi of these Organs associated with the yang brightness channels cannot descend, but reverses upward, causing the foul breath. Because deficiency of body fluids can lead to the rising of heat from deficiency, the patient has a dry mouth and yellow urine. She nonetheless does not drink much, which means that the injury to the body fluids is not yet severe. The absence of fever or aversion to cold indicates that there has been no invasion of pathogenic factors.

The pale tongue reflects the inability of the blood to circulate upward to nourish the tongue and give it its normal color. The thin, yellow coating indicates a pattern of heat. The thin pulse is characteristic of deficiency of blood and body fluids, and results from the blood vessels losing their normal shape.

Pattern of disease

All of the symptoms developed after labor. Because there is no evidence of invasion by external pathogenic factors (fever, aversion to cold), we may conclude that the pattern is of the interior.

The dry mouth, yellow urine, and thin, yellow tongue coating suggest a very mild pattern of heat.

Deficiency is evidenced here by the depleted body fluids and blood resulting in the lack of moisture in the Large Intestine.

Additional notes

1. What is the evidence of blood deficiency in this case?

Typical symptoms of blood deficiency include a pale and lusterless complexion, pale skin, lips, and nails, dizziness, palpitations, insomnia, numbness in the hands and feet, and blurred vision. Female patients can have menstrual disorders such as diminished quantity of bleeding, or even amenorrhea in severe cases. The site of disease is often the Heart and Liver. In this case, by contrast, the site of disease is the Large Intestine, and the patient has none of the typical symptoms listed above. The primary evidence is the patient's labor, which marked the onset of symptoms. She does not have symptoms typical of blood deficiency, but of deficiency (or insufficiency) of blood and body fluids.

2. What is the cause of the heat?

The patient has a dry mouth, yellow urine, and a yellow tongue coating—symptoms of heat. Yet what is the source of this pathogenic heat?

The blood and body fluids both pertain to the yin aspect of the body. When there is deficiency or injury to the blood and body fluids, the yin of the body becomes deficient and the balance of yin and yang is disturbed. Heat from deficiency is caused by a preponderance of yang, but in this case the heat is very mild compared with that of rising fire from deficiency, which is caused by yin deficiency.

3. Is there any evidence of Spleen deficiency?

We know that the patient's appetite is reduced, which was caused by the constipation obstructing the qi in the yang Organs associated with the yang brightness channels (Stomach and Large Intestine). This obstruction has affected the middle burner's function in regulating the upward and downward movement of qi. Because the turbid yin is thereby prevented from descending, and the clear yang from rising, they combine in the middle burner where they impede the Spleen's transportive and transformative functions, suppressing the appetite. Because this is only a side effect of the obstruction in the yang brightness Organs, there is no pattern of Spleen deficiency.

Conclusion

1. According to the eight principles:
   Interior, heat, deficiency.

2. According to theory of qi, blood, and body fluids:
   Deficiency of blood and body fluids.

3. According to Organ theory:
   Deficiency of body fluids in the Large Intestine.

Treatment principle

Moisten the Large Intestine and unblock the bowels.

Explanation of treatment principle

For each of the causes of constipation there is a different treatment. Moistening the Large Intestine can be achieved by:

- nourishing the yin
- nourishing the blood
- increasing the body fluids.

The basic principle is to increase the body fluids in order to moisten the Large Intestine and thereby soften the feces. If this can be achieved, the bowel movements will return to normal and the feces will be easily removed from the body.

Strong purgatives are used for reducing fire and pushing out the stool, a method that is appropriate for expelling pathogenic factors. By contrast, moistening the Large Intestine and unblocking the bowels is a very different and much gentler method. The herbs that are used for this purpose are juicy and oily. They moisten the Large Intestine and increase the body fluids, which helps strengthen the antipathogenic factors while moving the stool.

Basic herbal formula

Increase the Fluids Decoction *(zeng ye tang)* is a formula used to treat deficiency of body fluids. The ingredients include the following:

Radix Scrophulariae Ningpoensis *(xuan shen)* 30g
Tuber Ophiopogonis Japonici *(mai men dong)* 25g
Radix Rehmanniae Glutinosae *(sheng di huang)* 25g

Explanation of basic herbal formula

The indications for this prescription include dryness and a hot sensation in the throat and mouth, constipation with dry stools, a dry, red tongue, and a thin, rapid pulse. This formula was originally used for epidemic febrile diseases in which pathogenic heat has injured the body fluids, depriving the Large Intestine of nourishment and moisture, and thereby leading to constipation.

In the formula, Radix Scrophulariae Ningpoensis *(xuan shen)* is the chief herb. It is bitter, salty, and cold, and is associated with the Stomach and Kidney channels. It clears heat and nourishes the yin of the body.

The other two are herbs serve as deputies. Tuber Ophiopogonis Japonici *(mai men dong)* is sweet and cold, and is associated with the Stomach channel. It promotes the Stomach functions and the production of body fluids, nourishes the Intestines, and facilitates the removal of stool. Radix Rehmanniae Glutinosae *(sheng di huang)* is sweet, bitter, and cold, and is associated with the Heart and Kidney channels. It clears heat, nourishes the yin of the body, and generates body fluids.

There are no strong purgatives in this formula since it is not focused on unblocking the bowels directly, but tries to increase the overall body fluids, particularly in the Intestines, in order to nourish and moisten the Intestines; this will indirectly facilitate the movement of stool. If the constipation becomes severe, purgatives may be added, but caution must be exercised. If the dosage of the purgatives is too large, the antipathogenic factors will be injured.

Modified herbal formula

Radix Angelicae Sinensis *(dang gui)* 10g
Radix Polygoni Multiflori *(he shou wu)* 10g
Radix Scrophulariae Ningpoensis *(xuan shen)* 20g
Radix Rehmanniae Glutinosae *(sheng di huang)* 20g
Tuber Ophiopogonis Japonici *(mai men dong)* 10g
Radix et Rhizoma Rhei *(da huang)* 8g

Explanation of modified herbal formula

Because the patient is suffering from a deficiency of blood due to labor, and dryness in the Large Intestine, which has led to the constipation, the focus of treatment is to nourish the yin of the body. Increase the Fluids Decoction *(zeng ye tang)* was therefore chosen as the basic formula, with the addition of herbs that nourish and increase the blood to suit this particular patient's condition.

Thus, in addition to the herbs in the basic formula that nourish the body fluids, Radix Angelicae Sinensis *(dang gui)* and Radix Polygoni Multiflori *(he shou wu)* were added to nourish the blood, moisten the Large Intestine, and unblock the bowels. These herbs are appropriate when, as here, the constipation specifically involves blood deficiency. In addition, Radix et Rhizoma Rhei *(da huang)* was added to help unblock the bowels, purge, and hasten the result; however, this herb must not be used too long, as it may injure the antipathogenic factors.

Follow-up The patient was given one packet of the herbs daily, divided into two doses. After four days she was able to have one bowel movement a day, and was very pleased with the result. The dosage was then reduced to one packet every other day, divided into two daily doses. Three days later, Radix et Rhizoma Rhei *(da huang)* was removed from the formula, which was then restored to the original dosage (one packet daily) for another two weeks. The patient had one bowel movement every day or every other day, although on one occasion there was a two-day interval between bowel movements. She suffered no abdominal distention and her appetite returned to normal. At this stage the herbs were terminated and for four weeks she was given a prepared medicine called Eight-Treasure Pill to Benefit Mothers *(ba zhen yi mu wan)*. She took two pills every day. These pills continued to nourish the blood, and moisten and nourish the Large Intestine. The result was very satisfactory: the frequency of bowel movements was maintained, and the patient's general condition was restored to normal.

This kind of constipation following labor, which is caused by a lack of body fluids in the Large Intestine, can be treated very effectively with herbs, especially if the condition is treated at an early stage. Early treatment, ideally between two weeks and one month of the symptoms' appearance, can accelerate the body's recovery after labor, and will be more effective in nourishing and increasing the quantity of blood, and promoting the production of body fluids. Delayed treatment will often leave the patient with a chronic condition of blood deficiency, or both blood and qi deficiency, or habitual constipation. Since many women have no idea what to expect after labor, they often ignore themselves in their excitement to look after the baby, or else they resort to very strong chemical or other herbal laxatives. These can be very dangerous and can aggravate the deficiency of body fluids, which can lead to a chronic condition that lasts for several years, or, in severe cases, even for the rest of one's life. The patient in this case already had constipation for two months and therefore was not treated in time. This explains why the duration of treatment was relatively long; nonetheless, the results were very satisfactory. It is important that the practitioner take note of this.

Diagnostic Principles for Abnormal Bowel Movements

The most commonly encountered abnormalities of bowel movements are diarrhea and constipation. As both disorders are associated with a dysfunction of the Large Intestine, they have been grouped together for discussion in this chapter.

DIARRHEA

Diarrhea means an increase in the frequency of bowel movements, and changes in the quality of stools, which become loose and soft, watery, and accompanied by particles of undigested food, pus, blood, or a sticky liquid secretion. Some patients also experience abnormal sensations when they pass stools, such as a burning, hot sensation around the anus, straining, or tenesmus.

Etiology, pathological change, and site of disorder The causes of diarrhea include exposure to or invasion by pathogenic factors from the environment, such as damp-cold, damp-heat, summer dampness, or epidemic toxic factors. Diarrhea can also be caused by such problems as improper diet or dysfunction in the Organs.

Fig. 5-11

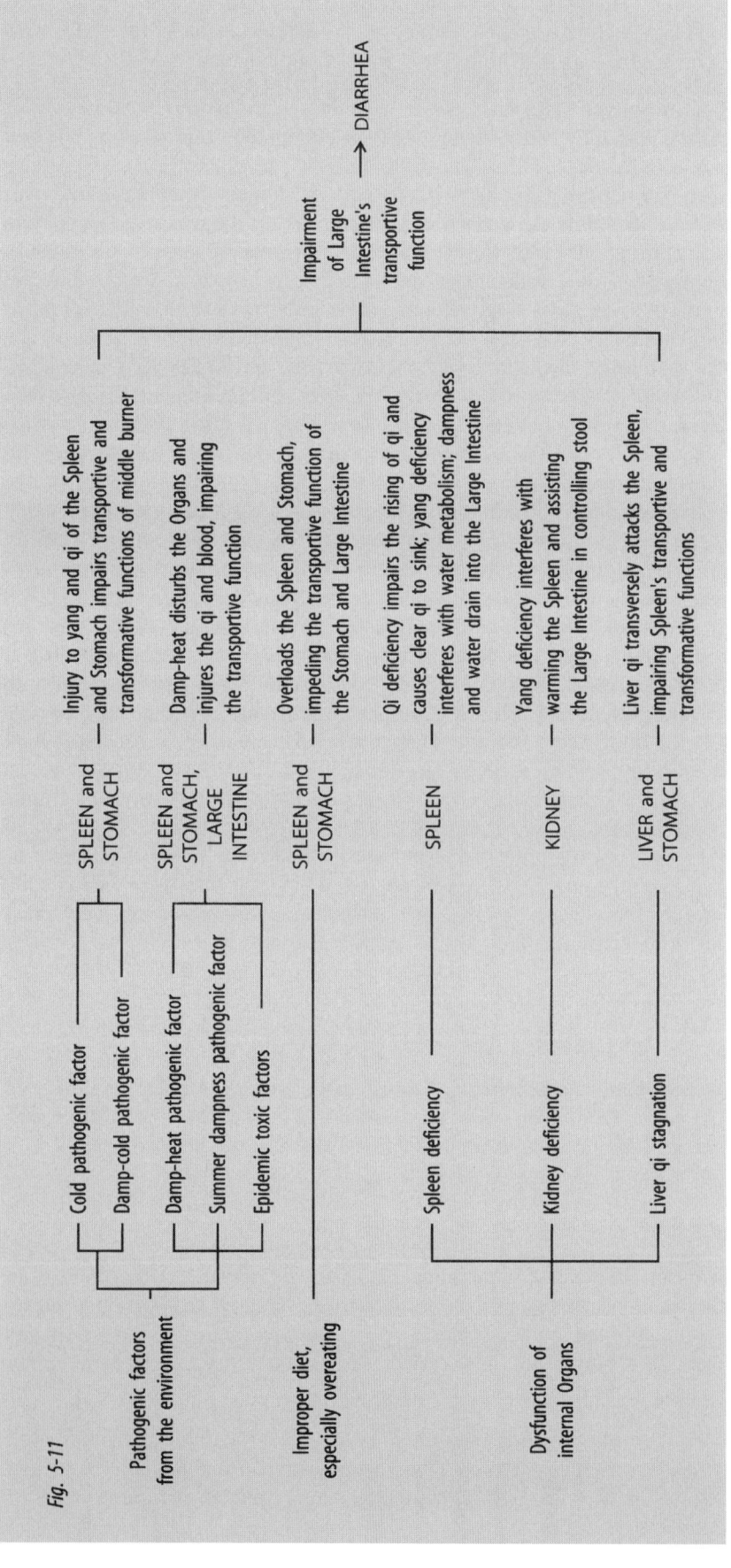

The physiological function of the Large Intestine is the transportation of waste after digestion, and the formation and removal from the body of the feces after metabolism. Diarrhea is therefore directly associated with the Large Intestine. However, the Spleen's and Stomach's function in the transportation and transformation of food, the Kidney yang's warming function, and the Kidney's function in controlling urination and defecation also have a close relationship with the digestion of food and the formation of the feces. Thus, disorders of the Spleen, Stomach, or Kidney can also result in diarrhea, as is often seen in clinical practice. In addition, disharmony between the Liver and Spleen, which is associated with dysfunction of the Liver in governing the free-flow of qi, can also cause diarrhea *(Fig. 5-11)*.

Symptoms and patterns

DIARRHEA CAUSED BY RETENTION OF DAMP-COLD: Pale face, cold limbs, heaviness around the body, poor appetite, no thirst, clear urine, coldness and severe pain in the abdomen which improves with warmth, clear and loose or watery feces without severe smell, white and greasy tongue coating, soggy pulse

DIARRHEA CAUSED BY RETENTION OF DAMP-HEAT: Fever, thirst with little inclination to drink, poor appetite, nausea, reduced quantity of urine that is brownish in color, abdominal pain, yellow, sticky, thick, and foul-smelling feces, a hot, burning sensation around the anus, red tongue with yellow and greasy coating, slippery and rapid pulse

If there is an invasion of summer dampness, the symptoms usually include an obvious fever, red complexion, excessive sweating, dry mouth, and desire to drink a lot of liquids. These are symptoms involving heat excess.

If there is an invasion of epidemic toxic factors in the Large Intestine, the stools will be accompanied by blood and a white discharge; there will also be tenesmus.

DIARRHEA CAUSED BY RETENTION OF FOOD: Very poor appetite with little desire to eat, belching, regurgitation, distention, fullness, and pain in the epigastric and abdominal regions that is relieved after diarrhea, sticky, thick, and foul-smelling feces containing undigested food, thick, greasy, or loose tongue coating, slippery pulse

DIARRHEA CAUSED BY LIVER QI STAGNATION: Stifling sensation in the chest, distention in the hypochondrial region, belching, frequent sighing, poor appetite.

Diarrhea can often be induced by anxiety or an emotional upset, and frequently starts with rumbling in the stomach. Feces are usually soft but loose, without any other type of change. Pain generally diminishes after diarrhea. Wiry, or sunken and wiry, pulse.

DIARRHEA CAUSED BY SPLEEN DEFICIENCY: Poor appetite, abdominal distention after eating, general lassitude, fatigue, dull pain in the epigastric and abdominal regions, preference for warmth and pressure, loose stools, diarrhea readily aggravated by improper diet or irregular food, pale tongue with a white coating, forceless, or a sunken and thin, pulse.

If the Spleen qi is sinking, there is generally a very long and chronic history of diarrhea, and a straining sensation around the anus.

DIARRHEA CAUSED BY KIDNEY DEFICIENCY: History is usually very long, and there is a chronic feeling of coldness. Also cold limbs, and cold and pain in the back. Urine becomes clear and increases in quantity, and there is urinary frequency at night. Cold and pain in the abdomen. Stools are loose and watery. In severe cases, there can be incontinence of bowel movement.

The tongue is pale, swollen, and soft, the coating is white and moist, and the pulse is sunken and thin *(Fig. 5-12)*.

Fig. 5-12

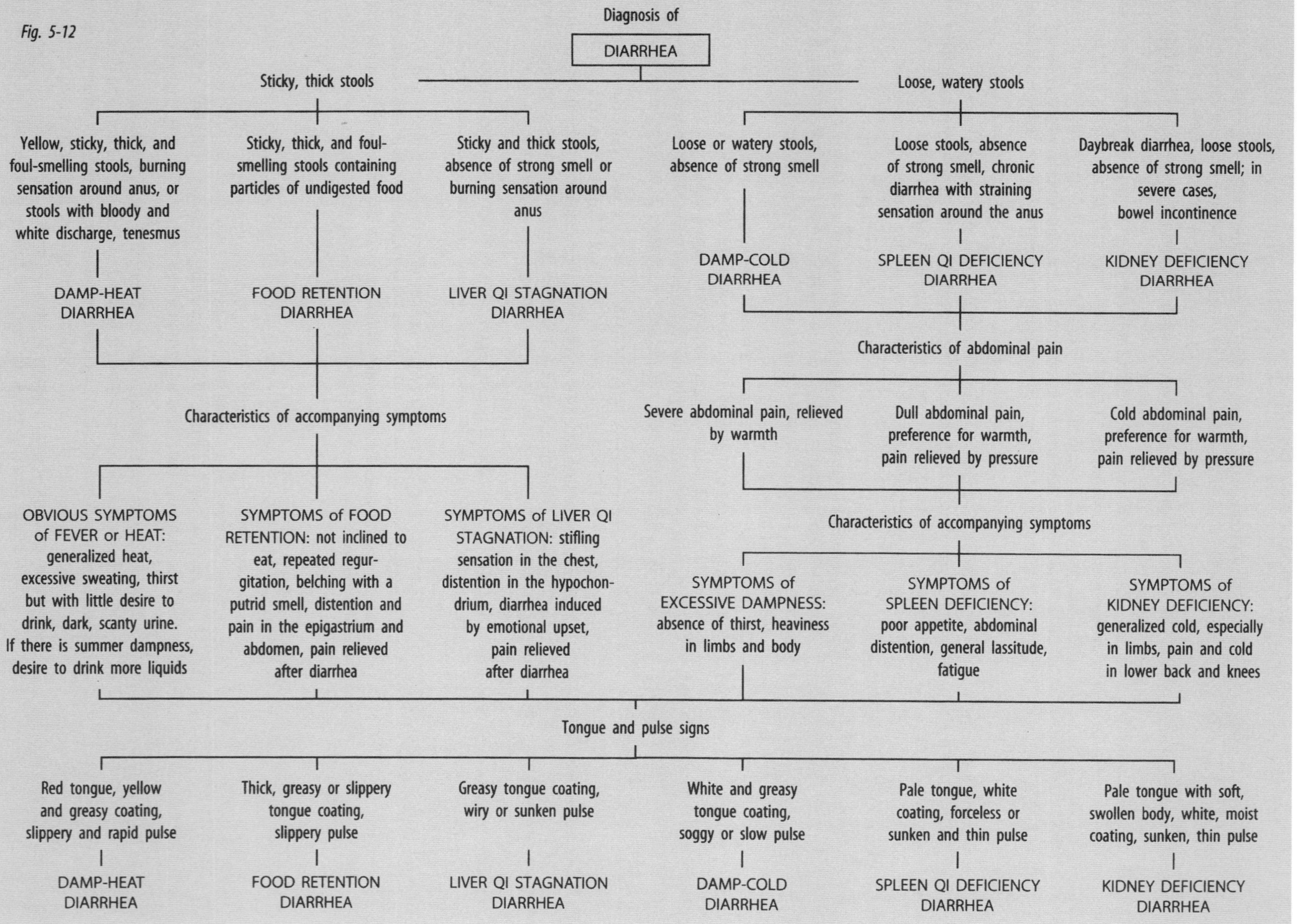

Diagnosis of
DIARRHEA

Sticky, thick stools

- Sticky, thick, and foul-smelling stools containing particles of undigested food
  - Characteristics of accompanying symptoms
    - SYMPTOMS OF FOOD RETENTION: not inclined to eat, repeated regurgitation, belching with a putrid smell, distention and pain in the epigastrium and abdomen, pain relieved after diarrhea
    - SYMPTOMS OF LIVER QI STAGNATION: stifling sensation in the chest, distention in the hypochondrium, diarrhea induced by emotional upset, pain relieved after diarrhea
  - Sticky, thick, and foul-smelling stools containing particles of undigested food
    FOOD RETENTION DIARRHEA
  - Sticky and thick stools, absence of strong smell or burning sensation around anus
    LIVER QI STAGNATION DIARRHEA

- Yellow, sticky, thick, and foul-smelling stools, burning sensation around anus, or stools with bloody and white discharge, tenesmus
  DAMP-HEAT DIARRHEA

- Tongue and pulse signs
  - Red tongue, yellow and greasy coating, slippery and rapid pulse
    DAMP-HEAT DIARRHEA
  - Thick, greasy or slippery tongue coating, slippery pulse
    FOOD RETENTION DIARRHEA
  - Greasy tongue coating, wiry or sunken pulse
    LIVER QI STAGNATION DIARRHEA

- OBVIOUS SYMPTOMS of FEVER or HEAT: generalized heat, excessive sweating, thirst but with little desire to drink, dark, scanty urine. If there is summer dampness, desire to drink more liquids

Loose, watery stools

- Loose or watery stools, absence of strong smell
  - Characteristics of abdominal pain
    - Severe abdominal pain, relieved by warmth
    - Dull abdominal pain, preference for warmth, pain relieved by pressure
  - Characteristics of accompanying symptoms
    - SYMPTOMS of EXCESSIVE DAMPNESS: absence of thirst, heaviness in limbs and body
    - SYMPTOMS of SPLEEN DEFICIENCY: poor appetite, abdominal distention, general lassitude, fatigue
  - Loose or watery stools, absence of strong smell
    DAMP-COLD DIARRHEA
  - Cold abdominal pain, preference for warmth, pain relieved by pressure

- Loose stools, absence of strong smell, chronic diarrhea with straining sensation around the anus
  SPLEEN QI DEFICIENCY DIARRHEA

- Daybreak diarrhea, loose stools, absence of strong smell; in severe cases, bowel incontinence
  KIDNEY DEFICIENCY DIARRHEA

- Tongue and pulse signs
  - White and greasy tongue coating, soggy or slow pulse
    DAMP-COLD DIARRHEA
  - Pale tongue, white coating, forceless or sunken and thin pulse
    SPLEEN QI DEFICIENCY DIARRHEA
  - Pale tongue with soft, swollen body, white, moist coating, sunken, thin pulse
    KIDNEY DEFICIENCY DIARRHEA

- SYMPTOMS of KIDNEY DEFICIENCY: generalized cold, especially in limbs, pain and cold in lower back and knees

CONSTIPATION

Constipation involves an increase in the interval between one bowel movement and the next, from more than one day to several days between bowel movements; it is usually accompanied by dry stools. There can be bleeding and varying degrees of pain around the anus, occasioned by the dryness and hardness of the feces, and the difficulty in passing them.

Etiology, pathological change, and site of disease

Whether the feces can be removed smoothly from the Large Intestine where they have been formed depends on whether the body fluids or qi in the Large Intestine are sufficient, as these two factors can directly affect bowel movements. The body fluids moisten the inner surface of the Intestines, and the qi in the Large Intestine pushes the feces out of the body. In clinical practice, if either of these two conditions is deficient, then constipation can easily occur.

Pathogenic heat, which consumes the body fluids, is a very common cause of constipation. It is frequently encountered in febrile diseases caused by an invasion of pathogenic factors or retention of fire excess in the Organs.

Other common causes of chronic constipation include the later stages of febrile disease, chronic illnesses where the yin and blood have been injured, after childbirth, or the loss of a large quantity of blood, and elderly people who have a chronic deficiency of yin and blood.

In addition, Spleen qi deficiency may result in qi deficiency of the Large Intestine, which leads to constipation. This situation is frequently seen in severe cases of qi deficiency. Kidney yang deficiency leading to retention of internal cold can readily lead to diarrhea, often including loose and watery stools. Constipation may also result, but this is uncommon.

As can be seen, the Large Intestine is generally the site of disease for constipation, although it may also be the Spleen or Kidney.

Symptoms and patterns

PATHOGENIC HEAT: Red complexion, restlessness, generalized hot sensation, no aversion to cold, thirst with a preference for frequent and cold beverages, dry stools, bowel movement once every few days, abdominal fullness, distention, and pain, the pain worsens with pressure, foul breath, poor appetite, reduced quantity of darker-colored urine, red tongue with a yellow, dry, and cracked coating, and a sunken, slippery, and forceful pulse.

YIN AND BLOOD DEFICIENCY: Constipation with bowel movement once every few days, absence of hot sensations or excessive sweating, occasional low-grade feverish sensation, dry mouth, foul breath, poor (sometimes normal) appetite, thin tongue coating, thin pulse

For those with blood deficiency, there may also be pale lips and face, indicative of malnourishment. For those with yin deficiency, there may also be restlessness and insomnia, indicative of a disturbance of the Heart spirit.

QI DEFICIENCY: Constipation with dry (sometimes soft) stools, which are difficult to pass. Bowel movements take much longer than usual, and afterwards the patient can feel exhausted, experience shortness of breath and sweating. In general, patients suffer from shortness of breath, are not inclined to speak, and experience lassitude, which usually worsens after a bowel movement. The tongue is pale with a white coating, and the pulse is either forceless, or sunken and forceless.

YANG DEFICIENCY: Bowel movement only once every few days, stools are not very dry or loose, general feeling of coldness, coldness in the extremities, absence of thirst. There is abdominal pain and coldness, urine is clear and of increased quantity, tongue is pale, swollen, and soft with a white, moist coating, and pulse is sunken, slow, and forceless.

Fig. 5-13

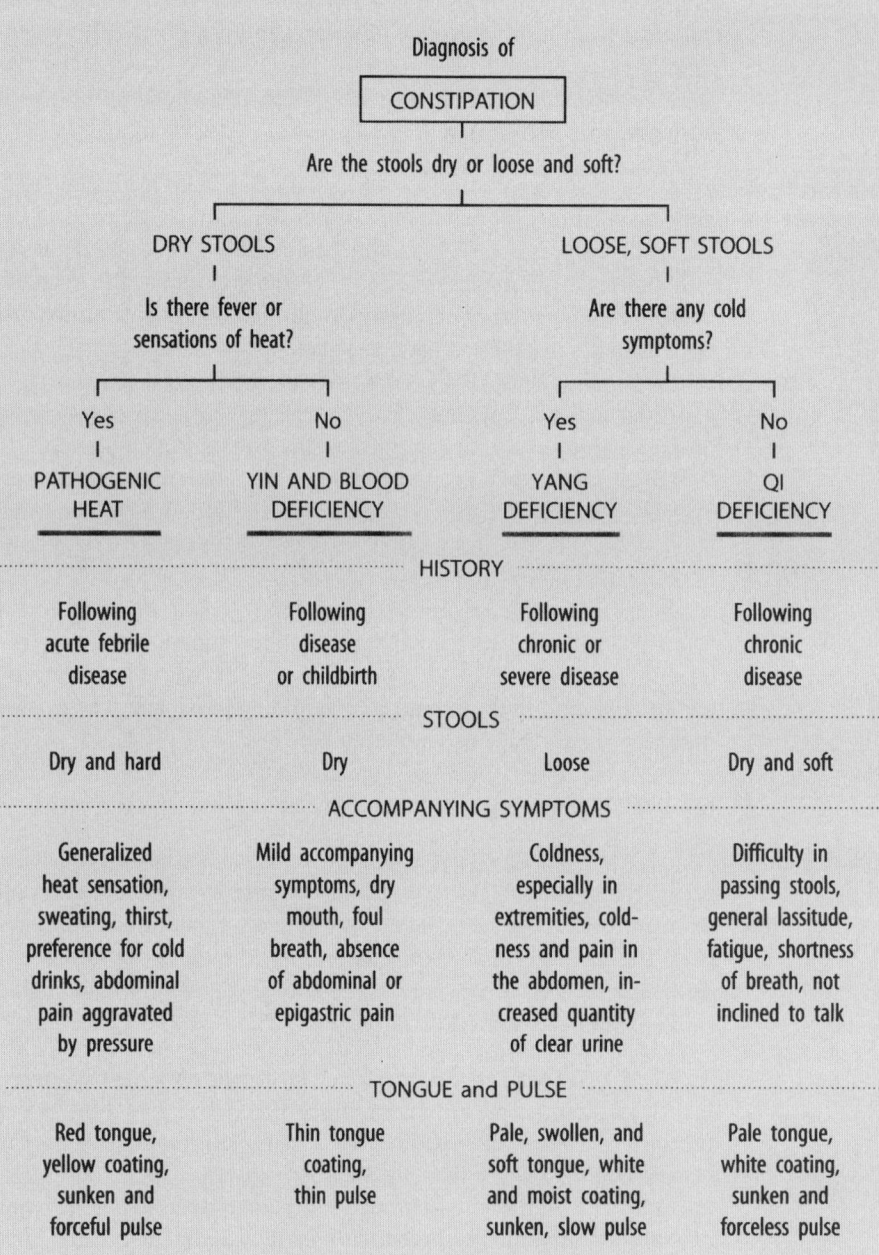

Diagnosis of

CONSTIPATION

Are the stools dry or loose and soft?

DRY STOOLS		LOOSE, SOFT STOOLS	
Is there fever or sensations of heat?		Are there any cold symptoms?	
Yes	No	Yes	No
PATHOGENIC HEAT	YIN AND BLOOD DEFICIENCY	YANG DEFICIENCY	QI DEFICIENCY

HISTORY

| Following acute febrile disease | Following disease or childbirth | Following chronic or severe disease | Following chronic disease |

STOOLS

| Dry and hard | Dry | Loose | Dry and soft |

ACCOMPANYING SYMPTOMS

| Generalized heat sensation, sweating, thirst, preference for cold drinks, abdominal pain aggravated by pressure | Mild accompanying symptoms, dry mouth, foul breath, absence of abdominal or epigastric pain | Coldness, especially in extremities, coldness and pain in the abdomen, increased quantity of clear urine | Difficulty in passing stools, general lassitude, fatigue, shortness of breath, not inclined to talk |

TONGUE and PULSE

| Red tongue, yellow coating, sunken and forceful pulse | Thin tongue coating, thin pulse | Pale, swollen, and soft tongue, white and moist coating, sunken, slow pulse | Pale tongue, white coating, sunken and forceless pulse |

Abnormal Urination

CASE 25: **Female, age 35**

Main complaint

Abnormal urination

History

Two years ago the patient developed retention of urine during pregnancy. The problem continued after childbirth. During the birth process she was catheterized several times, and after giving birth her urination seemed to gradually improve. She found that she could urinate normally, but sometimes she suffered slight urinary incontinence, especially when she coughed severely or used muscular force to lift anything.

Over the past six months she has found her first urination in the morning to be difficult. On waking she feels distention and fullness in the lower abdominal region, which, when severe, can be painful. She can only pass a very small quantity of urine at this time. When she tries to do something physical, the pressure in the lower abdominal region increases and the pain is aggravated. When she gets up, moves around, and massages the painful area, she can urinate freely and with a normal amount. These symptoms have been paroxysmal in nature, and have occurred on an irregular basis. The patient has been unable to identify any precipitating factors. In order to reduce the difficulty in urinating in the morning, she has controlled her intake of liquids during the evening. And because the symptoms have not been very severe, she thought it unnecessary to get a checkup.

This morning when she went out for the day the weather was very hot. She stopped later for lunch. She ate cold foods and had several cold drinks. She was unable to pass water after the meal, and following an afternoon nap, she tried moving around and massaging herself, but to no avail. At about 5 PM she checked into the emergency department of the hospital, where she was examined. Judging by her contorted face, she looked as though she were suffering badly. The lower abdominal region was very painful and distended. There had been slight incontinence of urine, but apart from this, the patient could not urinate at all.

Generally speaking, her health is otherwise good, and she both eats and sleeps well. Besides the paroxysmal difficulty in urinating described above, the quality and color of her urine are normal, and she does not have nocturia. Her bowel movements are regular, but the stools tend to be loose.

Tongue

Pale, with a white, greasy coating

Pulse

Sunken and thin

Analysis of symptoms

1. Onset of disorder after childbirth—insufficiency of antipathogenic factors.
2. Occurrence of recent onset after consumption of cold food and drink—obstruction of yang qi.
3. Slight urinary incontinence at times—impaired Bladder control.
4. Difficulty in urinating, with dripping incontinence—dysfunction in opening and closing of the Bladder.
5. Urination problem relieved by physical movement and massage—impaired qi activity.
6. No yellow urine or abnormal sensation when the patient urinates—absence of pathogenic heat.
7. Stools generally loose—Spleen qi deficiency.
8. Pale tongue and white coating—cold pattern.
9. Thin pulse—deficiency pattern.
10. Sunken pulse—interior pattern.

Basic theory of case

In Chinese medicine, urinary difficulty or blockage is called *lóng bì*. The word *lóng* indicates dripping of urination, while *bì* indicates a complete lack of urination. Although the two words are similar in meaning, *bì* is more severe than *lóng*.

As urine is stored in the Bladder, urinary blockage is directly associated with disorders of the Bladder itself. However, the formation and excretion of urine also depend on the functions of the three yin Organs associated with water metabolism—the Lung, Spleen, and Kidney—and also on the metabolic and transportation system of the three burners, which is referred to as qi transformation *(qì huà)*. It can thus be seen that the condition of urinary blockage may be associated with different Organs.

Common causes of urinary blockage include the following:

1. *Retention of substantial pathogenic factors in the Bladder, such as damp-heat or urinary calculus.* These types of pathogenic factors can directly block the passageway and affect the functioning of the Bladder, leading to urinary blockage.

2. *Obstruction of the Lung qi.* As the upper source of water metabolism, the Lung is responsible for the downward movement of water. When either external pathogenic factors or phlegm block the Lung qi, its function in facilitating the downward movement of water will be impeded, resulting in impaired qi activity in the three burners. It may also cause an imbalance in the metabolism of water.

3. *Spleen qi deficiency.* The Spleen is the source for the production of qi. Spleen qi deficiency can readily lead to qi deficiency in the lower burner, which can impair the qi activity and water metabolism in the Bladder, and thus the opening and closing of that Organ. This condition can cause urinary incontinence and blockage.

4. *Kidney deficiency.* The Kidney is responsible for urination and defecation. An injury to the Kidney, as well as Kidney deficiency, can interfere with the opening and closing of the Bladder, and can directly cause urinary blockage.

In addition to these factors, when the Liver qi's function in governing the free-flow of qi is impaired, this can also affect the qi activity in the lower burner, and sometimes lead to symptoms of urinary blockage.

Although symptoms of urinary blockage may be traced to different causes, there is very little difference in the actual symptoms. The practitioner must therefore look to the general presentation of the patient in order to determine the underlying cause.

Cause of disease | Deficiency of antipathogenic factors

The patient has no history of invasion by pathogenic factors, and there is also no evidence of a substantial pathogenic factor blocking the urinary passageway. She is not troubled by abnormal symptoms in the intervals between the paroxysmal attacks. The symptoms developed during pregnancy, and they wax and wane. This indicates deficiency of antipathogenic factors, resulting in dysfunction in both the lower burner and the Bladder.

Site of disease | Bladder

The patient has difficulty urinating, and also has slight incontinence of urine. There is distention, fullness, and pain in the lower abdominal region, which suggests that the site of disease is the Bladder.

Pathological change | According to Chinese medicine, the qi and blood are closely related, both physiologically and pathologically; each depends on the other. Blood or qi deficiency following childbirth is a common clinical occurrence. The patient in this case gave birth to her baby two years ago, and there are currently no symptoms of blood deficiency. Because the abnormal urination started before and continued after the baby was born, we can infer that injury to the qi was the primary mechanism, and that she never recovered properly thereafter. The normal opening and closing of the Bladder depend on the unhindered functioning of its qi. Deficiency of qi in the lower burner can impair Bladder control, leading either to incontinence of urine (inability of the Bladder to close) or urinary difficulty (inability to open), even to the point of complete retention of urine. In this case, the patient showed slight incontinence, but suffered mainly from difficulty in passing urine. This reflects a decline in the power needed to remove the urine from the Bladder, resulting from

Fig. 6-1 | qi deficiency in the lower burner.

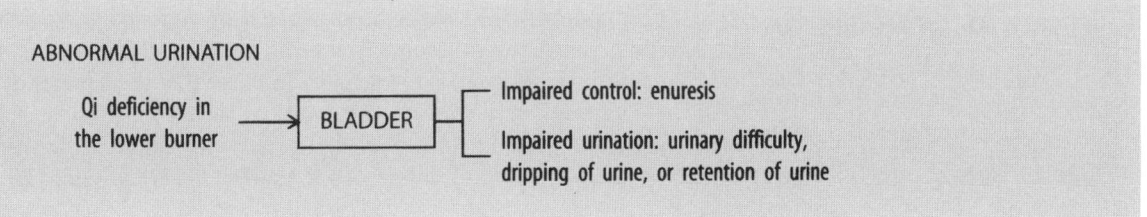

We know that the yang of the body enters the yin when we sleep, and that physical activity declines to its lowest level at this time. In the morning the yang qi of the body requires a certain period of time to regain its normal level. When there is qi deficiency, this recovery time is extended, and thus the first urination in the morning is difficult. Getting up and moving around stimulates the circulation of qi and blood throughout the body, including the lower burner. Local massage can directly stimulate the qi activity in the lower burner, and thus partially relieve the symptoms and assist urination. The symptoms do not occur during the daytime, because physical movement and normal work maintain the yang qi activity at a reasonable level.

Qi pertains to the yang aspect of the body, and characteristically circulates more freely with warmth; coldness, by contrast, impedes and obstructs the circulation of qi. The most recent onset in this case was induced by the over-consumption of cold food and drink. It is this cold that constricted and impeded the circulation of qi around the body, which led to the patient's difficulty in urinating. Because the urine remained in the Bladder where it obstructed the qi activity in the lower burner, the lower abdominal region became painful and distended, and there was a sensation of fullness. The involuntary dripping of urine can be attributed to the pressure of so much urine being stored in the Bladder.

The pale tongue here indicates that the blood is not circulating properly to the upper part of the body. The cause may be blood or qi deficiency, which impairs the circulation; in this case, it is qi deficiency. The white tongue coating tells us that there is no pathogenic heat, and the sunken, thin pulse indicates an interior, deficient pattern.

Pattern of disease

This is an interior pattern, wherein deficiency of the antipathogenic factors after childbirth led to the onset of the disorder.

There is an absence of any abnormal sensation of heat, either generally or locally. Nor is there a fever, and the patient's urine is not yellow. There is no problem with urination between the paroxysmal attacks. The most recent onset was induced by the consumption of too much cold food and drink. Evidence of a cold pattern can be found in the pale tongue and white coating, together with the absence of a rapid pulse.

Qi deficiency is the cause of the poor circulation. There is no substantial pathogenic factor blocking the urinary passageway, and no obstruction in the urethra.

Additional notes

1. What is the cause of the qi deficiency in the Bladder?

The source of qi for the Bladder comes from the Spleen, as well as the yang qi of the Kidney. The qi disorder in the Bladder is therefore associated either with the Spleen or the Kidney. In this case, although the disorder has lasted for two years, the symptoms have been intermittent and not very severe. The present onset is particularly severe, but was induced by ingesting improper food and drink, which would indicate that injury to the Spleen qi is the most likely explanation. Also, according to the history, the patient does not feel cold, has no soreness in the lower back, and does not need to urinate frequently during the night; were these symptoms present, it would point instead to a Kidney disorder. Moreover, the loose stools also supports the diagnosis of Spleen qi deficiency. And the fact that the patient finds it difficult to urinate first thing in the morning, but can do so after getting up and moving around, would also indicate that the Spleen qi is deficient, in that the clear yang is unable to rise, and the turbid yin to descend, properly. We may thus conclude that Spleen qi deficiency has inhibited the production of qi, which in turn has led to qi deficiency in the Bladder *(See Fig. 6-2)*.

2. What does the greasy tongue coating mean?

A greasy tongue coating usually indicates that there is retention of phlegm or dampness in the body. The patient's white and greasy tongue coating is associated

Fig. 6-2

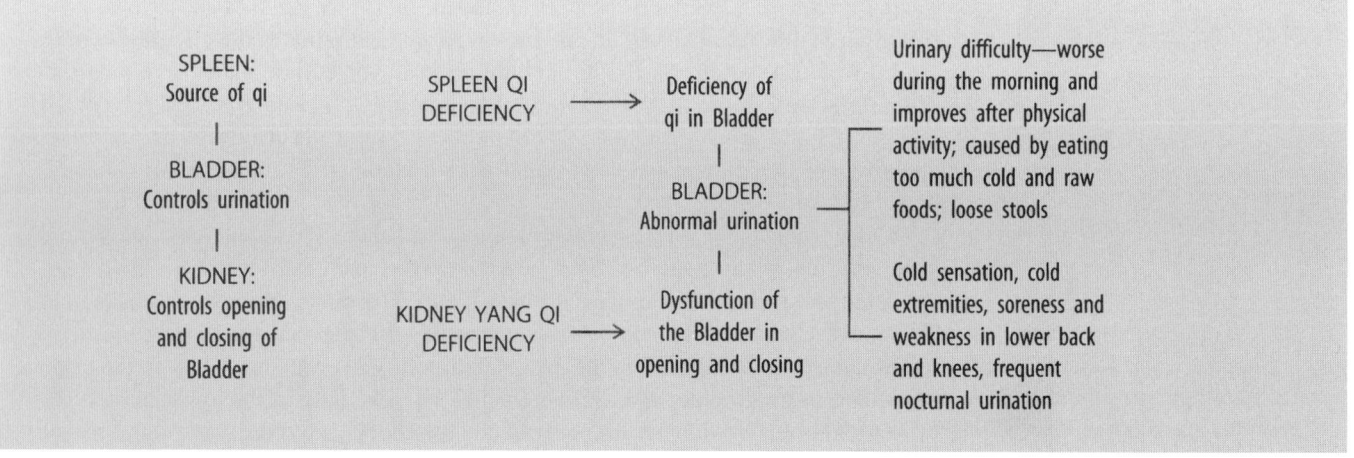

SPLEEN: Source of qi
|
BLADDER: Controls urination
|
KIDNEY: Controls opening and closing of Bladder

SPLEEN QI DEFICIENCY → Deficiency of qi in Bladder
|
BLADDER: Abnormal urination
|
KIDNEY YANG QI DEFICIENCY → Dysfunction of the Bladder in opening and closing

Urinary difficulty—worse during the morning and improves after physical activity; caused by eating too much cold and raw foods; loose stools

Cold sensation, cold extremities, soreness and weakness in lower back and knees, frequent nocturnal urination with Spleen qi deficiency, as impairment of the Spleen's transportive and transformative functions can lead to retention of water and dampness; in this instance, however, it is not very severe. Because there are no other related symptoms around the body, and because it is part of Spleen qi deficiency, it does not require special attention.

3. Is the pattern in this case one of deficiency or excess?

Excess refers to strong pathogenic factors of an excessive nature, including different types of obstruction and blockage, symptoms of which include the retention of feces in the Large Intestine, retention of urine in the Bladder, and retention of pathogenic water or fluids in either the chest or abdominal cavity. Although the patient's urination is obstructed in this case, from the analysis we know that this has been caused by qi deficiency. We may thus conclude that the pattern here is one of deficiency.

Conclusion

1. According to the eight principles:
   Interior, deficiency, cold.

2. According to theory of qi, blood, and body fluids:
   Qi deficiency resulting in retention of urine.

3. According to Organ theory:
   Spleen qi deficiency and retention of water in the Bladder.

Treatment principle

1. Strengthen the Spleen and regulate the qi.

2. Promote urination and remove the obstruction from the Bladder.

Explanation of treatment principle

When the lower burner is obstructed, urine can accumulate in the Bladder. Promoting urination is the main treatment principle for this type of condition. And, because the obstruction of the lower burner in this case was caused by qi deficiency in the middle burner, it is also important to strengthen the Spleen and regulate the qi.

This onset presents an emergency: we must use a method for relieving the symptoms immediately so that the patient can urinate. This is known as treating the manifestations during an emergency (*jí zé zhì qí biāo*). In addition, care must be taken to prevent further injury to the antipathogenic factors, and the Spleen qi must be strengthened. The advantage of acupuncture over herbal therapy is its ease of use and instant results. In this case, therefore, the first method of treatment is acupuncture and moxibustion.

Because the most recent onset was due to the over-consumption of cold food and drink, coldness and dampness are obviously present; the warming method (moxibustion) is therefore used to promote the metabolism of water and drain the dampness. The warming and heating method is used to dispel the cold, strengthen the yang, and regulate the metabolism of water.

Selection of points

First prescription:

BL-25 (*da chang shu*)
BL-32 (*ci liao*) [right side]
BL-33 (*zhong liao*)
SP-9 (*yin ling quan*) [right side]
SP-6 (*san yin jiao*)

Second prescription:

ST-28 (*shui dao*)
SP-9 (*yin ling quan*) [right side]
SP-6 (*san yin jiao*)

Explanation of points

BL-25 (*da chang shu*) is the back associated point of the Large Intestine. It regulates the Intestines and removes obstruction from the back. It is primarily used to treat disorders of the abdominal region, such as abdominal distention and pain, borborygmus, and diarrhea. It can also be used to treat lower back pain. In this case it is used to regulate the qi in the yang brightness Organs, and promote metabolism in the middle burner, in order to help regulate the qi in the lower burner.

BL-32 *(ci liao)* is located in the second posterior sacral foramen. It promotes the functioning of the lower back and knees. It regulates the Organs of the lower burner and treats difficulty in urination and defecation, dysmenorrhea, irregular periods, leukorrhea, pain in the lower back and sacral region, painful obstruction of the lower extremity, and muscular atrophy. Needling this point produces a very deep and strong sensation, and very effectively regulates the qi, removing severe obstruction of the qi and improving the functioning of both urination and defecation. It is one of the important points for the treatment of urinary retention. In this case it is used to promote urination and regulate the qi in order to relieve the abdominal distention. Sparrow-pecking moxibustion with a moxa stick is performed above this point for approximately thirty minutes.

BL-33 *(zhong liao)* is located in the third posterior sacral foramen. Its function is very similar to that of BL-32 *(ci liao)*: it promotes the functioning of the lower back and knees, regulates the Organs of the lower burner, and can be used to treat local pain. It is also utilized in the treatment of urinary and bowel dysfunction. Like BL-32 *(ci liao)*, needling this point can produce a very deep and strong sensation, which is very effective for regulating qi and removing stagnation. It is an excellent choice for relieving retention of urine. Sparrow-pecking moxibustion with a moxa stick is also performed above this point for approximately thirty minutes.

SP-9 *(yin ling quan)* strengthens the Spleen, unblocks the retention of water, and promotes the metabolism of water in the Triple Burner. According to Chinese medical theory, the Triple Burner is the passageway for the metabolism of water. Qi deficiency can impair the functioning of the Triple Burner, and if the waste water is not drained, it will be retained in the Bladder instead. This point is very effective in regulating qi and unblocking the retention of water. It is therefore a good choice in treating urinary difficulty, urinary incontinence, abdominal distention, edema, and related disorders. In this case it is used to strengthen the Spleen in order to promote the metabolism of water. The tonification method is used.

SP-6 *(san yin jiao)* is the meeting point of the three leg yin channels. It regulates the Spleen and Stomach, and tonifies the Liver and Kidney. This is one of the most commonly used points in clinical practice, and is an important point for treating disorders of the lower burner. It provides very effective relief from such urinary complaints as urinary difficulty, enuresis, painful urination, and lower abdominal pain.

ST-28 *(shui dao)*. The name of this point means pathway of water, and it is therefore suitable for regulating the metabolism of water and treating abdominal distention, and is an important point for treating retention of urine. It also regulates qi, dispels qi stagnation, and promotes the functioning of the Intestines. It is thus very effective in treating disorders of the Stomach and Intestines.

Combination of points

BL-32 *(ci liao)* and BL-33 *(zhong liao)* are situated very close to each other: the former is located in the second posterior sacral foramen, and the latter in the third posterior sacral foramen. Both the functions and needling sensations of these two points are very similar. When used together, this combination has an especially strong effect locally. They should be punctured to a depth of at least 15 to 25mm. The sensation produced by needling at both points is transmitted down the leg and radiates to the perineum. Both points can be used bilaterally, or one can be used on each side. In practice, there are no hard and fast rules as to which point should be used on the right, and which on the left: it depends on the position in which the patient lies, and what is more convenient for purposes of manipulation. Because the patient must lie on her right side in this case, BL-32 *(ci liao)* was needled on the right, and BL-33 *(zhong liao)* on the left.

SP-9 *(yin ling quan)* and SP-6 *(san yin jiao)* are both located on the Spleen channel, and both can be used to strengthen Spleen functions and promote the metabolism of water. However, SP-9 *(yin ling quan)* is better for promoting the functions of the Triple Burner, while SP-6 *(san yin jiao)* is better for promoting the functions of the lower burner, as well as nourishing and tonifying both the Kidney and Liver. Thus, both points can serve as distant points in treating retention of urine. This means that, besides the local points, which involve either the lower abdominal region or lower back area, these points can be used as assistant points. The two points can also be used independently when local points are not available. For example, if it is inconvenient to use points in the local area to treat urinary retention because of childbirth or surgery in the lower abdominal region or back, these two points can be utilized as distant points, producing very satisfactory results. As the patient in this case must lie on her right side, SP-9 *(yin ling quan)* is punctured only on the right, but SP-6 *(san yin jiao)* is punctured on both sides.

Follow-up   The patient came to the clinic for emergency treatment. The first acupuncture prescription was used, with heavy moxibustion at BL-32 *(ci liao)* and BL-33 *(zhong liao)*, for thirty minutes. Two or three minutes after withdrawing the needles, the patient passed about 500ml of urine, and the distention and pain in the lower abdominal region were immediately relieved.

The patient returned to the clinic the following morning to say that she had been unable to urinate since returning home the previous evening. Her abdomen had again become very badly distended, and she felt very uncomfortable in the lower back and lower abdominal regions. This time the second acupuncture prescription was used, and moxibustion applied to the lower abdominal area, in order to tonify the qi and warm the yang of the Triple Burner. The patient was again able to urinate after the treatment, and she subsequently suffered no further attacks of this complaint.

Although the patient had not urinated for one night and her lower abdominal region was very distended, the symptoms had diminished considerably by the time she came into the clinic on the following day. This case is characterized as a pattern of interior deficiency and cold, accompanied by retention of water, which is primarily a symptom of excess. On the previous day, acupuncture with strong needling was used to reduce the retention of fluids (a problem of excess). When the retention of water was relieved, a second strategy was chosen to prevent further injury to the antipathogenic factors. This is why, on the second day of treatment, the Bladder channel points were replaced by ST-28 *(shui dao)*. SP-9 *(yin ling quan)* and SP-6 *(san yin jiao)* were both needled bilaterally in order to tonify the qi and promote the metabolism of water. The use of this combination is quite appropriate for treating the main problem. What is more, as there is no danger of this formula injuring the antipathogenic factors, it is very safe.

Acupuncture can yield excellent results when used to treat urinary retention without physical blockage. It is imperative that the diagnosis be correct, and caution must be exercised when the retention of urine results from deficiency, as the needling method should not be too strong. Tonification (even movement) is frequently used. Obtaining qi, and enabling the qi to reach the area of the disoder, are both very important. Quite often patients can be cured after just one or two treatments. However, if a patient is unable to urinate properly after 40 to 50 minutes of treatment, catheterization should be used. This does not mean that acupuncture has failed: when the Bladder is filled again, acupuncture can once again be utilized. Many cases of deficiency must be treated several times before a satisfactory result can be achieved.

CASE 26: **Female, age 60**

Main complaint

Bloody urine (hematuria)

History

The patient has had recurrent cystitis for the past ten years. She experiences discomfort when urinating, and sometimes there is blood in the urine. A conventional medical checkup has ruled out cancer of the bladder. The cystitis and bloody urine generally occur once or twice yearly without any apparent precipitating event. During an attack, urination becomes frequent, urgent, and painful. When the patient urinates, she has a strong burning sensation in the urethra, and sometimes also suffers such general symptoms as pain in the lower back, fever, and lassitude. At the beginning of this disorder various antibiotics were prescribed, which left her with side effects including nausea, poor appetite, and abdominal pain. Because she could never finish a course of antibiotics, she started to use herbal remedies instead. She has taken remedies that clear heat and remove dampness, such as Guide Out the Red Pills *(dao chi wan)*.

Three days ago the patient experienced recurrent discomfort in urinating. She noticed that her urine had become a deep yellow, and the following day she found blood in the urine. Urination had become very frequent, urgent, and painful, and the symptoms gradually worsened. She complains of lower abdominal and lower back pain, and her temperature is between 37.5 and 38.0° C. She feels very thirsty, but is not inclined to drink much. Her appetite is poor and she is restless, but her energy level is still fairly good. She has had no bowel movements for two days, and has not taken any conventional medications.

The result of her blood exam is WBC 18,000 /mm^3, and her urine RBC ++++, WBC ++, PROT: +.

Tongue

Red with a yellow, greasy coating, which is thick at the middle and back of the tongue

Pulse

Slippery and forceful

Analysis of symptoms

1. Frequent, urgent, and painful urination, deep yellow urine, and a burning sensation in the urethra—damp-heat in the Bladder.

2. Bloody urine—injury to the vessels in the Bladder caused by pathogenic heat.

3. Lower abdominal pain and lower back pain—obstruction of qi activity in the lower burner.

4. Recurrent attacks and long duration of disorder—pathogenic dampness.

5. Fever, restlessness, and constipation—pathogenic heat.

6. Thirst, but not inclined to drink much—damp-heat.

7. Red tongue, yellow and greasy coating, and slippery pulse—damp-heat.

8. Forceful pulse—no insufficiency of antipathogenic factors.

Basic theory of case

In clinical practice there are several types of abnormal urination, more than one of which may be present in any given patient:

1. Abnormal quantity of urine—increased or decreased—or, at its worst, urinary blockage, which can lead to no urination at all (anuria).

2. Abnormal quality of urine, such as a change in color ranging from various shades of yellow to a dark, tea-like color. Red urine indicates the presence of blood (hematuria). The urine can also become mixed with various substances, like small particles of urinary calculus.

3. Abnormal sensations during urination, such as difficulty in urinating, a burning sensation in the urethra, or a cold sensation. In some cases this may be accompanied by a distending sensation in the very lower abdominal region.

In Chinese medicine one of the most common terms applied to abnormal urination is *lín zhèng,* or painful urinary difficulty. This is a very general concept that can be divided into smaller categories, one of which is hot painful urinary difficulty *(rè lín).* This term describes an abnormal sensation during urination, together with a change in color of the urine. There is a marked increase in the frequency of urination, but each time the quantity of urine decreases, sometimes to the extent that it only drips out. The color of the urine becomes either yellow or deep yellow. This type of urination is very urgent. There is a painful, burning sensation in the urethra, and after urinating, the patient feels that they should urinate again. In extreme cases the patient may be afraid to urinate because of these sensations. In other cases there may be blood in the urine, and it is then termed bloody painful urinary difficulty *(xuè lín).*

The main cause of hot painful urinary difficulty is retention of damp-heat in the lower burner, which impairs the qi activity in the Bladder. Because the dampness obstructs the qi activity it is classified as a turbid pathogenic factor. Retention of dampness in the Bladder can result in obstruction of qi in the Bladder and urethra, causing abnormal urination (such as dripping of urine) and distention of the Bladder, even after urination. Consumption of body fluids caused by pathogenic heat leads to concentration of urine; thus, the urine becomes yellow and even bloody, and there is a painful, urgent, and burning sensation in the urethra.

Fig. 6-3

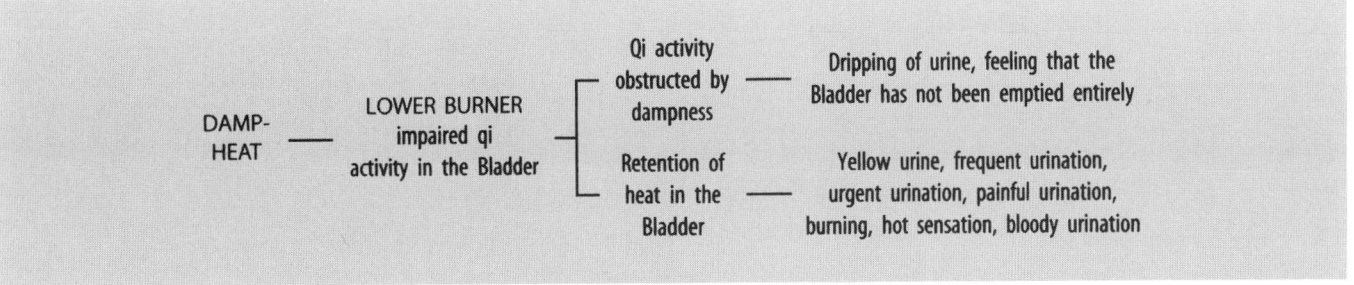

DAMP-HEAT — LOWER BURNER impaired qi activity in the Bladder

Qi activity obstructed by dampness — Dripping of urine, feeling that the Bladder has not been emptied entirely

Retention of heat in the Bladder — Yellow urine, frequent urination, urgent urination, painful urination, burning, hot sensation, bloody urination

If the pathogenic damp-heat is severe it can also affect the circulation of qi and blood through the entire body, giving rise to symptoms of a general nature.

Cause of disease

Damp-heat

The patient has frequent and urgent urination, a burning sensation in the urethra, bloody urine, is thirsty but not inclined to drink much, has a red tongue with a yellow, greasy coating, and a slippery pulse. All of this is evidence of a disturbance caused by pathogenic heat; that the qi activity has been blocked by pathogenic dampness; and that retention of dampness has resulted in the long, recurrent history of the disorder. Thus, damp-heat is the cause of the disease.

Site of disease

Bladder

The patient's main complaint is bloody urine with symptoms that are characteristic of abnormal urination and recurrent attacks of cystitis. All of this indicates that the Bladder is the site of the disease.

Pathological change

The history is fairly simple in this case, and the symptoms are both straightforward and obvious. The patient has symptoms which are typical of bloody painful urinary difficulty, as there is blood in the urine.

The disorder is recurrent, and has lasted for ten years. It was caused by dampness, a substantial pathogenic factor that remains in the body and is difficult to remove; the condition can therefore last a long time. Injury to the antipathogenic factors, however, is not severe: there are no strong symptoms of deficiency between attacks, and the symptoms occur only during attacks.

Dampness is heavy and turbid in nature. It sinks to the lower part of the body where it enters the Bladder, obstructing the qi activity in the Bladder and urinary tract as well. Meanwhile, the retention of heat can also disturb the qi activity in the Bladder, and lead to lower abdominal pain and abnormal urination. Hot painful urinary difficulty typically involves only a change in the color of the urine, and the disorder remains in the qi level; here, however, the urine is also bloody, which indicates that the pathogenic heat has penetrated more deeply and affected the blood system, resulting in an injury to the blood vessels in the Bladder. This means that there is bloody painful urinary difficulty.

The pathogenic heat in the lower burner has affected the circulation of qi and blood throughout the body, thus the patient suffers from other general symptoms, including fever. Her restlessness is caused by heat disturbing the Heart spirit, for which there are two possible explanations: either the pathological heat directly disturbed the Heart spirit; or, because of the Heart's interior/exterior relationship with the Small Intestine, the heat from the Bladder affected the Small Intestine, and, via the channels, the Heart spirit as well.

The thirst results from the retention of the pathogenic heat, which is consuming the body fluids; the retention of dampness, however, causes the patient to have little inclination to drink. The patient has had no bowel movements during the past two days because the heat has consumed the body fluids from the Large Intestine, causing constipation.

Fig. 6-4

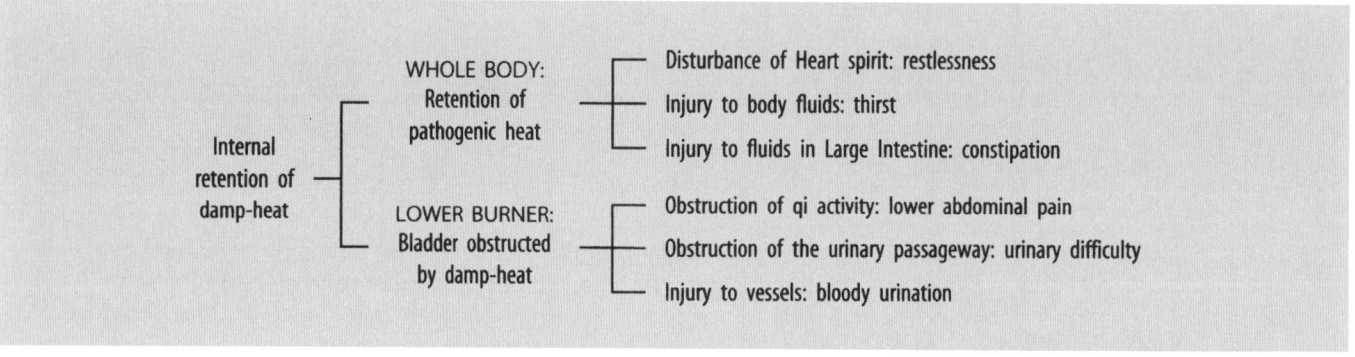

The red tongue and yellow coating are manifestations of heat. The yellow, greasy tongue coating reflects the presence of damp-heat. The middle part of the tongue corresponds with the middle burner, while the root corresponds with the lower burner. In this case, the middle and lower sections of the tongue coating are thick; in light of these symptoms, we may infer that the pathogenic factors are retained in the lower burner, and partially affect the middle burner. The slippery, forceful pulse reflects the retention of dampness in the body.

Pattern of disease

This is an interior pattern, as there are no symptoms of invasion by a pathogenic factor, and the disorder is located in the lower burner.

The deep red color of the urine, burning sensation when the patient urinates, restlessness, and the tongue and pulse signs are all indicative of heat.

The damp-heat in the lower burner, forceful pulse, and lack of injury to the antipathogenic factors indicate a pattern of excess.

Additional notes

1. What is the source of the pathogenic damp-heat?

Pathogenic damp-heat can be either of external or internal origin. For example, if one gets caught in the rain, spends a lot of time in the water, sleeps in a damp room, or lives in a damp climate or environment, dampness or damp-heat can enter through the surface of the body. In some instances damp-heat can directly affect the lower burner and cause illness. As an internal pathogenic factor, damp-heat—which can manifest as a dysfunction in the Spleen's transportation and transformation of water or body fluids, retention of dampness and water inside the body, or a constitutional tendency toward damp-heat—can travel downward to the lower part of the body, where it causes corresponding symptoms.

In this case the history is very long, and it is therefore difficult to ascertain exactly what happened at the very beginning. But we can be quite certain that damp-heat has been retained inside the body.

2. Is there any pattern of deficiency in this case?

Does the fact that the patient suffers from lassitude, a poor appetite, and lower back pain during attacks indicate Spleen or Kidney deficiency?

Actually, these symptoms are all very mild and occur only during attacks. The damp-heat has interfered with the qi and blood in the lower burner, resulting in the lower back pain. The damp-heat can also impede the upward and downward movement of normal qi in the middle burner, causing the patient to suffer from temporary lassitude and a poor appetite. With this in mind, together with the thick tongue coating and forceful pulse, we can conclude that there is not enough evidence to suggest a pattern of deficiency. Similarly, although there is damp-heat, there are not enough symptoms to connect the dampness with Spleen deficiency.

3. Which is stronger, the heat or the dampness?

When dampness and heat combine to form a pathogenic factor, we can say that there is both a yin factor (dampness) and a yang factor (heat). It is important to determine which of the two is stronger, or if both are of equal strength.

In this case the frequent and urgent urination, burning sensation in the urethra, and yellow, bloody urine all suggest that the heat in the Bladder is very strong. Also the patient's fever, constipation, red tongue, and yellow coating indicate that heat prevails overall in the body. Thus, in this instance the heat is stronger than the dampness.

4. How does one distinguish between hot painful urinary difficulty and bloody painful urinary difficulty?

Examine the symptoms and the pathological change. An important distinction is whether or not there is blood in the urine. Hot painful urinary difficulty mainly indicates that the heat is affecting the qi level; bloody painful urinary difficulty occurs when the pathogenic factor has penetrated more deeply and affects the blood system. Thus, bloody painful urinary difficulty is more severe and occurs more deeply at the site of the disease. Also, because they affect different systems of the body, the principles of treatment are different for each.

Conclusion

1. According to the eight principles:
   Interior, heat, excess.

2. According to etiology:
   Damp-heat.

3. According to theory of qi, blood, and body fluids:
   Heat at the blood level.

4. According to Organ theory:
   Damp-heat in the Bladder.

Treatment principle

1. Clear the heat and drain the dampness.

2. Cool the blood.

Explanation of treatment principle

The basic treatment principle is to clear the heat and drain the dampness. However, because the heat and dampness are of different natures, their relative strength is easily altered during the course of an illness. It is therefore important to determine whether clearing the heat or draining the dampness is to have priority.

In this case the heat is stronger than the dampness, therefore clearing the heat is the main principle that should govern treatment. If the dampness were stronger than the heat, or if the dampness and heat were of equal strength, the main treatment principle would change accordingly.

Damp-heat can affect different parts of the body. The method for removing it depends in part on the site of disease. If the dampness is situated on the surface of the body, the sweating method is used, releasing the dampness through the skin. If the dampness affects the middle burner, the Spleen can be strengthened in order to promote the Spleen's function in the transportation and transformation of water. If dampness affects the lower burner, we must promote urination (a diuretic method) to drain the excessive dampness from the body. In this case the damp-heat is retained in the lower burner (the Bladder), and thus the diuretic method was chosen to drain it.

Basic herbal formula

Eight-Herb Powder for Rectification *(ba zheng san)* is the basic formula used to treat hot and bloody painful urinary difficulty. The formula consists of the following ingredients:

Semen Plantaginis *(che qian zi)* 10g
Herba Dianthi *(qu mai)* 10g
Herba Polygoni Avicularis *(bian xu)* 10g
Talcum *(hua shi)* 10g
Fructus Gardeniae Jasminoidis *(zhi zi)* 10g
Caulis Mutong *(mu tong)* 10g
treated Radix et Rhizoma Rhei *(zhi da huang)* 10g
Medulla Junci Effusi *(deng xin cao)* 10g
Radix Glycyrrhizae Uralensis *(gan cao)* 10g

Explanation of basic herbal formula

The main indications of this formula are yellow, bloody, or cloudy urine, frequent urination, and difficulty in urinating combined with a burning sensation. Severe cases may present with urinary blockage *(lóng bì)* with difficulty in urination or inability to urinate, along with lower abdominal distention and pain. The tongue coating is yellow and greasy, the pulse is slippery and rapid. The basic pathological change in this pattern is that damp-heat in the Bladder has obstructed the urethra.

In this formula, Semen Plantaginis *(che qian zi)* is sweet and cold, Talcum *(hua shi)* is sweet, bland, and cold, and Caulis Mutong *(mu tong)*, Herba Dianthi *(qu mai)*, and Herba Polygoni Avicularis *(bian xu)* are bitter and cold. Each of these substances is associated with the Bladder, Small Intestine, or Kidney channel. They remove obstruction from the urinary tract and promote urination. All are cold in nature, and they are thus an important group of herbs for clearing heat. Here they are used to drain the dampness and heat in the Bladder through urination. Together they serve as both chief and deputy herbs in this formula.

There are two assistant herbs. Fructus Gardeniae Jasminoidis *(zhi zi)* is bitter and cold. It is associated with the Triple Burner channel, and thus drains the damp-heat through the Triple Burner. Radix et Rhizoma Rhei *(da huang)* is bitter and cold, and is associated with the Heart, Spleen, Stomach, and Large Intestine channels. It clears heat and quells fire; it also cools the blood.

The two envoy herbs are Medulla Junci Effusi *(deng xin cao)* and Radix Glycyrrhizae Uralensis *(gan cao)*. The former is sweet, bland, and slightly cold, and is associated with the Heart and Small Intestine channels. It clears heat and promotes the downward movement of the qi to guide out the heat. As most of the herbs in this formula expel the pathogenic factors, Radix Glycyrrhizae Uralensis *(gan cao)* is used to regulate and harmonize those herbs, preventing them from injuring the antipathogenic factors.

This formula is primarily used to treat hot painful urinary difficulty. It must be modified if used to treat other types of painful urinary difficulty.

Modified herbal formula

Semen Plantaginis *(che qian zi)* 10g
Talcum *(hua shi)* 10g
Fructus Gardeniae Jasminoidis *(zhi zi)* 10g
Radix et Rhizoma Rhei *(da huang)* 8g
Rhizoma Imperatae Cylindricae *(bai mao gen)* 10g
Herba Cephalanoplos Segeti *(xiao ji)* 12g
Medulla Junci Effusi *(deng xin cao)* 10g
Semen Coicis Lachryma-jobi *(yi yi ren)* 12g

Explanation of modified herbal formula

This case involves damp-heat in the lower burner. Eight-Herb Powder for Rectification *(ba zheng san)*, which is typically used for clearing heat from the qi level, was chosen to clear the heat, drain the dampness, and promote the Bladder functions. In this case, however, the damp-heat has already affected the blood. We therefore added herbs that cool the blood and stop the bleeding.

Herba Cephalanoplos Segeti *(xiao ji)* and Rhizoma Imperatae Cylindricae *(bai mao gen)* both cool the blood and promote urination; they are commonly used in treating bloody urine. Radix et Rhizoma Rhei *(da huang)* not only cools the blood, but also clears heat by purging, and treats constipation. We have reduced the number of herbs that expel pathogenic factors through the qi level in order to prevent those bitter and cold herbs from injuring the antipathogenic factors. Medulla Junci Effusi *(deng xin cao)* is retained in this modified prescription because its function is associated with the Heart channel. It can clear heat from the Heart, and thereby relieve the restlessness. In the original formula the only ingredient used to harmonize the herbs and strengthen the antipathogenic factors is Radix Glycyrrhizae Uralensis *(gan cao)*. In the modified formula it is replaced by Semen Coicis Lachryma-jobi *(yi yi ren)*, which not only promotes urination in order to expel the pathogenic factors, but also protects and prevents injury to the antipathogenic factors.

Follow-up

When the patient presented herself at the clinic, she stated very specifically that she did not wish to use antibiotics. Herbs were therefore prescribed, one packet taken daily, in two doses. Three days later, all of the symptoms had been alleviated. Apart from a slight burning sensation while urinating, all was well and there was no more blood in the urine. Both her blood and urine were checked, and were recorded as being normal. The patient took the herbal formula for a week thereafter, and then the treatment was terminated. She was very pleased with the result, and there were no more attacks on follow-up eighteen months later.

CASE 27: **Female, age 35**

Main complaint

Abnormal urination

History

Three days ago, for no apparent reason, the patient began to feel restless and developed a dry, hot sensation all over her body. Her urine became yellow and was greatly reduced in quantity, but there was no change in the frequency of urination. She experiences a burning, painful sensation when she urinates. She sweats excessively, has no aversion to cold, feels dizzy, very irritable, and thirsty, and drinks a large amount of cold beverages. Her appetite has declined. She also complains of dream-disturbed sleep. Her stools have become very dry over the past couple weeks, with one bowel movement every three or four days. She has no pain in the abdominal region, chest, or back.

The patient has always been in good health, and there is no personal or family history of Kidney disorders. The checkup revealed that there is no tenderness in the abdomen. The urine and blood are both normal, and her complexion is red.

Tongue	Red, with a slightly thick, dry, and yellow coating
Pulse	Thin, slippery, and rapid

Analysis of symptoms

1. Yellow urine, pain, and burning sensation while urinating—heat in the lower burner.

2. Hot sensation all over the body, and excessive sweating—pathogenic heat.

3. Thirst, strong inclination to drink cold beverages, reduced quantity of urine, and dry stools—injury to body fluids by pathogenic heat.

4. Restlessness, irritability, and dream-disturbed sleep—disturbance of Heart spirit by pathogenic heat.

5. Poor appetite—impairment of Spleen's transportive and transformative functions.

6. No aversion to cold—not an exterior pattern.

7. Red complexion, red tongue, and dry, yellow coating—heat pattern.

8. Slippery and rapid pulse—heat pattern.

Basic theory of case

In Chinese medicine the yang Organs that are related to the metabolism of water, and the production and excretion of urine, include the Triple Burner, the Small Intestine, and the Bladder.

The Triple Burner is the pathway of water metabolism. It is the biggest yang Organ in the human body, and includes all the yin and yang Organs. Although it is divided into three parts—upper, middle, and lower burners—it is regarded as one organic whole. Liquids enter the body and are transformed into body fluids. This is transported throughout the body via the Triple Burner. Water that is left over after metabolism, and excessive liquids, are then transported downward in the body through the Triple Burner.

The physiological function of the Small Intestine is to transport food and water. After digestion, a mixture of food and water enters the Small Intestine from the Spleen and Stomach. This mixture is composed of a clear component, the liquid, and a turbid component, which is the waste from food. The Small Intestine has a special and specific function of separating these clear and turbid components. The clear, liquid component is transported through the Triple Burner to the Bladder, where it becomes urine, and the turbid, solid component is transported to the Large Intestine and then out through the anus as feces.

The function of the Bladder is to store and excrete the urine. All excessive liquid and waste water eventually reaches the Bladder from various parts of the body, where it becomes urine. Urination depends upon the opening and closing of the Bladder *(Fig. 6-5)*.

Cause of disease

Pathogenic heat

The patient has a hot sensation over her entire body, excessive sweating, restlessness, thirst, yellow urine, a burning and painful sensation when she urinates, a red

Fig. 6-5

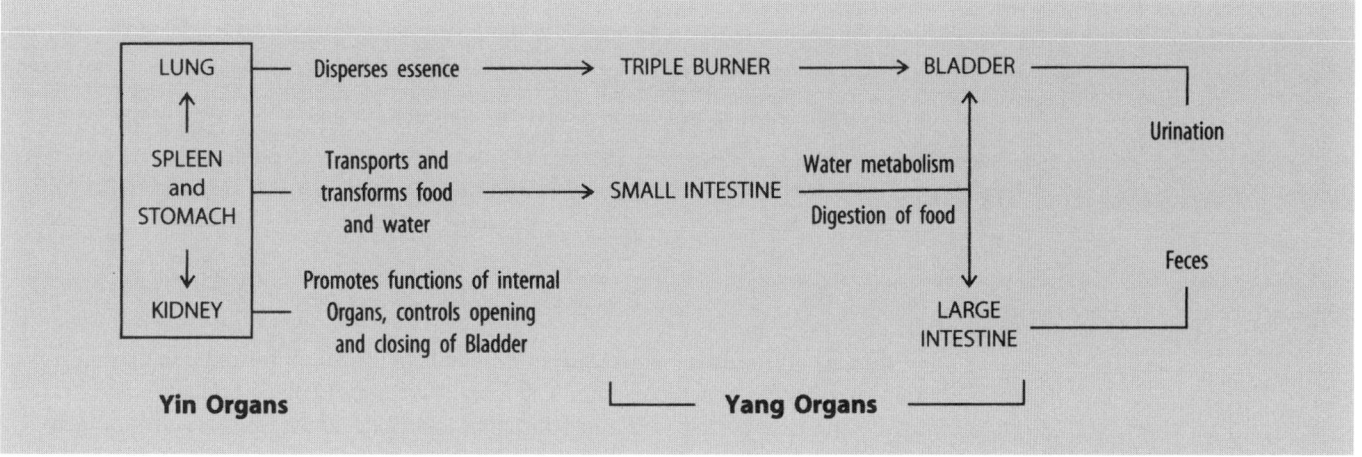

tongue with a yellow coating, and a rapid pulse. All of these symptoms reflect the presence of excessive heat and retention of fire in the body.

Site of disease

Heart and Small Intestine (which affects the Bladder)

The restlessness and irritability indicate that the site of disease is the Heart. The reduced quantity of yellow urine, as well as the burning and painful sensation during urination, points to the Small Intestine.

Pathological change

The restlessness and the dry, hot sensation over the entire body would indicate that the pathogenic heat and fire come from the upper part of the body. In this case they can be attributed to retention of Heart fire. Heat and fire have disturbed the Heart spirit, which is no longer peaceful; thus, the patient has become very restless and irritable, and experiences dream-disturbed sleep. The pathogenic heat and fire can also cause the body fluids to evaporate from the body, which accounts for the hot sensation throughout the body and the excessive sweating. Because the heat has injured the body fluids, the patient feels thirsty and has a strong desire to drink a lot of cold beverages. The heat rises and disturbs the head (literally *qīng gōng,* which means "clear palace"), resulting in the mixing together of clear yang and turbid qi in the head, causing dizziness.

The Triple Burner, Small Intestine, and Bladder are all associated with the production and excretion of urine. A disturbance in any of these yang Organs may lead to an abnormality in urination. Because the Heart and Small Intestine have an interior/exterior relationship, Heart fire can move downward through the channel system to the Small Intestine, where it can cause a pattern of heat excess. In the Small Intestine, the metabolism of water and body fluids can be affected by the pathogenic heat and fire. On one hand, they may be consumed by the heat, reducing the quantity of urine; on the other, the heat can follow the urine into the Bladder, causing the urine to become very hot. This accounts for the hot, burning sensation and pain felt by the patient when she urinates.

Superficially, it would seem that the problem lies within the Bladder, but on closer inspection we find that the disturbance in the Bladder results from the disorder in the Small Intestine. This, in Chinese medicine, presents a special pattern. The pathogenic heat resides mainly in the Small Intestine; it is not retained in the Bladder. We can tell that there is no localized pathogenic heat to stimulate the circulation of qi in the Bladder because, while there is a burning sensation and pain accompanying urination, the urination itself is neither urgent nor abnormally frequent.

Fig. 6-6

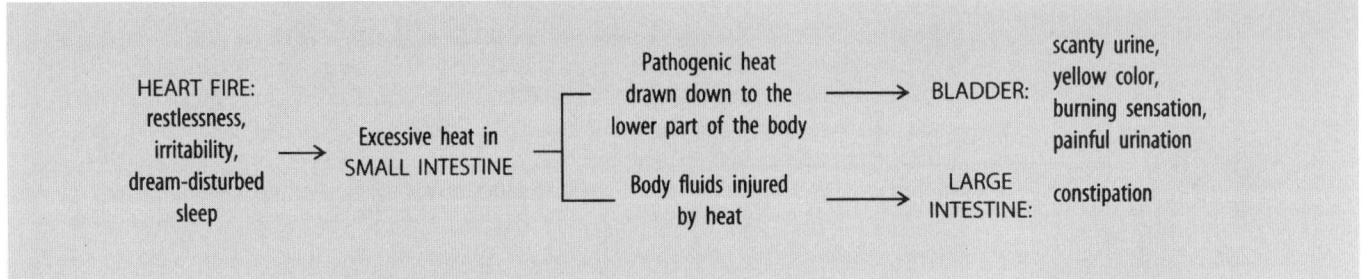

When Heart fire in the upper burner descends to the Small Intestine in the lower burner, it passes through the middle burner, where the Spleen and Stomach are located. The transportive and transformative functions of the Spleen and Stomach are thereby disturbed by the pathogenic heat, which depresses the appetite. However, this is the only symptom involving the middle burner, and is it not particularly severe. Thus, this symptom is not regarded as being especially significant.

Pattern of disease

The origin of the Heart fire is within the body, from whence it affected the Small Intestine and then the Bladder. Because the site of the disease is an internal Organ and not the surface of the body, the pattern is of the interior.

The patient feels hot all over her body and has a red complexion. She is thirsty, her urine is yellow, and her stools are dry. These symptoms reflect a pattern of heat.

As the pathogenic heat is very strong and excessive, and there is no evidence that the antipathogenic factors are deficient, the pattern is one of excess.

Additional notes

1. Is there evidence of Liver disorder in this case?

We know that the Liver governs changes in the emotions. Liver fire rising frequently causes restlessness, irritability, and emotional lability, especially with a tendency towards anger. Besides this type of symptom, there may be other Liver-related complaints involving impairment of the Liver's regulation of the free-flow of qi, such as pain and distention, or a burning sensation in the intercostal and hypochondrial regions. Liver fire can also rise through the channels and disturb the head, causing dizziness and tinnitus; the pulse will then be wiry, rapid, and forceful.

In this case, however, the restlessness and irritability are accompanied by insomnia; there are no other symptoms associated with the Liver. Instead, the other important symptoms involve abnormal urination. We may therefore conclude that it is Heart fire, and not Liver fire, that is the cause of the problem in this case.

2. What is the cause of the thin pulse?

All of the symptoms in this case are characterized by excess, which means that the pathogenic factors are very strong. The one exception is the thin pulse. The reason for this is that, while the pathogenic factor is very strong and has consumed the body fluids and injured the blood to a certain degree (thereby depleting the vessels), the injury is not very severe. Thus, the thin pulse can be disregarded. No special treatment is required, because as soon as the pathogenic heat is removed from the body, the consumption of body fluids and blood will then cease. Because the antipathogenic factors are not deficient in this case, the patient should make an easy recovery.

3. In cases of abnormal urination, how does one distinguish between Heart fire descending to the Small Intestine and damp-heat in the Bladder?

Both of these patterns are characterized by pain and a burning sensation during urination. The main distinguishing criteria are as follows:

• *Difference in urination.* In a pattern of Heart fire descending to the Small Intestine, the main symptoms are pain and a hot, burning sensation during urination. Usually, however, urination is neither frequent nor urgent.

By contrast, where there is damp-heat in the Bladder, urination is frequent, urgent, and painful, and is accompanied by a burning sensation. When the condition becomes severe, patients can suffer urinary blockage *(lóng bì).*

If either of these patterns is severe, there may also be bloody urine.

• *Difference in general symptoms.* A pattern of Heart fire moving down to the Small Intestine presents obvious symptoms of retention of excessive Heart fire, such as restlessness, irritability, insomnia, a red complexion, and ulcers on the tongue and in the mouth. However, there is an absence of lower back or lower abdominal pain.

With damp-heat in the Bladder, there is very obvious distention, pain, and a sensation of fullness in the lower abdominal region, as well as lower back pain, because the symptoms are primarily located in the lower burner. Although the patient may also suffer from such upper burner symptoms as fever and restlessness, they are usually not very severe, since they are caused by the heat in the lower burner affecting the upper burner.

Symptoms like thirst, constipation, a red tongue with a yellow coating, and a rapid pulse, can occur in both of these patterns. However, because the retention of Heart fire is a pure heat pattern, the patient will be thirsty and want to drink a lot of cold beverages, and the tongue coating will be yellow and dry. On the other hand, damp-heat in the Bladder occurs because of the presence of damp-heat; thus, although the patient will feel thirsty, he or she will have little inclination to drink much. Moreover, the tongue coating will not only be yellow, but also greasy.

Conclusion	1. According to the eight principles: Interior, heat, excess.
	2. According to etiology: Retention of pathogenic fire.
	3. According to Organ theory: Heart fire descending to the Small Intestine.
Treatment principle	1. Clear the Heart fire.
	2. Promote urination.

Explanation of treatment principle

In this case, while the symptoms have occurred in the Bladder, which is in the lower burner, the source of the pathogenic fire and heat is the Heart, in the upper burner. Thus, clearing Heart fire to treat the root of the disorder is the basic treatment principle. There are various methods for removing Heart fire, such as clearing the heat and draining the fire, or cooling the blood and clearing the heat. The Heart fire in this case has a very obvious tendency to move downward, where it affects the Small Intestine and the Bladder; treatment should likewise follow this tendency in order to remove the heat and fire. Thus, promoting urination is the principle that is utilized, so that the heat may follow the urine out of the body. One should also clear the heat from the upper burner by following the natural characteristic of heat, which is to rise.

Selection of points

PC-6 *(nei guan)*
CV-5 *(shi men)*
CV-3 *(zhong ji)*
ST-39 *(xia ju xu)* threading to BL-57 *(cheng shan)*
SP-6 *(san yin jiao)*

Explanation of points

PC-6 *(nei guan)* is the connecting point of the arm terminal yin channel. This point is well known for its ability to calm the Heart and spirit, treat disorders of the Heart, regulate qi, and alleviate pain. In addition, it is an important point for treating heat patterns, especially heat patterns involving the Heart channel, Heart fire or heat, as well as heat patterns associated with the Pericardium channel. In this case, because the Heart fire has moved downward to the Small Intestine, causing urinary difficulty, this point is used to regulate the qi, remove the fire, and clear the heat in order to allow the fire to be expelled from the upper burner, following its natural tendency. The reducing method is used so that heat may be cleared from the upper burner.

CV-5 *(shi men)* is very effective in removing obstruction, hence its Chinese name "stone gate," which means "gate of obstruction." In ancient times this point was used to treat amenorrhea, regarded as a typical form of obstruction. It is the alarm point of the Triple Burner; it tonifies the Kidney, strengthens basal qi, clears heat, and drains dampness. It is one of several points used to treat disorders of the urogenital system, such as urinary difficulty, edema, abdominal distention, involuntary seminal emissions, impotence, amenorrhea, excessive leukorrhea, and excessive uterine bleeding. The point is also used to treat other conditions like dysentery, diarrhea, abdominal pain, and hernia.

CV-3 *(zhong ji)* is located 4 units below the umbilicus in a region regarded as being the middle of the body, hence the name of the point, which means "middle pole." This is the alarm point of the Bladder, and the meeting point of the conception vessel and three leg yin channels. It clears heat, drains dampness, tonifies the Kidney, and strengthens basal qi. It is one of the most commonly used points for disorders of the urogenital system, such as retention of urine, enuresis, burning and painful urination, and urinary difficulty. It can also be used to treat many disorders of the reproductive system such as impotence, amenorrhea, leukorrhea, excessive uterine bleeding, and infertility. In this case, where there is a pattern of interior excessive heat, the reducing method is used to clear the heat. Because this point is located in the very lower abdominal region, it serves as a local point for this area, and is very effective in clearing the heat from the lower burner (Bladder) that has come from Heart fire in this case.

ST-39 *(xia ju xu)* threading to BL-57 *(cheng shan)*. This is the lower uniting point of the Small Intestine. It reduces heat, removes qi obstruction, and regulates the functions of the Intestines. A 2.5 or 3 unit needle is used to puncture this point, threading toward BL-57 *(cheng shan)*, which is on the lower part of the calf. The purpose of threading the needle in this manner is to drain the heat, which has come, via the leg yang brightness channel and the Small Intestine, from the Heart fire. Because ST-39 *(xia ju xu)* is threaded toward the Bladder channel, puncturing this point can also help regulate that channel, removing the heat from, and regulating the qi in, the Bladder. This, then, is an example of using one needle to affect two channels (Stomach and Bladder), and to regulate three Organs (Stomach, Small Intestine, Bladder).

SP-6 *(san yin jiao)* is the meeting point of the three leg yin channels. It regulates the Spleen and Stomach, strengthens the Kidney and Liver, regulates the qi in the lower burner, and removes obstruction from the channels and collaterals. This point is commonly used to treat urinary disorders, such as urinary difficulty, retention of urine, and enuresis. In this case it serves an assistant point, employed to regulate the qi, and, at the same time, strengthen the Spleen and thereby relieve the symptoms involving the impairment of that Organ's transportive and transformative functions.

Combination of points

PC-6 *(nei guan)*, ST-39 *(xia ju xu)*, and CV-3 *(zhong ji)*. These three points can be thought of as a small prescription for treating disorders involving urinary difficulty caused by the transference of Heart fire to the Small Intestine. The combination is especially good for patterns of pure interior excessive heat. The reducing method is used at all three points, but it is important to take into account the age and constitution of each patient when using the reducing method. Also, the antipathogenic factors must not be injured. CV-3 *(zhong ji)* serves here as a local point to clear the heat from the Bladder and lower abdomen. PC-6 *(nei guan)* clears heat from the upper burner, thereby reaching the source of the heat or fire in the Heart. ST-39 *(xia ju xu)* is used to clear the heat from the Small Intestine. Thus, these three points interact in treating this particular pattern in which heat moves downward from the Heart to the Small Intestine.

CV-5 *(shi men)* and CV-3 *(zhong ji)*. In this combination, two alarm points are used. The former is the alarm point of the Triple Burner, and the latter is the alarm point of the Bladder. Because the Triple Burner is the pathway for the metabolism of water, promoting the function of the Triple Burner will help drain dampness and promote urination. The Bladder is the Organ that stores urine. These two points are used to promote the functioning of these two Organs and to strengthen the regulation of the qi. Alarm points serve generally to remove excess and regulate qi. Here the two points are used together to regulate the qi and remove the obstruction from the lower burner.

Both points are located on the conception vessel, and there is a distance of only 2 units between them. A special method (threading) is used to link them together. The points are punctured horizontally, with the tips of the needles angled toward the lower abdominal region. The angle of insertion is based on the patient's build. If the build is not too heavy and the surface around the abdomen is thin, the angle of insertion is about 15°, but if the patient is large and has a heavy build, the angle is about 20°. The purpose is to link one needle to the other, in order to strengthen the action of regulating the qi and removing the heat. CV-5 *(shi men)* is 2 units below the umbilicus (close to the location of the Small Intestine), and CV-3 *(zhong ji)* is 4 units below the umbilicus (close to the Bladder); threading the two points is used to strengthen the draining of heat from the Small Intestine and Bladder in order to promote urination, remove the heat, and ameliorate the symptoms.

Follow-up

No herbs were prescribed for this patient, just acupuncture, which was administered once daily for three days. By then the quantity of urine had increased, the color was normal, the hot sensation during urination was alleviated, and the feeling of general feverishness had diminished. The patient's appetite returned to normal, and she dreamed less at night. She experienced no dizziness. Her stools, however, were still dry, and she still felt thirsty and wanted to drink a lot.

The treatment was therefore continued for another week, treating every other day. ST-25 *(tian shu)* was substituted for CV-5 *(shi men)* in order to regulate the functions of the Large Intestine and relieve the constipation. By week's end, the feverishness had completely disappeared, her sleep and urination had returned to normal, she had bowel movements almost every other day, and her stools were not as dry as before. The treatment was then terminated, and the patient advised to eat more vegetables and spend more time outdoors with physical exercise.

One month later the patient returned for a checkup. She now had bowel movements once a day or once every other day, her urination was normal, and all the other symptoms had disappeared.

This patient's complaint lasted for just three days. She had previously enjoyed good health and had no history of chronic illness. Although she had the advantage of being fairly young, she had a constitutional tendency toward excessive yang. In view of the fact that the accumulation of Heart heat and fire had lasted much longer than three days, it was important not only to deal with the short-lived urinary disorder, but also to have the patience to treat the retention of Heart fire, which sometimes requires lengthy treatment. In this case the treatment lasted ten days. Although this is longer than the history of the urinary disorder, it is a very quick response to the treatment. Many patients need much longer treatment time, either with acupuncture alone, or both acupuncture and herbs. Herbs were not administered in this case because the acupuncture worked so well and the patient wanted to avoid the trouble of preparing and cooking the herbs.

CASE 28: **Male, age 34**

Main complaint

Abnormal urination and infertility

History

For three years the patient has been suffering from pain in the area between the anus and testes (perineum). Sometimes the pain radiates towards the testes. He has slight urinary frequency and incontinence. After urinating, there is often some white discharge. Urination is not urgent or painful, and there is no burning sensation in the urethra. At the outset, the patient did not pay much attention to this complaint.

Another problem is that the patient and his wife of five years have been unable to have children. Six months ago the couple went to the hospital for a checkup. A prostatic secretion test showed that the patient has an excessive amount of white blood cells. A sperm test revealed a large number of white blood cells and dead sperm. The diagnosis was chronic prostatitis.

At present the patient still has all the symptoms described above, and is also severely depressed, as his wife wants a divorce. The patient experiences mental fatigue, severe lassitude, dizziness, restlessness, and a hot sensation in the chest. He can be very irritable and has episodic sweating on his head, very bad insomnia, and a poor appetite. He does not feel thirsty. The lower back and knees feel sore and weak, a condition that worsens if he stands or walks for any length of time. His urine is yellow, and he has a bowel movement either once daily or once every other day. The stools tend to be dry. His complexion is dark and lusterless.

Tongue

Slim and thin body, red in color, with a thin, yellow coating

Pulse

Sunken and thin

Analysis of symptoms

1. Pain in the perineum radiating to the testes—impairment of the circulation of qi and blood in the channels and collaterals.
2. Slight urinary frequency and incontinence, and white discharge after urination—dysfunction of the Kidney in controlling the urination and essence.
3. No urgent urination, pain, or burning sensation during urination—absence of pathogenic heat in the Bladder.
4. Infertility after several years of marriage—probable Kidney deficiency.
5. Lassitude and dizziness—malnourishment of the marrow and brain.
6. Restlessness, irritability, and insomnia—disturbance of Heart spirit.
7. Episodic sweating around the head, yellow urine, and dry stools—injury to the body fluids by heat.
8. Soreness and weakness in the lower back—malnourishment of the lower back caused by Kidney deficiency.
9. Dark and lusterless complexion—Kidney deficiency.
10. Red tongue, slim body, and a thin, yellow coating—heat from yin deficiency.
11. Sunken, thin pulse—interior, deficient pattern.

Basic theory of case

Prostatitis is frequently encountered in middle-aged males, or even young men with healthy constitutions. In clinical practice the condition is usually chronic, and in severe cases the reproductive ability can be affected. The main symptoms of the disorder are a white discharge from the urethra and varying degrees of a painful, distending sensation or discomfort in the very lower abdominal region, perineum, lower back, sacrum, or around the testes. When acute, the patient will have frequent, painful, and urgent urination, but when the disorder is chronic, there is only frequent urination.

In Chinese medicine the Kidney is responsible for storing essence. Kidney deficiency can impair the Kidney's ability to control the essence, which may then be involuntarily secreted from the body as a white discharge after urinating. In severe cases the white discharge is secreted on its own, independent of urination. Usually the site of the disorder is in the Kidney, not the Bladder. Because it is not caused by pathogenic heat disturbing the Bladder, there is an absence of such symptoms as urgent or painful urination.

Fig. 6-7

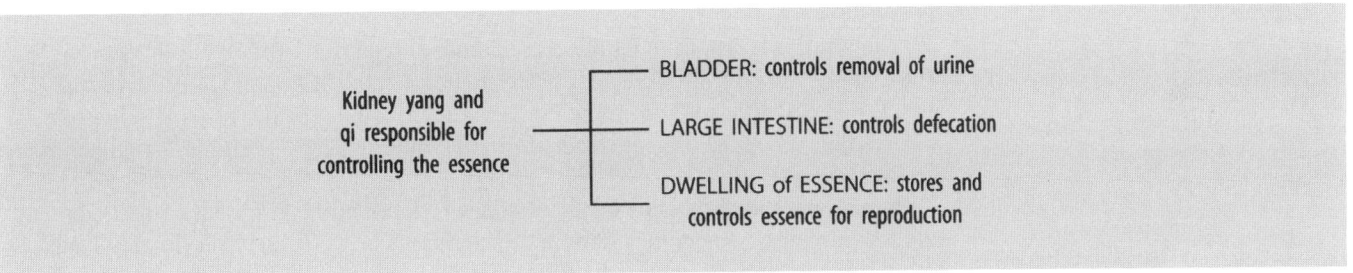

A common cause of the failure of the controlling function of the Kidney is deficiency of yin or yang in the Kidney. Deficiency of yin is usually accompanied by symptoms that are characteristic of heat from deficiency, such as a feverish sensation or tidal fever, malar flush, a burning sensation in the chest, palms, and soles, dryness in the mouth and throat, a red tongue with very little coating, and a thin and rapid pulse. Deficiency of Kidney yang is often associated with internal cold, with such symptoms as a feeling of being cold, general lassitude, fatigue, coldness in the limbs, clear urine, loose stools, a pale, lusterless tongue with a white and moist coating, and a sunken and slow pulse.

Very occasionally, the failure of the Kidney in controlling the essence and urination can be complicated by damp-heat in the Bladder. When this occurs, the symptoms can be very similar to hot painful urinary difficulty (see case 26).

Cause of disease

Deficiency of antipathogenic factors

In this case the patient has only very mild urinary frequency, which is neither urgent nor painful. The fact that there is no burning sensation in the urethra while urinating reflects the absence of an excessive pathogenic factor. The disorder has lasted a long time and the patient feels fatigued, experiences general lassitude, and has soreness and weakness in the lower back and knees. This, combined with the tongue and pulse signs, establishes the diagnosis of deficiency of antipathogenic factors.

Site of disease

Kidney

The patient has urinary frequency and incontinence, a white discharge after urination, soreness and weakness in the lower back and knees, and infertility. All of this evidence indicates that the site of disease is the Kidney.

Pathological change

Physiologically, the distinguishing functional characteristic of the five yin Organs is to store and retain (essence, for example), while that of the six yang Organs is to transport substances and fluids. The Kidney is a yin Organ that stores the essence of the body. It is important that the Kidney store the essence for important uses, rather than releasing it unnecessarily.

In this case the patient has mild urinary incontinence and frequency, but there is no abnormal sensation during urination. This indicates a dysfunction of the Kidney in controlling, with accompanying Bladder symptoms in opening and closing. The white discharge passing out through the urethra after urination suggests a dysfunction of the Kidney in controlling the essence. In other words, Kidney essence is leaking from the body.

The Kidney is located in the lower burner; Kidney yin provides nourishment to the tissues and Organs in the lower burner. When essence involuntarily leaks from the body it will injure the Kidney yin, which interferes with the delivery of local nutrition; hence the soreness and weakness in the lower back area. The knees are similarly affected. The pain in the perineum and testes is likewise caused by yin deficiency, which results in poor circulation of qi and blood in the local channels and vessels.

The brain, according to Chinese medicine, is regarded as the "sea of marrow." The essence and qi from the Kidney rises to nourish the brain, and to produce marrow. When essence leaks from the body, malnourishment of the brain and marrow also results; hence the patient suffers from very poor energy, lassitude, fatigue, and dizziness.

Because of the deficiency of yin, the face is deprived of sufficient nourishment, and the complexion becomes dark and lusterless. The deficiency of yin also leads to a preponderance of yang, which gives rise to heat from deficiency, which rises and disturbs the Heart spirit; hence the restlessness, hot sensations, insomnia, and irritability. Heat from deficiency can also expel fluids from the body in the form of excessive sweating. It may also injure the body fluids, causing yellow urine and dry stools.

The thin tongue body, red tongue, and thin, yellow coating reflect the malnourishment of fluids caused by yin deficiency, and also the retention of heat from deficiency. The sunken, thin nature of the pulse suggests a pattern of interior deficiency: because of the yin deficiency, the vessels are not properly filled.

Pattern of disease

This is an interior pattern because of its chronic nature, and the injury to the Kidney and antipathogenic factors.

There is deficiency of yin, and rising of heat from deficiency: the patient is restless, sweats excessively, and has a red tongue with a yellow coating, all of which reflect a pattern of heat.

The injury is to the yin and essence. There is no evidence of an excessive pathogenic factor. It is therefore a pattern of deficiency.

Additional notes

1. What is the cause of the infertility in this case?

It was noted earlier that chronic prostatitis is the cause of the infertility in this case. According to Chinese medicine, the essence, which is stored in the Kidney, is closely related to development, growth, and the reproductive functions. Severe injury to Kidney essence, therefore, can cause infertility.

In this case the patient has suffered from abnormal urination for the past three years, but in view of the fact that the couple has been unable to produce children after five years of marriage, the infertility has obviously been around longer than the abnormal urination. So, is there any relationship between the infertility and the chronic prostatitis?

Reviewing the history, we find that the patient came to the clinic six mouths ago, at which time he stated that he had been suffering from abnormal urination for about three years. From this we can deduce that the disorder had become increasingly obvious over the period of three years, and finally got his attention; in other words, it is very difficult to ascertain exactly when the abnormal urination actually began. Thus, it is fair to assume that the cause of the infertility is primarily associated with the disorder of the prostate gland. The conventional medical checkup verified this relationship between the two disorders.

2. Cases 26, 27, and 28 all concern abnormal urination, but what are the differences among them?

Case 26 involved damp-heat in the Bladder, case 27 a pattern of Heart fire moving downward to the Small Intestine, and case 28 a failure of the Kidney in controlling the essence. The main complaint in each of these cases was abnormal urination, but other than the variation in symptoms, the most important differences were the site of disease, pathological change, and nature of the underlying pattern.

• *Site of disease and pathological change*

In case 26 the pathogenic factors directly affected the Bladder, which led to the abnormal urination. In case 27 the pathogenic factors first affected the Heart, and from there moved downward to the Small Intestine, where they caused abnormal urination. In the present case (28) the site of disease is the Kidney; the disorder in this Organ has affected the Bladder, which has resulted in abnormal urination.

• *Nature of the patterns*

Cases 26 and 27 involved heat in patterns of excess; this case also involves heat, but from deficiency. Thus, the symptoms, principles of treatment, and methods will be different in each case *(Fig. 6-8)*.

3. Is there a Heart disorder in this case?

The patient suffers from symptoms involving a disturbance of Heart spirit: restlessness, a hot sensation in the chest, irritability, and insomnia. Aren't these symptoms evidence of Heart fire rising?

Fig. 6-8

	CASE 26	CASE 27	CASE 28
SIMILAR SYMPTOM	Abnormal urination	Abnormal urination	Abnormal urination
DISTINGUISHING SYMPTOMS (URINATION)	Yellow urine, bloody urine, urinary frequency and urgency, hot and painful urination	Yellow urine, hot and painful urination	Yellow urine, whitish discharge following urination, slightly frequent urination, incontinence of small quantity of urine, no urgency, burning or painful urination
ACCOMPANYING SYMPTOMS	High fever, dry mouth, strong desire to drink, restlessness, poor appetite, pain in the lower abdomen	Very severe restlessness, irritability and insomnia	Red tongue, slim and thin body, thin yellow coating, sunken, thin pulse
	Red tongue, yellow, thick, and greasy coating, slippery, forceful pulse	Red tongue, yellow, thick and dry coating, thin, slippery, rapid pulse	Dizziness, general lassitude, fatigue, accompanied by restlessness, irritability, soreness and weakness in the lower back
SITE of DISEASE	Bladder	Heart, Small Intestine	Kidney, Heart
DIAGNOSIS	Excessive heat pattern; damp-heat retention in the Bladder	Excessive heat pattern; Heart fire descends to Small Intestine	Heat from deficiency; impairment of Kidney's controlling function; disharmony between Heart and Kidney

As explained above, the basic pathological change in this case is Kidney yin deficiency, which has led to the rising of heat from deficiency. This type of heat disturbs the Heart spirit. Under normal conditions a state of harmony exists between the Heart and Kidney, that is, between fire and water. The rising heat from Kidney yin deficiency has disturbed this harmonious relationship. But since the disturbance of the Heart spirit manifested after the appearance of Kidney yin deficiency, it is considered secondary to the Kidney disorder. We may therefore dismiss Heart fire rising as the underlying diagnosis.

Conclusion

1. According to the eight principles:
   Interior, heat, deficiency.

2. According to Organ theory:
   Impairment of the Kidney's controlling function,
   Kidney yin deficiency, and disharmony between the Kidney and Heart.

Treatment principle

1. Promote the Kidney function of controlling the essence.

2. Nourish the Kidney yin.

Explanation of treatment principle

Since there is yin deficiency, the yin of the body requires nourishment. And since the yin deficiency is accompanied by internal heat, the cooling method is used in order to prevent further injury to the yin from heat.

The most important treatment principle for this patient is promotion of the Kidney function in controlling the essence. Only this can prevent further loss of yin and essence. Thus, strengthening the controlling function is essential to the treatment of the root of this disorder *(zhì běn)*.

It is unnecessary to treat the infertility directly. The Kidney function will improve over time, and, at a later period, the reproductive function will gradually be restored.

Basic herbal formula

Mantis Egg-Case Powder *(sang piao xiao san)* is the principal formula used in the treatment of Kidney deficiency leading to involuntary seminal emissions and enuresis. The formula contains the following ingredients:

Ootheca Mantidis *(sang piao xiao)* 30g
Radix Polygalae Tenuifoliae *(yuan zhi)* 30g
Rhizoma Acori Graminei *(shi chang pu)* 30g
Os Draconis *(long gu)* 30g
Radix Ginseng *(ren shen)* 30g
Sclerotium Poriae Cocos *(fu ling)* 30g
Radix Angelicae Sinensis *(dang gui)* 30g
Plastrum Testudinis *(gui ban)* 30g

Explanation of basic herbal formula

The indications for this formula are urinary frequency, white, cloudy urine or enuresis, involuntary seminal emissions, fatigue, poor energy, appetite, and memory, a pale tongue with a white coating, and a sunken, forceless pulse.

The underlying pathogenesis of this pattern is deficiency of the Kidney and Heart, and disharmony between water and fire. Because of the Heart qi deficiency and thus the loss of proper nourishment for the Heart spirit, the patient's memory and mental condition are very poor. Kidney qi deficiency has interfered with the Kidney's ability to control urination and seminal emissions, and thus the patient suffers from involuntary seminal emissions or enuresis, frequent urination, and white, cloudy urine.

This formula regulates and tonifies the Heart and Kidney, and promotes the Kidney function of controlling seminal emissions and urination. The chief herb is Ootheca Mantidis *(sang piao xiao)*, which is sweet, salty, and neutral, and is associated with the Liver and Kidney channels. It promotes the controlling function of the Kidney, and thereby relieves the associated symptoms of involuntary seminal emissions and enuresis.

There are two deputy herbs. Os Draconis *(long gu)* is sweet, astringent, and slightly cold. It is associated with the Heart channel and promotes the restraining function of the body. It is used in treating disorders like involuntary seminal emissions and spontaneous sweating. It settles the emotions and benefits the Heart spirit, relieves absentmindedness and lack of concentration, palpitations, and insomnia. The other deputy, Plastrum Testudinis *(gui ban)*, is sweet, salty, and cold, and is associated with the Heart and Kidney channels. It nourishes the yin of the body in treating Kidney deficiency, as well as the blood in treating Heart deficiency.

There are three assistant herbs. Radix Ginseng *(ren shen)* is sweet and slightly warm. It is associated with the Spleen and Lung channels, and is very effective in strengthening the source qi of the body. Sclerotium Poriae Cocos *(fu ling)* is sweet, bland, and neutral, and is associated with the Heart and Kidney channels. It soothes the Heart spirit. Radix Angelicae Sinensis *(dang gui)* is sweet, acrid, and warm, and is associated with the Heart and Liver channels. It nourishes the Heart blood.

Rhizoma Acori Graminei *(shi chang pu)* and Radix Polygalae Tenuifoliae *(yuan zhi)* serve here as both assistant and envoy herbs. Both substances are acrid and warm, and are associated with the Heart channel. They soothe the Heart spirit and promote harmony between the Heart and Kidney.

This formula focusses on the Heart and Kidney, especially in the treatment of qi deficiency.

Modified herbal formula	Ootheca Mantidis *(sang piao xiao)* 15g
	Radix Rehmanniae Glutinosae Conquitae *(shu di huang)* 20g
	Plastrum Testudinis *(gui ban)* 15g
	Fructus Corni Officinalis *(shan zhu yu)* 15g
	Rhizoma Coptidis *(huang lian)* 5g
	Tuber Ophiopogonis Japonici *(mai men dong)* 8g
	Sclerotium Poriae Cocos *(fu ling)* 8g
	Semen Nelumbinis Nuciferae *(lian zi)* 8g

Explanation of modified herbal formula

Because the Kidney's control over seminal emissions and urination is impaired in this case, Mantis Egg-Case Powder *(sang piao xiao san)* is used as the basic formula to promote the controlling function of the Kidney. The emphasis of the basic formula is on restoring harmony to the Heart and Kidney, and the treatment of qi deficiency. In this case, however, there is no apparent qi deficiency. Rather, the primary complaint is Kidney yin deficiency, which has led to heat from deficiency and disturbance of the Heart spirit. Certain modifications of the basic formula are therefore required, focussing on the prevention of overheating.

In the modified formula, Radix Ginseng *(ren shen)*, which strengthens the source qi, is omitted, but Fructus Corni Officinalis *(shan zhu yu)* and Radix Rehmanniae Glutinosae Conquitae *(shu di huang)* are added, as both are very effective in nourishing the yin. Fructus Corni Officinalis *(shan zhu yu)* can also assist Ootheca Mantidis *(sang piao xiao)* in strengthening the controlling function of the Kidney, and thereby address the urinary frequency, incontinence, and white discharge after urination. Semen Nelumbinis Nuciferae *(lian zi)* is substituted for Os Draconis *(long gu)*, Rhizoma Acori Graminei *(shi chang pu)*, and Radix Polygalae Tenuifoliae *(yuan zhi)* in the group of herbs that treats the Heart disorder, because Semen Nelumbinis Nuciferae *(lian zi)* promotes the controlling function of the Kidney, soothes the Heart spirit, and promotes the functions of the Heart and Kidney. In effect, then, this single herb does the work of three.

Tuber Ophiopogonis Japonici *(mai men dong)* nourishes the yin and clears the Heart fire, and Rhizoma Coptidis *(huang lian)* is used purely to clear the Heart fire.

Thus, this combination not only nourishes the Heart yin, but also clears the heat from deficiency. The dosage of Rhizoma Coptidis *(huang lian),* however, must be small to prevent injury to the yang.

Although the basis of this formula is Mantis Egg-Case Powder *(sang piao xiao san),* the direction of treatment has been changed from that of a neutral property and function in order to tonify the qi, to a cold property and function in order to nourish the yin.

Follow-up   The patient was given one packet of the herbal formula daily, divided into two doses, and was advised to visit the clinic once a week. After one month the urinary frequency and incontinence were both cured. The white discharge from the urethra had decreased significantly, but not completely. Nor was there much improvement in the symptoms related to the heat from deficiency; the patient still complained of the pain in the perineum, his appetite was still poor, and he felt very thirsty. The tongue was red and the coating yellow. Both the thirst and the thickening of the yellow tongue coating reflected a weakness in the Spleen's transportive and transformative functions, which led to damp-heat. Because this could have been attributed to the astringent and yin-nourishing herbs, whose effect may be to reduce the qi activity in the middle burner, the prescription was modified. Fifteen grams of Radix Rehmanniae Glutinosae *(sheng di huang)* were substituted for the Radix Rehmanniae Glutinosae Conquitae *(shu di huang),* as the former is quite effective in clearing heat, and has less impact on the digestive system, although it is also weaker in nourishing the yin. All in all, the former herb is a much better choice than the latter in this case, and was therefore used in the modified formula. In addition, 2g of Fructus Amomi *(sha ren)* were added to promote the Spleen qi (through its aromatic qualities), but because this herb is acrid and warm, only a small amount was used.

The patient took the modified formula for a month, as before. He was then given another prostatic secretion test, which showed that the amount of white blood cells had decreased dramatically.

The herbal remedy was then stopped for a period of two weeks, to allow the patient's condition to stabilize. This was done because the main symptoms had already improved, just like the laboratory results. Stopping the herbs enabled him to take a break. It also allowed us to see if the symptoms would return. While there was no recurrence, we restarted the herbal treatment to consolidate the result. The patient took the same formula, with some minor changes appropriate to his condition, for four more months, during which all the symptoms were gradually alleviated. The final prostatic secretion test revealed that everything was normal, but the sperm test showed that sperm activity was still low, although other aspects were normal. The next step, therefore, was the treatment for infertility, which is not discussed here, except to note that a year later, the patient's wife became pregnant.

Diagnostic Principles for Abnormal Urination

Painful urinary difficulty *(lín zhèng)* is the most commonly seen urinary disorder in the clinic. Basic symptoms include urinary frequency and pain. Different types of painful urinary difficulty are identified in accordance with the cause of disease and the symptoms: qi painful urinary difficulty *(qì lín),* stony painful urinary difficulty *(shí lín),* hot painful urinary difficulty *(rè lín),* bloody painful urinary difficulty *(xuè lín),* cloudy painful urinary difficulty *(gāo lín),* and consumptive painful urinary difficulty *(láo lín,)* which is associated with physical exhaustion. In addition, some patients with abnormal urination do not experience pain. Although such patients do not fit into any of the categories of painful urinary difficulty, we will also discuss this condition below.

Cause of disease	In general, there are two primary causes of painful urinary difficulty: invasion by an external pathogenic factor, and dysfunction of the internal Organs. The disorder is mainly associated with the Bladder, which is located in the lower burner. A dysfunction in an internal Organ is the usual cause; an invasion by a pathogenic factor is not as common.
Damp-heat	Dampness may either come from the external environment or arise internally as a result of dysfunction in an internal Organ. The characteristics of the dampness in either case are the same: heavy and turbid, with a tendency to drain to the lower part of the body. Thus, symptoms will generally consist of heaviness and pain in the lower back, edema, swelling in the lower limbs, and diarrhea. If damp-heat is retained in the Bladder, abnormal urination will result. This is the most common cause of painful urinary difficulty.
Pathogenic heat	Urine is derived from the body fluids. Both retention of fire in the internal Organs (excessive fire) as well as heat from deficiency of yin or body fluids can consume the body fluids, which in turn affects the production and excretion of urine. In severe cases there may also be bloody urine.
Qi stagnation	In certain circumstances, Liver qi stagnation, or stagnation of qi activity in general, can affect the qi activity and metabolic functions in the lower burner, especially in the Bladder; this in turn can affect urination. In this event, besides urinary difficulty, patients may also have symptoms involving qi stagnation in general.
Qi deficiency or yang deficiency	Qi or yang deficiency of the internal Organs can interfere with the metabolism of water in the lower burner, and prevent the proper opening and closing of the Bladder. This is the main factor underlying abnormal urination in patterns of deficiency, and is very commonly encountered in the clinic.

Fig. 6-9   *Causes of abnormal urination*

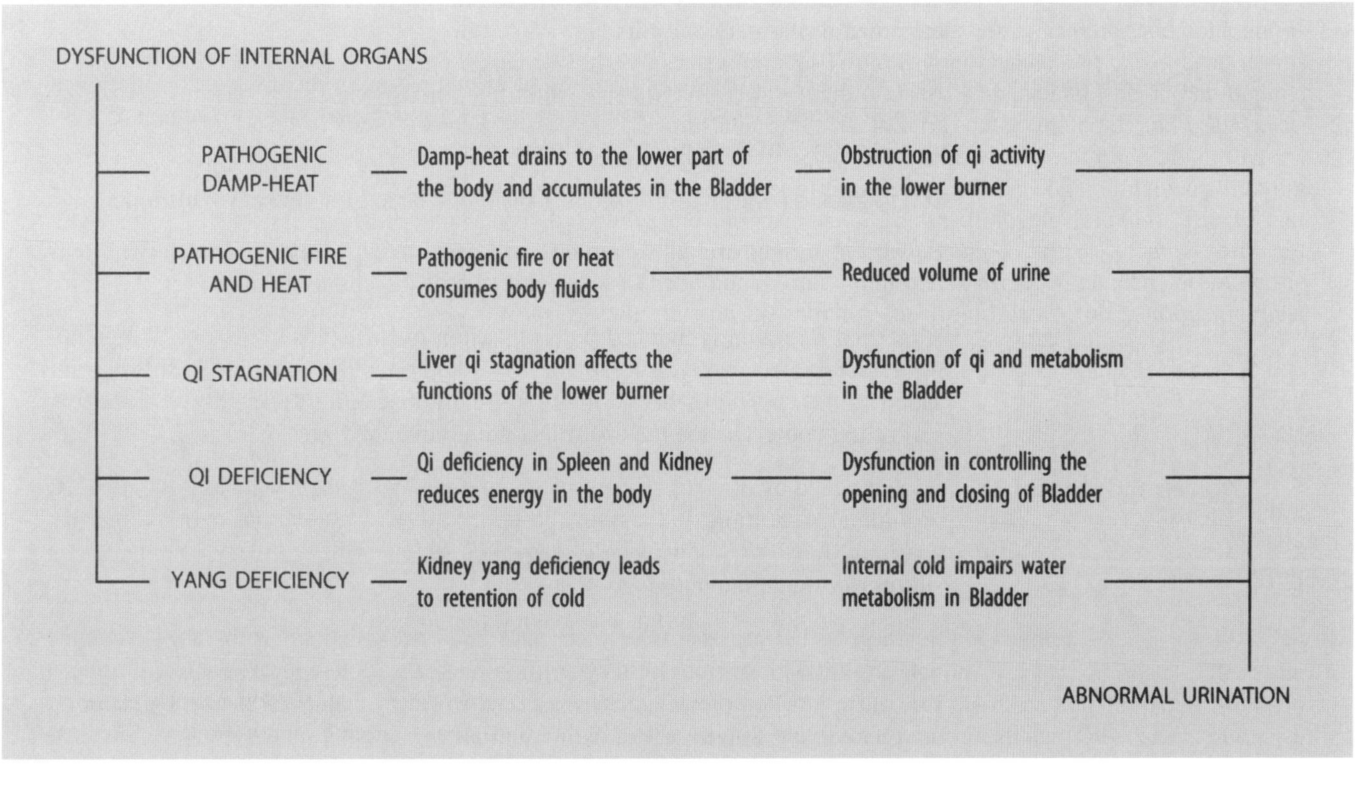

DYSFUNCTION OF INTERNAL ORGANS

PATHOGENIC DAMP-HEAT	Damp-heat drains to the lower part of the body and accumulates in the Bladder	Obstruction of qi activity in the lower burner	
PATHOGENIC FIRE AND HEAT	Pathogenic fire or heat consumes body fluids	Reduced volume of urine	
QI STAGNATION	Liver qi stagnation affects the functions of the lower burner	Dysfunction of qi and metabolism in the Bladder	
QI DEFICIENCY	Qi deficiency in Spleen and Kidney reduces energy in the body	Dysfunction in controlling the opening and closing of Bladder	
YANG DEFICIENCY	Kidney yang deficiency leads to retention of cold	Internal cold impairs water metabolism in Bladder	

ABNORMAL URINATION

Site of disease and pathological changes

In Chinese medicine the metabolism of water depends on the proper interaction of three Organs: the Lung, Spleen, and Kidney. Liquid from food and drink is transformed into body fluids, which nourish and moisten the internal Organs, tissues, and all the other organs of the body. The body fluids support the physiological functions of the entire body. The metabolism of water is a very complicated process that includes warming, dispersing, transporting, and spreading the body fluids throughout the body. After metabolism, the waste or excess liquid travels through the water passageway in the Triple Burner and Small Intestine, and eventually enters the Bladder, where it becomes urine. The Bladder's control of storage and excretion of urine relies on the Kidney qi.

In addition, a pathological change in any of the internal Organs will affect some part of the water metabolism, with corresponding symptoms *(Fig. 6-10)*.

The Liver and Heart are not directly associated with the metabolism of water. However, the Liver governs the free-flow of the body's qi, and thus Liver qi stagnation can result in an obstruction to qi activity in the lower burner; that is, it can influence urination to a certain degree. The Heart has an interior/exterior relationship with the Small Intestine. In Chinese medicine the Small Intestine is regarded as the pathway of urination. Therefore, certain Heart and Liver disorders can also affect urination.

Diagnostic Indicators

I. Diagnosing the nature of the disorder based on urinary symptoms

Heat pattern

Yellow or bloody urine, reduced quantity of urine, foul-smelling urine, hot, burning, and painful sensation during urination

Cold pattern

Clear urine with little color, increased quantity of urine, no obvious smell from urine, no abnormal symptoms accompanying urination

Excess pattern

Difficulty and severe pain in passing urine, with distention in the lower abdomen, urinary frequency and urgency, accompanied by yellow urine; no obvious nocturnal urination; urinary calculus

Deficiency pattern

Urination lacking in power, dripping of urine or urinary incontinence, urinary frequency with clear, watery urine and no pain, nocturnal urinary frequency, very cloudy urine, but containing no calculus

II. Diagnosing the site of a urinary disorder based on general symptoms

Besides abnormal urination, patients will present with certain general symptoms depending on which of the Organs is the site of the underlying disorder.

Lung

Abnormal urination is induced by an invasion of, or exposure to, external pathogenic factors, frequently accompanied by symptoms like coughing, a stifling sensation in the chest, and occasionally puffiness or edema, especially in the upper part of the body. The tongue coating is thin, white, and greasy.

Spleen and Stomach

Accompanied by obvious symptoms of the digestive system, such as poor appetite, abdominal distention, fullness in the epigastric and abdominal regions, nausea, vomiting, loose or watery stools, a swollen tongue with a greasy coating, and a slippery or moderate pulse.

Kidney

Soreness and weakness in the lower back and knees. Patients with yang deficiency will present with obvious cold symptoms, such as a cold appearance, cold limbs, a pale, lusterless complexion, absence of thirst, watery, loose stools or early morning diarrhea, a pale tongue with a white and greasy coating, and a sunken, forceless

Fig. 6-10   Abnormal urination

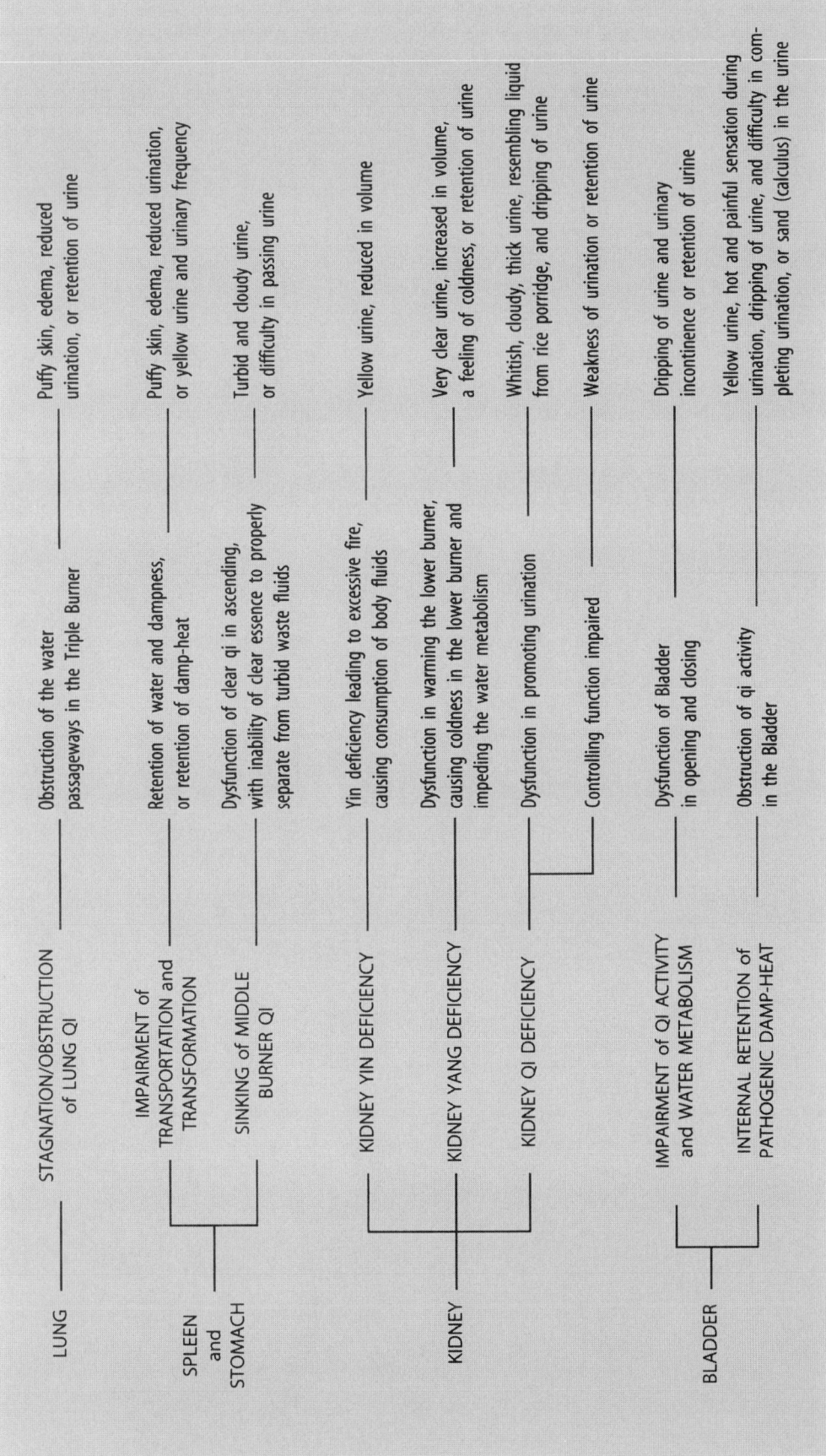

LUNG —— STAGNATION/OBSTRUCTION of LUNG QI —— Obstruction of the water passageways in the Triple Burner —— Puffy skin, edema, reduced urination, or retention of urine

SPLEEN and STOMACH

IMPAIRMENT of TRANSPORTATION and TRANSFORMATION —— Retention of water and dampness, or retention of damp-heat —— Puffy skin, edema, reduced urination, or yellow urine and urinary frequency

SINKING of MIDDLE BURNER QI —— Dysfunction of clear qi in ascending, with inability of clear essence to properly separate from turbid waste fluids —— Turbid and cloudy urine, or difficulty in passing urine

KIDNEY

KIDNEY YIN DEFICIENCY —— Yin deficiency leading to excessive fire, causing consumption of body fluids —— Yellow urine, reduced in volume

KIDNEY YANG DEFICIENCY —— Dysfunction in warming the lower burner, causing coldness in the lower burner and impeding the water metabolism —— Very clear urine, increased in volume, a feeling of coldness, or retention of urine

KIDNEY QI DEFICIENCY —— Dysfunction in promoting urination —— Whitish, cloudy, thick urine, resembling liquid from rice porridge, and dripping of urine

Controlling function impaired —— Weakness of urination or retention of urine

BLADDER

IMPAIRMENT of QI ACTIVITY and WATER METABOLISM —— Dysfunction of Bladder in opening and closing —— Dripping of urine and urinary incontinence or retention of urine

INTERNAL RETENTION of PATHOGENIC DAMP-HEAT —— Obstruction of qi activity in the Bladder —— Yellow urine, hot and painful sensation during urination, dripping of urine, and difficulty in completing urination, or sand (calculus) in the urine pulse. Patients with yin deficiency usually have accompanying symptoms of heat from deficiency, such as tidal fever, night sweats, feeling of being hot in the afternoon, restlessness, hot sensation in the palms, chest, and soles, malar flush, dry mouth, dry stools, red tongue with a slender body, dry, thin tongue coating, and a thin, rapid pulse.

Bladder

The symptoms are located mainly in the lower abdominal area, and very seldom in the middle or upper burners. They include fullness, distention, and pain in the lower abdominal area, red tongue with a yellow, greasy coating, and a slippery, rapid pulse.

Constraint Disorders

CASE 29: **Female, age 45**

<table>
<tr><td>**Main complaint**</td><td>Depression, insomnia, and pain over the entire body</td></tr>
<tr><td>**History**</td><td>The patient has been suffering from insomnia, general pain, and discomfort over the entire body for a long time. Quite often these symptoms occur when she is depressed or has had some emotional upset. The symptoms can be mild or severe, and the duration of the attacks can be very irregular.</td></tr>
</table>

Main complaint

Depression, insomnia, and pain over the entire body

History

The patient has been suffering from insomnia, general pain, and discomfort over the entire body for a long time. Quite often these symptoms occur when she is depressed or has had some emotional upset. The symptoms can be mild or severe, and the duration of the attacks can be very irregular.

Four days ago the patient felt depressed and suffered from insomnia. Since then she has slept for only a few hours every night: five hours at most, but usually less. Her sleep is light and dream-disturbed. In the mornings she experiences pain, soreness, and general discomfort over her entire body. Her muscles feel tight and her nape and head feel sore and swollen.

She has episodic hot flushes on the face, but does not sweat. Her appetite has been very poor for a few years. She has excessive saliva and a feeling of tastelessness in the mouth. Bowel movements are difficult: they are sluggish, and when she is finished, she feels that there is more to come, even though she cannot pass anything more. Her stools are soft, loose, and improperly formed. The patient's stools were examined repeatedly at a local hospital for appearance, occult blood, mucago, cells (including RBC, WBC, epithelial cells, phagocyte), bilirubin, stercobilinogen, stercobilin, as well as for ova and parasites. No abnormalites were found. The cycle of her periods is prolonged, and the bleeding is scanty.

Tongue

Pale and swollen with a thin, white, and moist coating

Pulse

Thin and slippery

Analysis of symptoms

1. Attacks associated with emotional upset and depression—impairment of the Liver's control of the free-flow of qi.

2. Insomnia, light and dream-disturbed sleep—disturbance of Heart spirit.

3. Discomfort over the entire body, tightness in the muscles, and swelling and soreness in the nape and head—impaired circulation of qi and blood in the channels and collaterals.

4. Poor appetite, excessive saliva, tasteless sensation in the mouth, soft and loose stools—Spleen's transportive and transformative functions impaired.

5. Prolonged menstrual cycle with scanty bleeding—insufficiency of blood.

6. Swollen tongue with a white and moist coating, slippery pulse—retention of water and dampness.

7. Pale tongue and thin pulse—deficiency of qi and blood.

Basic theory of case

Constraint disorder *(yù zhèng)* is a special Chinese medical term. *Yù* has many different meanings, the most appropriate of which in this context are constrained, depressed, melancholy, and pent-up. The word *zhèng* means a disorder or pattern. This term is used to classify a group of disorders, such as anxiety and depression, which have been caused by emotional upset and qi stagnation. There are various symptoms associated with constraint disorder, and they can be divided into two major groups. The first group consists of psychological symptoms, that is, abnormal emotional manifestations, and the second consists of various physical symptoms associated with emotional upset.

In clinical practice one may encounter many different types of emotional or psychological symptoms, the most common of which are the following:

- *Depression.* These patients generally feel very low, have no confidence at work or in everyday life, and think in a negative manner. They feel useless, oppressed with worry, and sad for no particular reason. Some patients may weep or cry. In severe cases they lose interest in everything and everyone around them, including their own family.
- *Anxiety.* These patients can feel anxious for no particular reason, and are restless. They are unable to relax, or even sit down in comfort. They worry endlessly or find things to worry about, be they big or small. They think about things obsessively, are constantly on the move, and nothing can satisfy them.
- *Irritability and bad temper.* These patients know that there is something wrong with themselves. Although they become irritable or angry for no particular reason, or for some unimportant reason, they feel that it is their own fault, and that they cannot control themselves. Something very small, such as a minor upset in the family or at work, will be enough to make them angry or quarrelsome.

The emotions of people suffering from these disorders can change very quickly from positive to negative. They are moody and their symptoms can vary. They can be easily affected by their environment or by the pace of their lives, which may be too hectic. Too much intensive work over a long period of time, long hours, pursuing only one type of activity, putting pressure on themselves because of being single or too independent, and not enough rest because of late nights due to either work or entertainment, can all be contributing factors. When they become overtired, they can easily turn quarrelsome. Movies or TV programs that offer strong stimulation can be the cause of erratic emotions and emotional upset.

Yet, no matter how severe these emotional or psychological symptoms may be, such patients do not lose their normal sense of judgment. After an emotional outburst, patients often feel regret and criticize themselves for what they have said or done. This type of self-criticism often adds psychological pressure on the patient, aggravating other emotional symptoms.

With respect to physical symptoms associated with emotional disturbance, in Chinese medicine each Organ is associated with a different emotional aspect. Included in the Liver's governance of the free-flow of qi is the regulation, control, and moderation of emotional disturbance. Thus, constraint disorders are closely related to Liver ailments. The Heart is responsible for the spirit. If an illness disturbs the Heart spirit, this may affect emotional stability—another source of constraint disorders. Among the Organs, the Liver and Heart are most vulnerable to emotional and psychological distress. In clinical practice, which of the Organs will be affected is very much dependent upon the patient, the precipitating factors, and the individual symptoms. It is important to remember that Organs other than the Liver and Heart may account for emotional and psychological disturbances.

Fig. 7-1

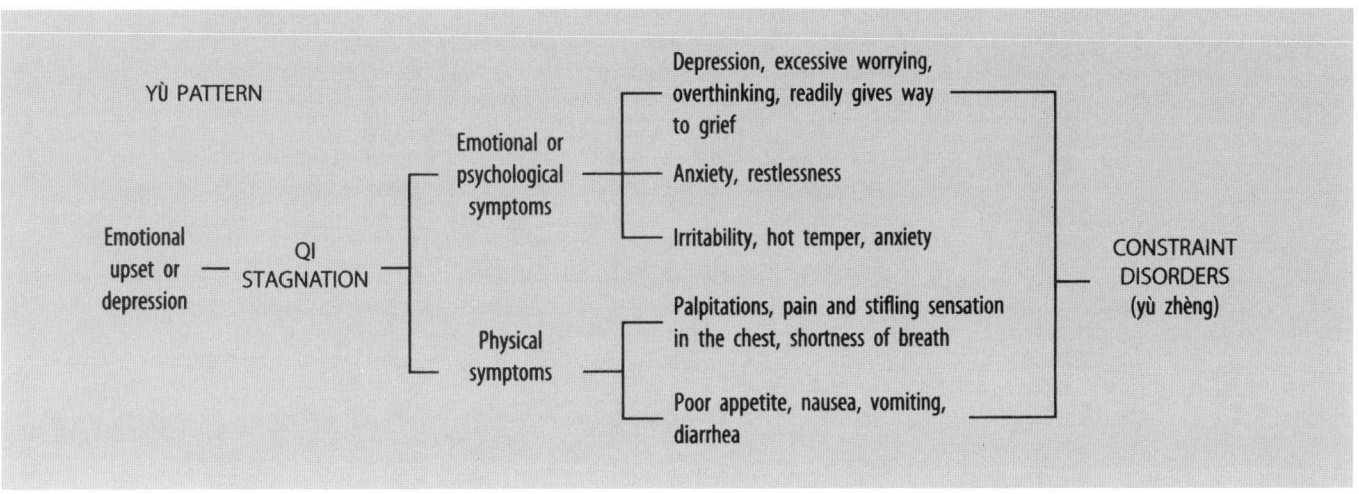

Cause of disease	Qi stagnation
	The patient has no history of an invasion by an external pathogenic factor, and the main symptoms in this case were induced by an emotional disturbance which led to the discomfort, soreness and generalized pain — evidence of an obstruction of qi activity and the free-flow of qi. Qi stagnation is therefore the cause of disease.
Site of disease	Heart and Spleen
	The patient has insomnia and dream-disturbed sleep, indicating that the site of disease is the Heart.
	Poor appetite, the sensation of tastelessness in the mouth, and the unformed stools suggest a dysfunction of the Spleen.
Pathological change	According to five-phase theory, the Heart pertains to fire and the Spleen to earth, so the relationship between the Heart and Spleen is one of generation between mother and child. In its physiological aspect, the Spleen is the source of production for qi and blood. The replenishment of Heart qi and blood relies on the Spleen and Stomach; thus, a dysfunction of the Heart can be induced by a disorder of the Spleen and Stomach.

The patient in this case has had a long-term disorder related to the Spleen and Stomach. Her poor appetite reflects a problem with the transportive and transformative functions of the Spleen. The sensation of tastelessness in the mouth, and the excessive saliva, indicate retention of dampness in the Spleen, and the soft, unformed stools point to retention of dampness in the Large Intestine. All of this evidence suggests that the Spleen's transportation and transformation of water has been impaired. And because of the relationship between the Heart and Spleen, the deficiency of Spleen qi has impaired the production of qi and blood, which led to malnourishment of the Heart spirit.

It should also be noted that, as the patient is nearing menopause, there is a natural insufficiency of qi and blood. The production of qi and blood at its source, the Spleen, is also reduced. The Liver therefore does not receive an adequate supply of blood from the Spleen and Stomach, causing deficiency of Liver blood; that is, there will be an insufficiency in the "sea of blood" in general, which will lead to a prolonged menstrual cycle and scanty bleeding. This deficiency can also impair the Liver's regulation of the free-flow of qi; thus, stagnation of Liver qi ensues. The patient's emotions then become very unstable, and the various symptoms appear.

Fig. 7-2

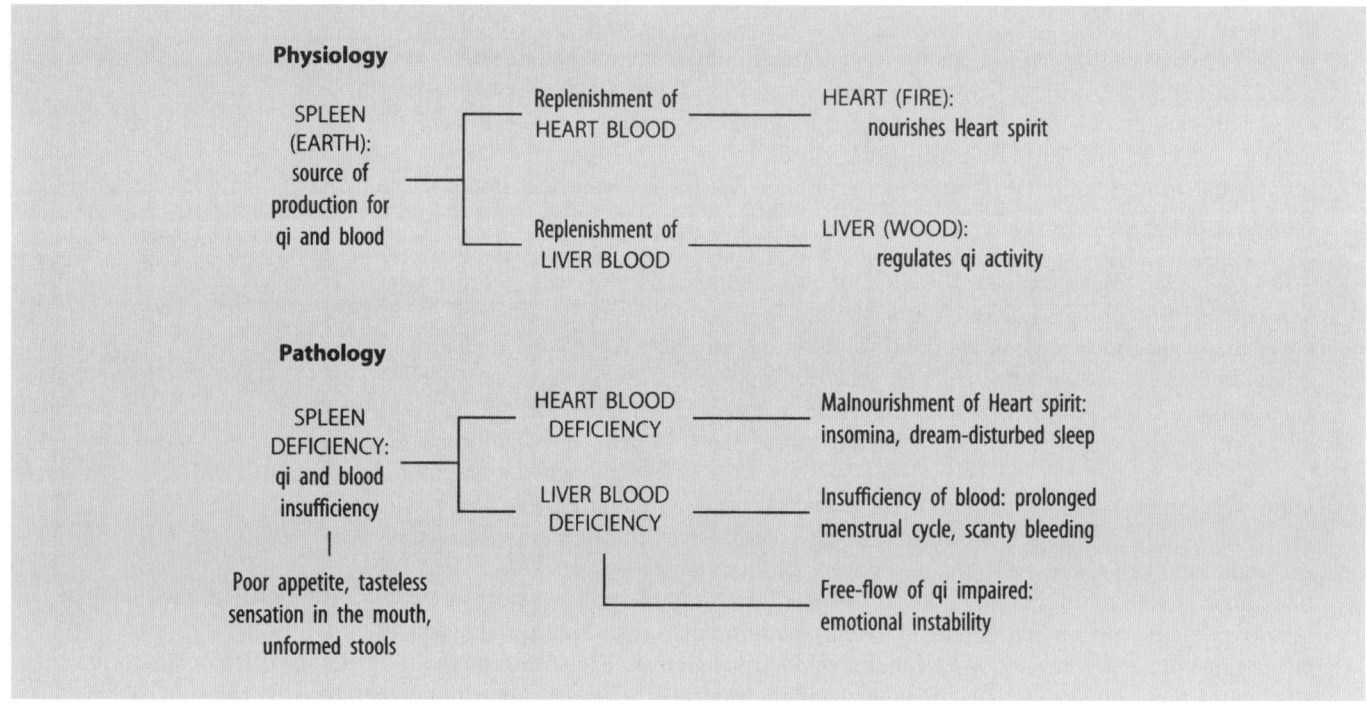

Physiology

SPLEEN (EARTH): source of production for qi and blood

Replenishment of HEART BLOOD — HEART (FIRE): nourishes Heart spirit

Replenishment of LIVER BLOOD — LIVER (WOOD): regulates qi activity

Pathology

SPLEEN DEFICIENCY: qi and blood insufficiency

Poor appetite, tasteless sensation in the mouth, unformed stools

HEART BLOOD DEFICIENCY — Malnourishment of Heart spirit: insomina, dream-disturbed sleep

LIVER BLOOD DEFICIENCY — Insufficiency of blood: prolonged menstrual cycle, scanty bleeding

Free-flow of qi impaired: emotional instability

Insomnia and dream-disturbed sleep suggest that the Heart spirit has been disturbed, and the pain and discomfort felt throughout the body reflect poor circulation and stagnation of qi activity in the vessels, channels, and collaterals (*See Fig. 7-2*).

The false urge to defecate after a bowel movement signifies stagnation of qi in the Intestines. The storage and removal of feces from the Intestines is associated with the qi activity of the Large Intestine and the whole body in general. In this case, because the qi activity is disturbed by the stagnation of qi, the qi in the Large Intestine cannot move properly, and its ability to remove the feces is thereby impaired. Thus, the patient's bowel movement is unsatisfactory: the stools move out sluggishly, and there is a feeling of more to come, even when the bowel movement has ceased. This sensation is due to qi stagnation in the Large Intestine, not to the presence of feces still in the Intestines.

The pale tongue and thin pulse reflect a deficiency of qi and blood. The tongue body has lost its normal shape, color, and luster, and the vessels do not have their normal fill of blood. The tongue is swollen, the coating is white and moist, and the pulse is slippery, all of which indicate the presence of dampness and retention of water in the body.

To summarize, the illness in this case has affected the Heart, Liver, and Spleen, but the Spleen disorder is the root of the problem.

Pattern of disease

The patient has an interior pattern because, according to the history, there has been no invasion by an external pathogenic factor. The soreness throughout the body is associated with an emotional upset, which further rules out an external pathogenic factor.

The patient has a poor appetite, loose stools, a feeling of tastelessness in the mouth; she does not feel thirsty, and has a pale tongue with a white coating. This is therefore a cold pattern. However, because she has episodic hot flushes on the face, the presence of pathogenic heat is also indicated. (For further discussion, see "Additional notes", item 2 below.)

The poor appetite, unformed stools, prolonged menstrual cycle, pale tongue, and thin pulse are indicative of a pattern of deficiency. However, there is also qi stagnation, which means that there is an accompanying problem of excess.

Additional notes

1. Is there Spleen yang deficiency in this case?

The patient has a pale and swollen tongue with a thin, white, and moist coating. This kind of tongue is often encountered in a pattern of Spleen yang deficiency. However, because there is no complaint of cold limbs or a feeling of coldness throughout the body, Spleen yang deficiency must be ruled out. The tongue signs here merely reflect retention of damp-cold.

2. What is the pathogenesis of the episodic hot flushes?

The hot flushes on the face suggest that heat or fire has risen. This can be attributed to heat—either in the upper or lower burner— from deficiency. In this instance, the cause of the flushes is likely to be deficiency of yin and blood, which causes heat from deficiency of the Heart to rise upward to the face.

Other than this, there are no symptoms associated with heat; rather, the other symptoms reflect the retention of damp-cold in the Spleen and Stomach. There is thus a combination of heat and cold patterns in this case—heat above and cold below—but the heat is not severe.

3. Is there any relationship between qi deficiency and qi stagnation?

Qi deficiency is a symptom of deficiency, and qi stagnation a symptom of excess. As both of these conditions are present in this case, what is the proper analysis?

Based on the presentation, this patient's primary pathology—qi and blood deficiency—is associated with Spleen deficiency. The cause of the qi stagnation in this case is qi deficiency, which reduces the force needed to circulate the qi, accompanied by Liver blood deficiency, which impairs the Liver's regulation of the free-flow of qi. In other words, the stagnation of qi was caused by the deficiency of qi; deficiency is the root of the excess. The problem associated with excess is not a major concern at this time.

Conclusion

1. According to the eight principles:
   Interior, combination of heat and cold (heat above, cold below, with cold predominant), combination of deficiency and excess (excess within deficiency).

2. According to theory of qi, blood, and body fluids:
   Qi and blood deficiency accompanied by qi stagnation.

3. According to Organ theory:
   Deficiency of Spleen qi, malnourishment of Heart spirit, and insufficiency of Liver blood.

Treatment principle

1. Tonify the Spleen and nourish the blood.

2. Nourish the Heart and calm the spirit.

3. Regulate the qi.

Explanation of treatment principle

The deficiency of Spleen qi in this case has deprived the Heart spirit of its nourishment; thus, tonifying and strengthening the Spleen qi, nourishing the Heart, and calming the spirit are essential for this patient. If the deficiency of Spleen qi can be improved, the source of production for the qi and blood will become richer. The qi and blood can then easily be replenished, and the Heart spirit will be nourished and become calm.

As earlier noted, apart from the precipitating factor, there are no particular symptoms associated with Liver qi stagnation. However, since qi stagnation is one of the pathological changes in this case, regulating the qi can reduce the frequency of recurrence, improve the condition of the Liver, and accelerate recovery.

Selection of points

N-HN-54 *(an mian)*   SP-8 *(di ji)*
CV-17 *(shan zhong)*   ST-36 *(zu san li)*
CV-15 *(jiu wei)*   LR-3 *(tai chong)*
PC-5 *(jian shi)*

Explanation of points

N-HN-54 *(an mian)* has a tranquilizing effect and is used chiefly to treat disturbances of the spirit, including the Heart spirit. This is why its name in Chinese is "calm sleep." It can be used in the treatment of insomnia, dizziness, epilepsy, manic disorders, and hysteria. In this case the point is used in treating the patient's insomnia, disturbance of spirit, and unsettled emotional condition.

CV-17 *(shan zhong)* is located at the center of the chest, or more poetically (as the Chinese name implies) in the "center of the temple." It is the alarm point of the Pericardium, and is one of the eight meeting points *(bā huì xuè)* for the qi in general. In addition, it is a meeting point of five channels: the leg greater and lesser yin channels, the arm greater and lesser yang channels, and the conception vessel. The function of this point is to regulate qi, promote the movement of qi to relieve chest symptoms, and promote the downward movement of qi in the treatment of rebellious qi (reversal of qi) in the chest. Besides its local function, this is an important point in the treatment of qi stagnation. Here the point is used to regulate the qi, relieve the depression, and clear the heat from the upper burner. The reducing method is used *against* the direction of the channel, that is, the tip of the needle is angled downward.

CV-15 *(jiu wei)*. *Bān jiū* is the Chinese word for turtle dove, and *wěi* means tail. The point is located below the xiphoid, which resembles the tail of a turtle dove, hence the name. This is the connecting point of the conception vessel. It harmonizes the functions of the middle burner, promotes the downward movement of qi in the middle burner, clears heat, and resolves phlegm. It is used to calm the spirit in the treatment of disturbances of the emotions and spirit such as manic disorders, restlessness, anxiety, panic attacks, and epilepsy. In this case the point is used to regulate the qi and remove heat from the upper part of the body. The reducing method is used, as with CV-17 *(shan zhong)* above.

PC-5 *(jian shi)*. The word *jiān* means gap, and *shǐ* means messenger. This point is located in the gap between the tendons in the forearm, and its function is to transfer the qi energy in the channels, like a messenger; hence its name. This is the river point of the arm absolute yin channel. It settles the emotions, calms Heart spirit, and harmonizes the functions of the middle burner. In particular, it regulates Stomach functions.

This is an important point in the treatment of depression, which, according to Chinese medicine, is a constraint disorder. It is also used in the treatment of a very important type of depressive illness called restless Organ disorder *(zàng zào)*, which is similar to severe anxiety and hysteria. The disorder is usually characterized by very severe depression and loss of interest in most everything. In this case, the point is used to nourish the Heart and calm the Heart spirit. Because the patient not only has an emotional problem but also symptoms involving the middle burner, this point is most appropriate. It can be used to regulate the qi in the middle burner, which here is deficient, and to relieve such symptoms as poor appetite and excessive saliva.

SP-8 *(di ji)*. *Dì* means earth, and *shēng jī* means life. This point can be used in treating involuntary seminal emissions as well as menstrual disorders; thus, it promotes the reproductive functions, that is, the production of new life, just as the earth assists in the growth of plant life. This is the accumulating point of the Spleen channel. It promotes the functions of the Spleen, and regulates the blood. It can be used in the treatment of both qi and blood disorders, but especially blood. It can also be used in treating such Spleen disorders as abdominal distention, poor digestion, and poor appetite. In this case, because the patient suffers from Spleen qi deficiency as well as blood deficiency, a prolonged menstrual cycle, and scanty bleeding, the point is used to strengthen the functions of the middle burner and regulate the blood. Even needle manipulation is indicated.

ST-36 *(zu san li)* is used to regulate the Stomach and Spleen, strengthen the antipathogenic factors, and promote the functions of source qi in general. This point is very effective in treating deficiency, and in tonifying the qi and yang of the middle burner, especially the Spleen qi. It is used in treating the symptoms associated with impairment of the Spleen's transportive and transformative functions. In this case it is used for the problem in the middle burner, and to promote the digestive function. The tonification method is indicated.

LR-3 *(tai chong)* is both the stream and source point of the Liver channel. It soothes Liver qi, treats both the rising of Liver qi and constraint of Liver qi, and regulates blood. In this case, the point is used in treating the patient's general condition due to qi stagnation; and since she readily suffers from attacks of the disorder, it is used to regulate not only the Liver qi, but also the qi in general, and to promote the free-flow of qi throughout the body. The patient's prolonged menstrual periods and scanty bleeding reflect blood deficiency, especially of Liver blood; this point is used to regulate blood. Even needle manipulation is utilized.

Note on needling methods

The main needling method used for the points on the upper burner of the trunk is the reducing method; even (balanced) needle manipulation is used at only one of these points. The primary method used for the points on the limbs is the tonification method. Overall, the purpose is to clear the heat from the upper burner, remove the depression and disturbance of spirit from the head, and tonify the qi of the middle burner in order to support the Heart spirit.

Combination of points

PC-5 *(jian shi)* and LR-3 *(tai chong)* is a combination of points on the arm and leg terminal yin channels. The former is the river point of the Pericardium channel, and the latter is the stream and source point on the Liver channel. PC-5 *(jian shi)* removes qi stagnation from the upper and middle burners, and offers significant relief for problems associated with depression: it calms the Heart spirit and also treats symptoms of the head and emotions. LR-3 *(tai chong)* regulates Liver qi, promotes the free-flow of qi throughout the body, treats qi stagnation patterns, relieves heat, and regulates blood. It promotes the functions of both qi and blood.

This combination of points can be used in treating such symptoms as depression, anxiety, and panic. It can also be used in treating severe problems such as epilepsy and manic-depression. Because both the Heart and Liver feature prominently in a constraint disorder, this combination is chosen to regulate both of these Organs, and to relieve the qi stagnation and depression.

ST-36 *(zu san li)* and SP-8 *(di ji)*. The first of these points is on the Stomach channel, which is yang in nature. It is very suitable for strengthening the functions of the Spleen and Stomach, and for promoting the antipathogenic factors. It can also regulate and harmonize the functions of the middle burner, regulate the qi, and alleviate pain. Because this point is on a yang brightness channel, it can exert a strong influence on the qi and yang levels. SP-8 *(di ji)* is the accumulating point of the Spleen channel, which is yin in nature. It strengthens the Spleen and regulates qi and blood, although the emphasis is on the blood and yin. It is especially useful in treating disorders pertaining to menstruation and involuntary seminal emissions. It can also be used in treating dysfunctions of the Spleen and Stomach. This combination of points therefore draws on both yin and yang, qi and blood. Because of its effectiveness in removing obstruction from the qi and blood, it is a very useful and important combination in clinical practice.

Herbal formula   Although herbs could have been used in this case to strengthen the Spleen and regulate the qi, they were not because the patient did not like to take herbs orally.

Follow-up   The patient was treated once daily for five days, after which she had become much calmer emotionally. Her sleep was normal, and the generalized pain had disappeared. Her bowel movements were slightly improved. It was suggested that she take an herbal remedy in order to strengthen the Spleen and regulate the qi and blood, but as she did not like to take anything orally, and preferred instead to continue with acupuncture, she was treated for another week, every other day. After the second week of treatment her appetite was very good, her bowel movements were more or less normal, and treatment was therefore terminated.

During the following one-and-a-half years, the patient only had a few minor attacks due to emotional upset, but she followed the advice that had been given to her and came for treatment in a timely manner. These treatments were basically the same as those discussed above, and the attacks were relieved fairly quickly.

In clinical practice, many patients do not like to take any type of oral medication, either conventional or herbal. This may be for personal reasons, or because some patients have experienced good results from acupuncture in the past. In any event, it is unnecessary to force oral medication on patients. However, it is necessary to extend the treatment time for such patients after the main problem has resolved, in order to strengthen the result and prevent future attacks. This should be explained to patients so that they can understand why the treatment must continue, and to ensure their cooperation. This particular patient was treated for a week after her problem had more or less been resolved, as it was necessary to focus more on the deficiency in order to consolidate the result of the treatment.

CASE 30: **Male, age 39**

Main complaint   Irritability and excessive episodic sweating

History   About six months ago, the patient started to feel very irritable, and often, for no apparent reason, he would get "butterflies" and a hot sensation in the chest, which he found was beyond his control. He became restless and developed a hot sensation all over the body. He sweated, had palpitations, and could not sit or stand still. These symptoms have continued to the present. Each episode lasts from a few minutes to about half an hour, and then gradually resolves. The patient cannot recall anything that might have precipitated this condition, but the attacks are often associated with arguments or situations with a strong emotional component.

The patient also complains that his concentration and memory are poor; he experiences dizziness, general lassitude, and blurred vision. However, when he was checked by an ophthalmologist, his vision was declared normal. His appetite is sometimes good and sometimes bad, and he has no discomfort in the epigastric or abdominal regions. His sleep is dream-disturbed, and his urine output has decreased. His stools are slightly dry; he has bowel movements once a day or once every other day. Several medical checkups, including ECG and blood pressure, revealed no abnormality.

Tongue   Slightly red with a thin, white coating

Pulse   Thin and slightly wiry

Analysis of symptoms   1. "Butterflies" in the chest, palpitations, and dream-disturbed sleep—disturbance of Heart spirit.

2. Hot sensation all over the body, excessive sweating, and extreme restlessness—disturbance by internal heat and fire.

3. Irritability, attacks associated with emotional situations—impairment to the free-flow of Liver qi.

4. Poor concentration and memory, dizziness—malnourishment of the spirit.

5. Blurred vision—malnourishment of the eyes.

6. Reduced quantity of urine, slightly dry stools—injury to body fluids by heat.

7. Thin pulse—depletion of body fluids.

8. Slightly wiry pulse—impairment of qi activity.

Basic theory of case

In Chinese medicine, qi and fire are separate concepts. Qi, in its various manifestations, is one of the body's antipathogenic factors. Fire is pathogenic, and includes both pathogenic heat and pathogenic fire, which consume the qi and injure the body fluids. It can also stir up internal wind and disturb the blood. Of course, the term "fire" in the concept of "fire at the gate of vitality" *(mìng mén huǒ)* is in a different category from the pathogenic fire discussed here.

As a general matter, then, qi has no relationship to pathogenic heat or fire; yet in certain circumstances it does. This condition is referred to as surplus qi transforming into fire. In other words, when qi becomes stagnant and constrained and the qi activity is thereby obstructed, the surplus or pent-up qi can accumulate in a certain part of the body, where it produces heat and eventually internal fire.

The basis of this pathological change is that qi pertains to the yang aspect of the body, which is associated with heat. Under normal circumstances, qi-related heat is not very obvious, but when a surplus of qi builds up in the one place, heat too will gradually accumulate and eventually lead to fire. This constrained qi is then no longer normal, but has transformed into the pathogenic factor known as qi stagnation. This is one of the most common reasons for internal fire in the five yin Organs, and especially in the Liver and Heart.

Humans have developed many different emotions and emotional states. Sometimes our emotions are mild, and at other times intense. Since the Liver and Heart are closely associated with emotional or psychological factors, strong emotions can affect the qi activity in the body, causing poor circulation or even stagnation of qi in the Heart and Liver. The pathological accumulation of surplus qi may then manifest as Heart or Liver fire. Because this type of internal fire is caused by qi constraint, the condition is often referred to as qi constraint transforming into fire *(qì yù huà huǒ).*

Fig. 7-3

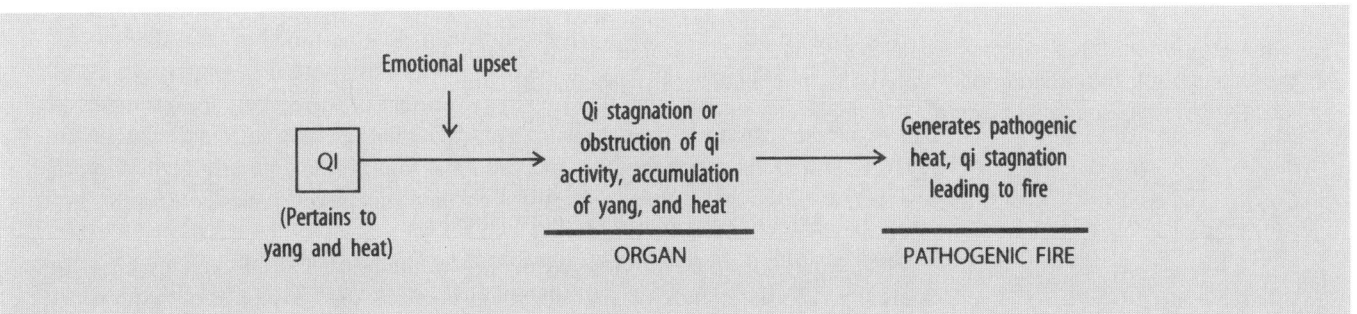

Emotional upset

QI (Pertains to yang and heat) → Qi stagnation or obstruction of qi activity, accumulation of yang, and heat — ORGAN → Generates pathogenic heat, qi stagnation leading to fire — PATHOGENIC FIRE

In order to treat this disorder, it is important to regulate the qi as well as remove the heat, since this is the only way to resolve the root of the problem.

Cause of disease

Internal pathogenic fire

Fire rises and disturbs the spirit, affecting the Heart and consuming body fluids. The patient is restless, irritable, sweats excessively, and has dry stools. All of these are symptoms of fire, which is the cause of disease here.

Site of disease

Heart

The patient is anxious, has palpitations, episodic "butterflies" in the chest, and dream-disturbed sleep. The locus of all these symptoms is the Heart, which is the site of the disease.

Pathological change

In the discussion of the basic theory of the case it was explained how stagnant qi transforms into fire. The early stage of a qi stagnation pattern can occur without the presence of heat or fire, but when the pattern persists for a long time or changes dramatically, the heat symptoms will gradually become more apparent, and eventually lead to a pattern of heat from excess.

The patient has been feeling irritable and restless for about six months. This suggests that Heart fire is already present, and, because it is strong, has disturbed the Heart spirit. The patient therefore suffers attacks of restlessness, "butterflies" in the chest, palpitations, anxiety, and dream-disturbed sleep. The pathogenesis of this disorder was previously described in the chapter on insomnia in our book *Acupuncture Patterns and Practice.*

Heat and fire tend to disperse from the inside of the body toward the outside, and to rise upward. This explains why the patient feels hot on the surface of the body. In addition, heat pushes the body fluids from the inside to the outside, causing excessive sweating. The symptoms are episodic because pathogenic heat and fire are invisible and unformed, like qi; they move and change very quickly, rising upward where they manifest in various symptoms. As heat disperses from the body, this reduces the heat that remains, and the symptoms may temporarily disappear. However, until the underlying pathological change that caused the qi stagnation has been resolved, the symptoms can recur.

The Liver governs the free-flow of qi and regulates the emotions. When these functions are impaired, the patient will become very moody and irritable. In this case, episodes of constraint disorder are very often associated with emotional upset; this indicates a dysfunction of Liver qi, although it is not severe.

The Heart is the Organ that houses the spirit, which depends for its nourishment on Heart blood. In this case, the pathogenic heat has disturbed the Heart spirit, causing restlessness and anxiety. The heat is also consuming the yin and blood of the Heart, resulting in malnourishment of the Heart spirit, which accounts for the patient's poor concentration and memory. And because the functioning of the eyes depends on nourishment from the yin and blood, their injury from heat has blurred the patient's vision.

The middle burner's transportive and transformative functions are also associated with the general qi activity of the body. When this activity is impaired, it will interfere with the upward and downward movement of the Spleen and Stomach qi. This is why the patient's appetite is irregular. The patient also suffers dizziness and general lassitude because the heat and fire have injured the antipathogenic factors; however, at the moment these symptoms are not very severe, and therefore qi and blood deficiency cannot be diagnosed.

Heat injures the body fluids, reducing the quantity of urine and making the stools dry. The deficiency of yin and blood prevents the vessels from being properly filled, hence the thin pulse. The wiry quality of the pulse can be attributed to the dysfunction in qi activity.

Pattern of disease

There is no history of invasion by an external pathogenic factor, but there is internal heat and fire. It is therefore an interior pattern.

Heat has disturbed the Heart spirit and consumed the qi and body fluids, indicating that this is a heat pattern.

The patient is restless, has "butterflies" in the chest, and is anxious, all of which are symptoms of excess. However, pathogenic fire has injured the antipathogenic factors, and there is thus some deficiency, but it is not very severe. The pattern here is therefore a combination of deficiency and excess.

Additional notes

1. Is there Liver fire rising in this case?

If a patient's qi becomes stagnant following a sudden emotional upset or change, it can lead to obstruction of qi, which can transform into fire. This can be either Heart or Liver fire rising. In this case the patient is restless, irritable, feels hot all over, and sweats excessively. Do these symptoms reflect Heart or Liver fire?

With Heart fire rising or excessive Heart fire, there will be palpitations and insomnia; these are symptoms associated with a disturbance of the Heart spirit. But with Liver fire rising, the patient will be quick to anger, and there will be distention and pain in the intercostal and hypochondrial regions; these are symptoms associated with a dysfunction of Liver qi. In this case, it is very obvious that there is Heart fire rising, but there is not much evidence of Liver fire rising.

Fig. 7-4

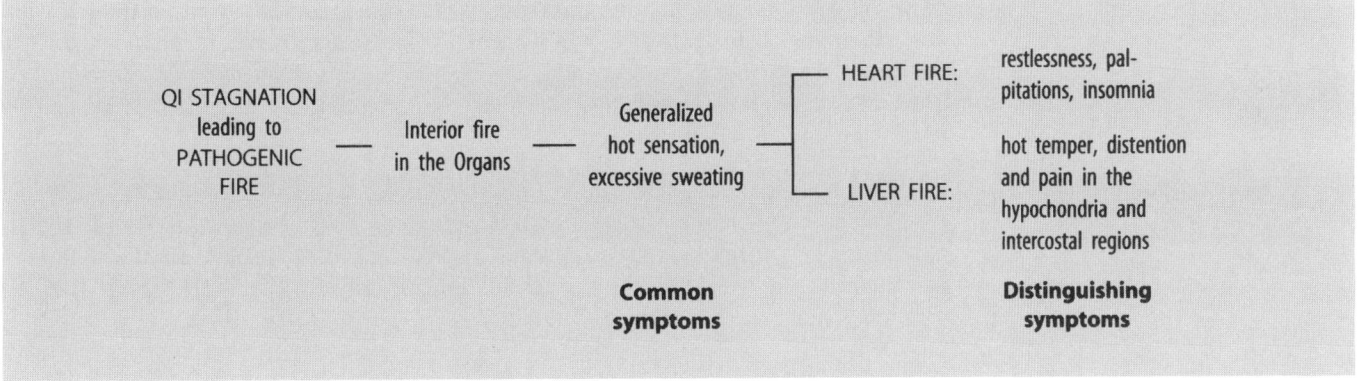

Common symptoms — **Distinguishing symptoms**

QI STAGNATION leading to PATHOGENIC FIRE — Interior fire in the Organs — Generalized hot sensation, excessive sweating — HEART FIRE: restlessness, palpitations, insomnia — LIVER FIRE: hot temper, distention and pain in the hypochondria and intercostal regions

2. Is there Liver blood deficiency?

Heart fire rising or excessive Heart fire can injure the blood and yin of the body, depriving the spirit of nourishment; this in turn can affect the memory, concentration, and mental energy. The patient here also has blurred vision, which reflects malnourishment of the eyes. Does this evidence indicate Liver blood deficiency in this case?

Apart from the blurred vision, there are no other symptoms which could be attributed to Liver blood deficiency, such as pale complexion, numbness of the hands and feet, or malnourishment of the nails. For this reason, only blood deficiency in general can be diagnosed; there is too little evidence to support a diagnosis of Liver blood deficiency in particular.

3. What do the pulse and tongue signs indicate?

It has been established that there is a heat pattern in this case. With heat patterns the tongue should be red with a yellow coating, and the pulse should be rapid, but these signs are nowhere to be found. The reason is that the heat and fire are not yet severe, and the disease is situated in only one Organ (the Heart) and has not spread to the remainder of the body.

Conclusion

1. According to the eight principles:
   Interior, heat, and excess, accompanied by mild deficiency.

2. According to etiology:
   Pathogenic fire.

3. According to Organ theory:
   Excessive Heart fire, injuring the yin and blood.

Treatment principle

1. Clear the Heart fire and settle the Heart spirit.
2. Regulate the qi.
3. Nourish the blood.

Explanation of treatment principle

The basic treatment principle for a heat pattern is to clear the heat and drain the fire. With acupuncture, use the reducing and cooling methods of needle manipulation; with herbal therapy, use bitter and cold herbs.

Fire resulting from stagnant qi pertains to an internal heat pattern in the Organs. In Chinese medicine the treatment principle relies on using fire's natural characteristics: dispersing, moving outward, and rising. This is summarized in the treatment adage, "When the fire is [from] constraint, disperse it *(huǒ yù fā zhī)*". Thus, the fire in cases such as this one is treated by letting it disperse, or removing the heat-inducing obstruction so as to allow the heat to move out of the body. It is *not* treated by draining the fire downward. This is because the heat or fire is caused by qi constraint, and the natural tendency of qi—like heat and fire—is to rise and move outward. If only the draining method is used in an effort to drain the heat downward, the obstruction of qi will worsen. When the obstruction is removed and the qi activity is thereby unimpeded, the heat and fire will resolve very quickly. Thus, clearing heat and regulating qi activity is essential in the treatment of fire or heat resulting from qi obstruction.

Basic herbal formula #1

Clear the Nutritive Level Decoction *(qing ying tang)* is one of the formulas from the Qing dynasty classic *Systematic Differentiation of Warm Diseases (Wen bing tiao bian)*. This formula is used in treating epidemic febrile diseases, at the stage in which the pathogenic factor has already entered the nutritive *(yíng)* level. The formula contains the following ingredients:

Cornu Rhinoceri (xi jiao)[1] 2g
Radix Rehmanniae Glutinosae *(sheng di huang)* 15g
Radix Scrophulariae Ningpoensis *(xuan shen)* 9g
Herba Lophatheri Gracilis *(dan zhu ye)* 3g
Tuber Ophiopogonis Japonici *(mai men dong)* 9g
Radix Salviae Miltiorrhizae *(dan shen)* 6g
Rhizoma Coptidis *(huang lian)* 4.5g
Flos Lonicerae Japonicae *(jin yin hua)* 9g
Fructus Forsythiae Suspensae *(lian qiao)* 6g

Explanation of basic herbal formula #1

The indications of this formula include fever, which worsens during the night as the temperature rises, severe restlessness, delirium (in very severe cases), insomnia, mild subcutaneous hemorrhage, dry tongue with a deep red body, and a rapid pulse. The basic pathological change is that pathogenic heat has entered the nutritive level from the qi level, wherein the Heart blood and Heart spirit have been affected by the pathogenic heat, giving rise to symptoms associated with the early stage of a nutritive level pattern. At this stage, the pathogenic heat has caused the blood circulation to become overactive, and has disturbed the Heart spirit.

There are two chief substances in the formula. Cornu Rhinoceri *(xi jiao)* is bitter, salty, and cold, and is associated with the Heart and Liver channels. Radix Rehmanniae Glutinosae *(sheng di huang)* is sweet, bitter, and cold, and is associated with the Heart, Liver, and Kidney channels. Both substances clear heat from the nutritive level and cool the blood. The latter substance also nourishes the yin and promotes the body fluids.

---

1. Because of its endangered status, Cornu Rhinoceri *(xi jiao)* is no longer used. Instead, Cornu Bubali *(shui niu jiao)* is substituted, usually with a six-fold increase in dosage.

There are two deputy herbs: Radix Scrophulariae Ningpoensis *(xuan shen)*, which is bitter, salty, and cold, and is associated with the Lung, Stomach, and Kidney channels, and Tuber Ophiopogonis Japonici *(mai men dong)*, which is sweet and cold, and is associated with the Lung, Heart, and Stomach channels. Both herbs assist Radix Rehmanniae Glutinosae *(sheng di huang)* in clearing the heat and nourishing the yin.

There is a group of five assistant herbs in this formula. Radix Salviae Miltiorrhizae *(dan shen)* and Rhizoma Coptidis *(huang lian)* are both bitter and cold, and are associated with the Heart and Liver channels. The former cools the blood and dispels blood stasis in order to remove the heat from the blood system. The latter clears heat and drains fire in order to clear pathogenic heat from the qi level. Herba Lophatheri Gracilis *(dan zhu ye)* is sweet, bland, and cold, Flos Lonicerae Japonicae *(jin yin hua)* is sweet and cold, and Fructus Forsythiae Suspensae *(lian qiao)* is bitter and cold; these three herbs are associated with either the Lung and Stomach channels, or the Heart and Lung channels. They clear heat, relieve toxicity, expel heat or fire from constraint, and promote the expulsion of heat through the skin by moving the heat from the nutritive to the qi level, and then out of the body.

Basic herbal formula #2

Gardenia and Prepared Soybean Decoction *(zhi zi dou chi tang)* is drawn from the *Discussion of Cold-induced Disorders (Shang han lun)* and is used in treating patterns of heat from constraint in the chest. The formula contains the following ingredients:

Fructus Gardeniae Jasminoidis *(zhi zi)* 10g
Semen Sojae Praeparatum *(dan dou chi)* 10g

Explanation of basic herbal formula #2

The indications for this formula include a stifling sensation in the chest, restlessness, and insomnia. The pathological change for this pattern reflects that of an exterior pattern of a febrile disease, when treatment is not given in time, or when improper treatment is administered. The external pathogenic factors have entered the body and transformed into heat, which accumulates in the chest, disturbing the Heart spirit.

In this formula, Fructus Gardeniae Jasminoidis *(zhi zi)* is bitter and cold, and is associated with the Heart, Lung, and Triple Burner channels. It clears heat, drains fire, and relieves restlessness, and therefore serves as the chief herb. The deputy, Semen Sojae Praeparatum *(dan dou chi)*, is acrid, bitter, and cold, and is associated with the Lung and Stomach channels. It removes external pathogenic factors, and relieves restlessness. The first of these herbs promotes the downward-moving function of the body, and the second, the upward-moving function. The former clears heat, while the latter induces the pathogenic factor to be move outward through the surface of the body. Thus, both herbs, acting in concert, promote the body's upward- and downward-moving functions, expel the pathogenic heat through the body surface, and remove heat from constraint in the chest.

Modified herbal formula

Rhizoma Coptidis *(huang lian)* 8g
Fructus Gardeniae Jasminoidis *(zhi zi)* 8g
Herba Lophatheri Gracilis *(dan zhu ye)* 6g
Radix Rehmanniae Glutinosae *(sheng di huang)* 15g
Plumula Nelumbinis Nuciferae *(lian xin)* 3g
Tuber Ophiopogonis Japonici *(mai men dong)* 12g
Semen Sojae Praeparatum *(dan dou chi)* 6g

Explanation of modified herbal formula

The prescription used in this case is based on a combination of Clear the Nutritive Level Decoction *(qing ying tang)* and Gardenia and Prepared Soybean Decoction *(zhi zi dou chi tang)*, with certain modifications. This case is neither a warm-febrile disease *(wēn rè bìng)* nor a cold-induced disease *(shāng hán bìng)*. It involves qi stagnation transforming into fire, which has disturbed the Heart spirit. Clear the Nutritive Level Decoction *(qing ying tang)* is used to cool the blood and clear the heat from the Heart. It is combined with Gardenia and Prepared Soybean Decoction *(zhi zi dou chi tang)*, a mild diaphoretic that disperses and removes the obstruction to the qi activity, thereby allowing the heat from constraint to leave the body.

Most of the herbs in Clear the Nutritive Level Decoction *(qing ying tang)* are omitted because in this case, the heat in the blood system is not severe. Thus, it is unnecessary to use Cornu Rhinoceri *(xi jiao)*, Radix Scrophulariae Ningpoensis *(xuan shen)*, and Radix Salviae Miltiorrhizae *(dan shen)*, which are cold and serve to cool the blood. Radix Rehmanniae Glutinosae *(sheng di huang)* and Tuber Ophiopogonis Japonici *(mai men dong)* are retained in the modified formula to clear heat from the Heart and to nourish the blood. Semen Sojae Praeparatum *(dan dou chi)* is substituted for Flos Lonicerae Japonicae *(jin yin hua)* and Fructus Forsythiae Suspensae *(lian qiao)* in order to dispel and disperse the stagnant fire, and also to strengthen the expulsion of heat by use of the diaphoretic method. Rhizoma Coptidis *(huang lian)* and Herba Lophatheri Gracilis *(dan zhu ye)* are also retained, and Plumula Nelumbinis Nuciferae *(lian xin)* is added. Together, these three herbs strongly act to clear heat from the Heart. Thus, the functions of this modified formula are to clear heat from the Heart, promote the qi activity, and remove the obstruction to the qi. The main focus of the formula is directed at the qi level.

Follow-up

The patient was given one packet of the herbal formula daily, divided into two doses. After one week, the restlessness had declined a good deal, as had the sweating. Only occasionally did he become restless and experience palpitations, although his sleep was still dream-disturbed, and his concentration and memory were still poor. This indicated that although the Heart fire had already diminished, the symptoms of Heart blood deficiency had become more apparent.

Fructus Gardeniae Jasminoidis *(zhi zi)*, Semen Sojae Praeparatum *(dan dou chi)*, and Plumula Nelumbinis Nuciferae *(lian xin)* were therefore removed from the formula, and 10g of Radix Angelicae Sinensis *(dang gui)*, 6g of Radix Paeoniae Lactiflorae *(bai shao)*, and 8g of Radix Polygalae Tenuifoliae *(yuan zhi)* were added to nourish the Heart and soothe the spirit. A sufficient number of the original herbs were left in the formula to clear the remaining heat. Treatment was continued for another two weeks, after which there were no further episodes of restlessness and palpitations. The patient was able to sleep soundly, and by this stage his memory and concentration were greatly improved. He was very pleased with the result and stopped taking the herbs for one week, during which there were no ill effects. The patient was advised to continue taking the herbs for another two weeks in order to strengthen the result.

After a couple of months the patient returned to the clinic for a checkup. He reported that only occasionally did he experience short episodes of palpitations and restlessness. The patient was told to resume taking the herbal formula, with some minor modifications, for another month, at which time the treatment was successfully concluded.

CASE 31: **Female, age 48**

Main complaint

Recurrent depression, pain, and a stifling sensation in the chest

History

For at least the past five years, the patient has suffered recurrent depression and chest disorders. At the beginning of each episode, she suddenly feels very depressed and experiences tension in the back, along with heaviness, stiffness, and a stifling sensation in the chest, as well as difficulty in breathing. Sometimes this becomes very severe and she can lose consciousness. After just a few minutes, the symptoms are relieved and the patient feels no after effects. Her blood pressure has been checked several times, and ECGs have been taken, but the results are always normal. The symptoms often occur after an emotional upset, or in situations of social tension.

The patient feels that her physical and mental energy have been very poor over the past few years, and that her sleep has been unsound. Consequently, she feels exhausted during the day, and any sort of mental activity makes her feel quite dizzy. Her moods can swing from one extreme to the other. When she experiences the stifling sensation in the chest, relief is afforded by somebody beating on her back with their fists. Her appetite is poor, but her bowel movements and urination are normal. She has been taking Valium intermittently, and vitamin tablets for the past five years, but has never received any traditional Chinese medical treatment, such as acupuncture or herbal therapy.

Tongue	Pale and lusterless with a thick, white, greasy coating
Pulse	Lax

Analysis of symptoms

1. Pain and stifling sensation in the chest, relieved by beating the back with fists—impaired qi activity in the chest.

2. Difficulty in breathing—impaired Lung qi.

3. Unconsciousness—loss of control of the spirit.

4. Onset associated with emotional upset or tension—Liver's regulation of the free-flow of qi is impaired.

5. Depression, moodiness, and dramatic mood swings—Liver's regulation of the free-flow of qi is impaired.

6. Poor mental energy, unsound sleep, exhaustion during the day, and dizziness caused by any mental activity—malnourishment of the spirit.

7. Poor appetite—Spleen's transportive and transformative functions are impaired.

8. Pale and lusterless tongue with a thick, white, and greasy coating; lax pulse—poor circulation of qi and blood.

Basic theory of case

In Chinese medicine the term inversion *(jué zhèng)* is applied to a group of disorders characterized by unconsciousness. The word *jué* means to stop or end (it also appears in the term *jué yīn*, or terminal yin); *zhèng* means pattern. The main symptoms of inversion include sudden shock or unconsciousness accompanied by extreme coldness in the extremities. A pattern of inversion may develop during certain diseases, or it can arise independently. The basic pathological change pertaining to this pattern is a severing or separation of yin and yang, leading to a severe disorder of qi and blood circulation, as well as the loss of control of the spirit. There are different types of inversion, which are classified on the basis of the underlying cause of the severance of yin and yang. The main patterns are those due to qi, phlegm, blood, and summerheat. Each of these patterns has its own cause, pathogenesis, and symptoms.

Qi inversion is caused by severe stagnation of qi, leading to an obstruction of qi and blood circulation in the Organs, channels, and collaterals. This results in the severing of yin and yang. Because the Liver governs the free-flow of qi and the regulation of qi activity in the body generally, the most common cause of qi inversion is severe qi stagnation in the Liver. The patient is very often affected by external factors, such as emotional upset or changes in the social environment. At the onset, a patient will fall and lose consciousness, but the breathing and heartbeat remain normal. After a while the symptoms resolve and the patient will regain consciousness; there are no sequelae. Qi inversion is a mild form of inversion, but even so, patients can suffer from recurrent attacks.

The other types of inversion are usually accompanied by after effects, such as motor impairment, hemiplegia, paresthesia, or psychological disorders. Severe cases can present with a deep coma and even death. Thus, it is vital to correctly distinguish among the different types of inversion.

Fig. 7-5

INVERSION:	CAUSES	SYMPTOMS
QI	Emotional upset or over-stimulation	Sudden onset of unconsciousness and coldness in the limbs, recurrent onsets, no sequelae after the attacks
PHLEGM	Obstruction in head and brain caused by phlegm retention	Sudden onset of unconsciousness, gurgling in the throat, very rough breathing, possible sequelae after attacks
BLOOD	Abnormal blood circulation caused by reversal of qi	Sudden onset of unconsciousness and trismus, red complexion, very rough breathing, constipation or retention of feces and urine, sequelae after attacks
SUMMERHEAT	Summerheat attacking the Heart	Dizziness and headaches following sudden onset of unconsciousness, red complexion, generalized hot sensation or trembling of the muscles, no sequelae after attacks

Cause of disease

Qi stagnation

During the onset of an attack the patient finds breathing to be difficult, and experiences a stifling sensation in the chest. When the symptoms become severe she can lose consciousness. The symptoms go away after a short time, and she suffers no after effects. This pattern of symptoms suggests severe stagnation of qi in the chest, which has impaired the upward and downward movement of qi activity. This pattern is characteristic of severe qi stagnation, and is the cause of the disorder in this case.

Site of disease

Liver and Heart

The patient has recurrent episodes which are associated with emotional upset and change, and the stifling sensation in the chest is the main symptom. These symptoms indicate that the site of disease is the Liver.

The patient loses consciousness because of loss of control of the spirit, thus the Heart is also a site of the disease.

Pathological change

This case serves as a good example of qi collapse. Liver qi stagnation can impede the free-flow of qi, giving rise to disorders in the general qi activity in the body; the upward and downward movement of pectoral qi (*zōng qì*) can thereby be affected. In its normal state, the function of pectoral qi is to assist the Lung with respiration and the Heart with the circulation of blood. In this case, however, the normal circulation of pectoral qi is impeded by the stagnation of qi in the chest, reflected in the feeling of tension in the chest and back. The poor circulation of pectoral qi can certainly lead to an obstruction of Lung qi, and thus the patient finds breathing to be very difficult, and suffers a stifling sensation in the chest. By beating on the back with fists, the physical vibration assists in the circulation of qi in the chest, and in the removal of the obstruction. The symptoms are thereby relieved for a short period of time.

Similarly, as the Heart qi cannot circulate properly, the circulation of qi and blood becomes stagnant. Qi cannot ascend to the upper part of the body, the normal relationship between yin and yang is disturbed, and the spirit loses control. The Heart spirit, now severely obstructed, is unable to carry on its normal psychological activities, and the patient thus suffers a sudden loss of consciousness. However, because there is only stagnation of qi, and no accumulation of substantial pathogenic factors such as phlegm, dampness, or blood stasis, as soon as the qi activity improves, the obstruction of qi will be relieved, and the patient will regain consciousness. The symptoms will then disappear by themselves, without sequelae.

The frequency of qi obstruction experienced by this patient means that the upward movement of clear yang and the downward movement of turbid yin is impaired. The brain and Heart spirit are thereby deprived of proper nourishment from the clear yang and qi. This diminishes the patient's mental energy and causes dizziness after any kind of mental activity; it also accounts for her lack of energy during the day, and her inability to sleep soundly at night. The poor appetite is due to impaired qi activity in the middle burner, which affects the transportive and transformative functions of the Spleen and Stomach.

Fig. 7-6

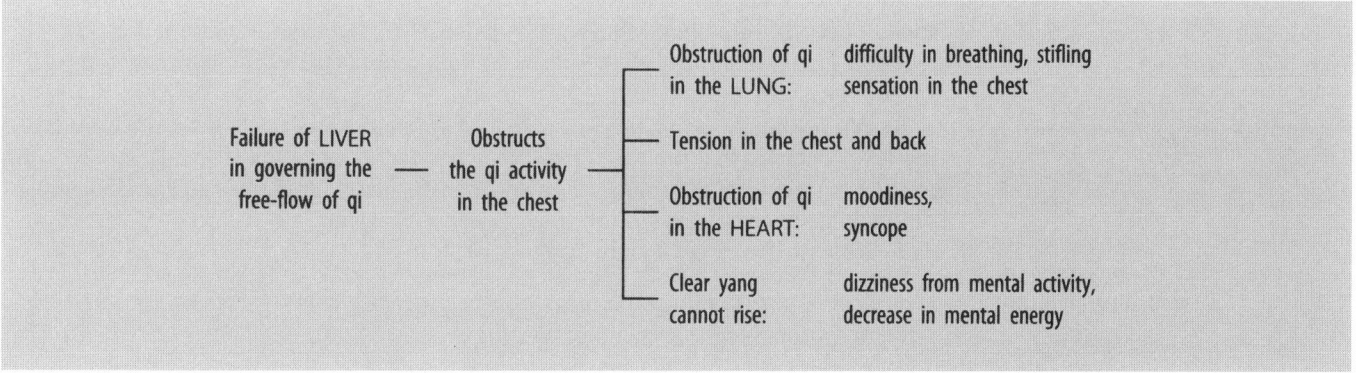

Failure of LIVER in governing the free-flow of qi — Obstructs the qi activity in the chest —

Obstruction of qi in the LUNG: difficulty in breathing, stifling sensation in the chest

Tension in the chest and back

Obstruction of qi in the HEART: moodiness, syncope

Clear yang cannot rise: dizziness from mental activity, decrease in mental energy

Qi provides the underlying energy for the circulation of blood. When the qi cannot circulate properly, blood circulation becomes sluggish; as a result, the tongue becomes pale and lusterless, and the pulse will be lax. The tongue coating is white, indicating the absence of heat. It is also thick and greasy, suggesting the retention of dampness in the middle burner. This is caused by the dysfunction in the transportive and transformative functions of the Spleen.

Pattern of disease

There is no evidence in the history of invasion by an external pathogenic factor. The pathogenesis suggests stagnation of qi activity, and this is accordingly an interior pattern.

There are no abnormal feelings of heat, coldness, or thirst; the bowel movements and urination are normal, the tongue coating is white and not yellow, and the pulse is lax and not rapid. Thus, there is no tendency toward either heat or cold.

The stagnation of qi in the chest, which has obstructed the pectoral qi and thereby impaired the Heart spirit, indicates a pattern of excess.

Additional notes

1. Why is the Liver diagnosed as the site of disease?

The history of this case indicates that the patient suffers episodes of syncope. Because this is obviously connected with a dysfunction of Heart spirit, and in the absence of symptoms associated with the hypochondrial and intercostal regions, why is the diagnosis Liver qi stagnation?

The main evidence supporting this conclusion lies in the qi inversion pattern. Qi inversion is caused by a failure of the Liver to regulate the free-flow of qi. Moreover, the episodes are associated with emotional upset, the symptoms disappear after a short period of time, and there are no sequelae. Thus, there is stagnation of qi alone, which is associated with the Liver, but no stagnation of phlegm, dampness, or blood, or retention of food. We may therefore conclude that the Liver is the site of disease.

2. Is there any general qi, Heart, or Spleen qi deficiency?

The patient complains of poor mental energy, and of feeling dizzy after any mental activity. Her sleep is unsound, her energy during the day is inadequate, and her appetite is poor. These symptoms are caused by the failure of clear yang to rise, leading to malnourishment of the spirit, and interfering with the transportive and transformative functions of the Spleen. These symptoms are very often found in patterns of Heart qi or blood deficiency, as well as Spleen qi deficiency. How, therefore, is one to distinguish these patterns?

In terms of general manifestations, the symptoms of qi or blood deficiency of the Heart usually includes palpitations, restlessness, and "butterflies" in the chest; Spleen qi deficiency is often accompanied by loose stools and other symptoms associated with the digestive system. In addition, Heart or Spleen qi deficiency will often involve symptoms of general qi deficiency, such as physical fatigue and shortness of breath, which are aggravated by physical activity. Patients with Heart blood deficiency often have a pale complexion, lips, and nails—symptoms associated with malnourishment of the blood. In this case, these very important symptoms do not exist.

Based on the symptoms associated with qi stagnation in the chest, we may therefore conclude that the patient suffers from malnourishment of the Heart spirit and impairment of the transportive and transformative functions of the Spleen, both of which are secondary to the qi stagnation, which is a disorder of excess. There is no pattern of deficiency in this case.

Conclusion

1. According to the eight principles:
   Interior, excess, neither heat nor cold.

2. According to theory of qi, blood, and body fluids:
   Qi stagnation.

3. According to Organ theory:
   Liver qi stagnation, qi inversion.

Treatment principle

Regulate the qi and promote Liver function.

Explanation of treatment principle

The treatment of inversion can be divided into two parts. The first occurs during the onset or acute stage, when the principle of treatment should be to recapture the spirit and revive consciousness. The second part occurs in the intervals between the episodes, when it is essential to treat the underlying cause of the illness.

During the onset or acute stage, when the spirit must be recaptured and the patient revived from unconsciousness, acupuncture is usually very successful. The selection of points is based on the type of inversion. In this case, GV-26 *(ren zhong)*, PC-6 *(nei guan)*, and LR-3 *(tai chong)* can be used with strong stimulation in order to activate the circulation of qi and blood in the channels, collaterals, and vessels, remove the obstruction of qi, restore the relationship between yin and yang, and thus recapture the spirit. On this basis, the patient will quickly regain consciousness. This is a very strong method, and it is important that it be stopped immediately after the patient has regained consciousness, otherwise the yang qi of the body will be injured.

During the patient's visits to the clinic there were no episodes of qi inversion (that is, unconsciousness), and thus the method of regulating qi was utilized in order to promote Liver function. In this way, the root of the illness was tackled by regulating the qi activity of the body in general, as well as the circulation of qi and blood, in order to restore the upward and downward movement of qi, improve the delivery of nourishment in the form of clear yang to the Heart spirit, and promote the upward and downward actions of the middle burner. The stifling sensation in the chest and other symptoms were thereby relieved, and the recurrence of the qi inversion pattern avoided.

Basic herbal formula

Five Milled-Herb Decoction *(wu mo yin zi)* is one of several typical formulas for regulating, and removing obstruction from, the qi. The formula contains the following ingredients:

Radix Linderae Strychnifoliae *(wu yao)* 9g

Radix Aucklandiae Lappae *(mu xiang)* 6g

Lignum Aquilariae *(chen xiang)* 6g

Semen Arecae Catechu *(bing lang)* 9g

Fructus Citri seu Ponciri Immaturus *(zhi shi)* 9g

Explanation of basic herbal formula

The indications for this formula are sudden syncope caused by very severe anger, or a severe distending and radiating pain in the chest and abdominal region caused by emotional upset. The primary cause of these symptoms is emotional upset injuring the Organs, which results in severe qi stagnation in the Liver, and thus obstruction of qi in the body. In severe cases this can lead to the separation or disconnection of the yin from the yang.

Radix Linderae Strychnifoliae *(wu yao)* is the chief herb in this formula. It is acrid and warm, and is associated with the Lung, Spleen, and Kidney channels. It is very potent in regulating qi activity and removing obstruction from the system. It treats the stifling sensation in the chest, hypochondrial pain, and epigastric and abdominal distention and pain associated with different types of qi stagnation.

There are four deputy herbs. Lignum Aquilariae *(chen xiang)* and Radix Aucklandiae Lappae *(mu xiang)* are both acrid, bitter, and warm, and are associated with the Spleen and Stomach channels. Both substances regulate qi and remove pain. However, the former is used in treating pain and distention in the chest and abdominal region (that is, the upper and middle burners), and also in promoting the downward movement of qi. While the latter herb is used mainly in treating qi stagnation in the Spleen and Stomach, as well as in the Large intestine, it can also be used in treating disharmony between the Liver and Spleen (the middle and lower burners). Fructus Citri seu Ponciri Immaturus *(zhi shi)* is bitter, acrid, and slightly cold, and Semen Arecae Catechu *(bing lang)* is acrid, bitter, and warm. Both of these herbs are associated with the Stomach and Large Intestine channels, and are used to regulate qi, remove distention, and promote digestion.

Although there are no herbs in the formula specifically associated with the Liver channel, all of the herbs are very effective in regulating the qi, promoting the qi activity, and removing obstruction. The formula is therefore used in treating various types of qi stagnation and qi reversal, including Liver qi stagnation.

Modified herbal formula

Radix Bupleuri *(chai hu)* 8g

Radix Ligustici Chuanxiong *(chuan xiong)* 4g

Radix Linderae Strychnifoliae *(wu yao)* 6g

Lignum Aquilariae *(chen xiang)* 3g

Fructus Meliae Toosendan *(chuan lian zi)* 8g

Radix Polygalae Tenuifoliae *(yuan zhi)* 5g

Rhizoma Acori Graminei *(shi chang pu)* 5g

Pericarpium Citri Reticulatae *(chen pi)* 6g

Explanation of modified herbal formula

This patient is suffering from qi inversion. Because she is now between attacks, the focus of treatment is on regulating the Liver qi to promote its function in governing the free-flow of qi.

As can be seen, many modifications were made to Five Milled-Herb Decoction *(wu mo yin zi)* to adapt it to this case, which is primarily a Liver qi disorder. Thus, quite a number of herbs were added to strengthen its ability to regulate the Liver qi. In the modified formula, Radix Bupleuri *(chai hu)* and Fructus Meliae Toosendan *(chuan lian zi)* are used to regulate the Liver qi and remove qi stagnation. Not only can Radix Ligustici Chuanxiong *(chuan xiong)* regulate the Liver qi, it can also remove blood stasis; it is therefore a good choice in this instance since it can treat the poor circulation of blood caused by the stagnation of qi.

Besides qi stagnation, there are also symptoms here suggesting that the Spleen's transportive and transformative functions are impaired, but there is no apparent retention of food. Thus, Pericarpium Citri Reticulatae *(chen pi)* is substituted for both Fructus Citri seu Ponciri Immaturus *(zhi shi)* and Semen Arecae Catechu *(bing lang)* in order to prevent those herbs from possibly injuring the antipathogenic factors.

Radix Aucklandiae Lappae *(mu xiang)* was omitted from the modified formula as well, since the qi stagnation in the Stomach and Large Intestine is not very severe. Radix Polygalae Tenuifoliae *(yuan zhi)* and Rhizoma Acori Graminei *(shi chang pu)* were added to revive the spirit in the treatment of sudden syncope and loss of consciousness. Although the patient presently has no symptoms involving loss of consciousness, the clear yang is unable to properly nourish and support the brain and Heart spirit. These two herbs were added to promote the clear yang function in nourishing and supporting the Heart spirit and brain, and thereby treat the associated symptoms of dizziness, poor energy, and poor concentration.

Follow-up

Over the course of a month, the patient was given one packet of the herbal formula daily, divided into two doses. She came to the clinic once a week for a checkup, and minor adjustments were made to the formula based on her condition. By month's end, the patient reported that the stifling sensation had diminished considerably, that her moods and emotions were much improved, and that her appetite had picked up. A two-week break was taken, and then treatment was resumed for another month, by the end of which most of the symptoms had disappeared. At this stage, the patient's energy level was back to normal, and treatment was therefore terminated.

During the following two years the patient occasionally returned to the clinic for treatment of a mild stifling sensation in the chest, or depression caused by tension or emotional upset, but each time she needed only a very short course of treatment. No further syncope was reported during that time.

CASE 32: **Female, age 55**

Main complaint

Anxiety, easily frightened, and intermittent, alternating feelings of heat and cold over the entire body

History

The patient has suffered from anxiety, spontaneous sweating, a feeling of sadness, and being easily frightened (panic attacks) for a long time. She has used various conventional anti-anxiety medications and tranquilizers, but the results were never very satisfactory. Ten years ago she began to experience intermittent, alternating sensations of heat and cold all over her body. Both sensations could occur at the same time, but in different parts of her body. Her periods ended when she was 48, but these symptoms did not go away. She very often feels hot with a swelling sensation in her forehead, the lateral sides of the arms, the upper back, the front of the thighs, and both knees. She also feels cold in the lower back, the calves, and the soles of her feet. These feelings of hot and cold come and go on a very irregular basis; they can become aggravated after a strong emotional upset, like anger or fright.

Presently her symptoms are more or less the same as they always have been. She has a poor appetite, despite often feeling hungry. Her stomach is distended most of the time, and there is little change in this condition after eating. She has very bad breath, and sometimes her palms feel hot. She finds it difficult to fall asleep and frequently has nightmares. Her stools are greasy and unformed, and she has a bowel movement only once every three to four days.

Tongue

Dark red, with a white, slightly yellow, and greasy, though slightly dry, coating

Pulse

Sunken, lax, and markedly forceless at both proximal positions; the right proximal position is weaker than the left

Analysis of symptoms

1. Intermittent, alternating hot and cold sensations all over the body—disharmony of yin and yang.

2. Intermittent symptoms aggravated by anger or fright—qi stagnation.

3. Tendency to feel weepy, sad, and easily frightened—deficiency of qi in the Organs.

4. Poor appetite, despite feeling hungry, and abdominal distention—impairment of Spleen's transportive and transformative functions.

5. Very bad breath—reversal of Stomach qi.

6. Difficulty in falling asleep, nightmares—disturbance of Heart spirit.

7. Hot sensation in the palms—heat from deficiency.

8. Greasy and unformed stools, bowel movements once every three to four days—impairment of Large Intestine qi.

9. Slightly yellow and dry tongue coating—internal pathogenic heat.

10. Sunken, lax, and forceless pulse—insufficiency of antipathogenic factors.

11. Markedly forceless pulse at both proximal positions—Kidney deficiency.

Basic theory of case

Yin and yang is the fundamental concept underlying Chinese medicine and natural philosophy. All substances and objects inside and outside the human body are classified as either yin or yang. The surface of the body, for example, is yang and the inside yin, the back is yang and the abdomen yin, the upper part of the body is yang and the lower part yin, the qi is yang and the blood yin. Yang is characteristically warm and active, yin is cold and tranquil. Thus, everything in the body that is warm, active, functional, and moves upward and outward is regarded as yang, and their opposite as yin.

Under normal circumstances the yin and yang are balanced; their opposite and interdependent natures maintain the body in a state of equilibrium, that is, neither too hot nor too cold, and neither hyper- nor hypoactive. If this balance is upset, the body will develop various symptoms of pathology. If the yang is hyperactive, there may be a pattern of heat with such symptoms as a generalized feeling of heat, irritability, red complexion, and red eyes. If there is too much yin, patients will develop a pattern of cold with such symptoms as a feeling of cold in the body, aversion to cold, depression, and a pale complexion.

Some patients may develop intermittent and alternating sensations of heat and cold, or a combination of heat and cold at the same time. An imbalance of yin and yang is also the cause of these symptoms, but here neither the yin nor yang is predominant; each dominates in its turn. When this happens, the body will alternate between heat and cold on an irregular basis. In clinical practice, these symptoms often occur in conjunction with disharmony between the qi and blood. This type of disharmony can cause obstructions in the channel and collateral system, which will interfere with the rebalancing of yin and yang. When the qi activity is obstructed, there can be an accumulation of stagnant qi, which will generate heat in certain parts of the body. As the qi cannot circulate beyond the blockage, a feeling of coldness is produced in other areas of the body. Because qi stagnation is changeable in its location and degree of severity, the patient will experience various combinations of hot and cold symptoms.

Fig. 7-7

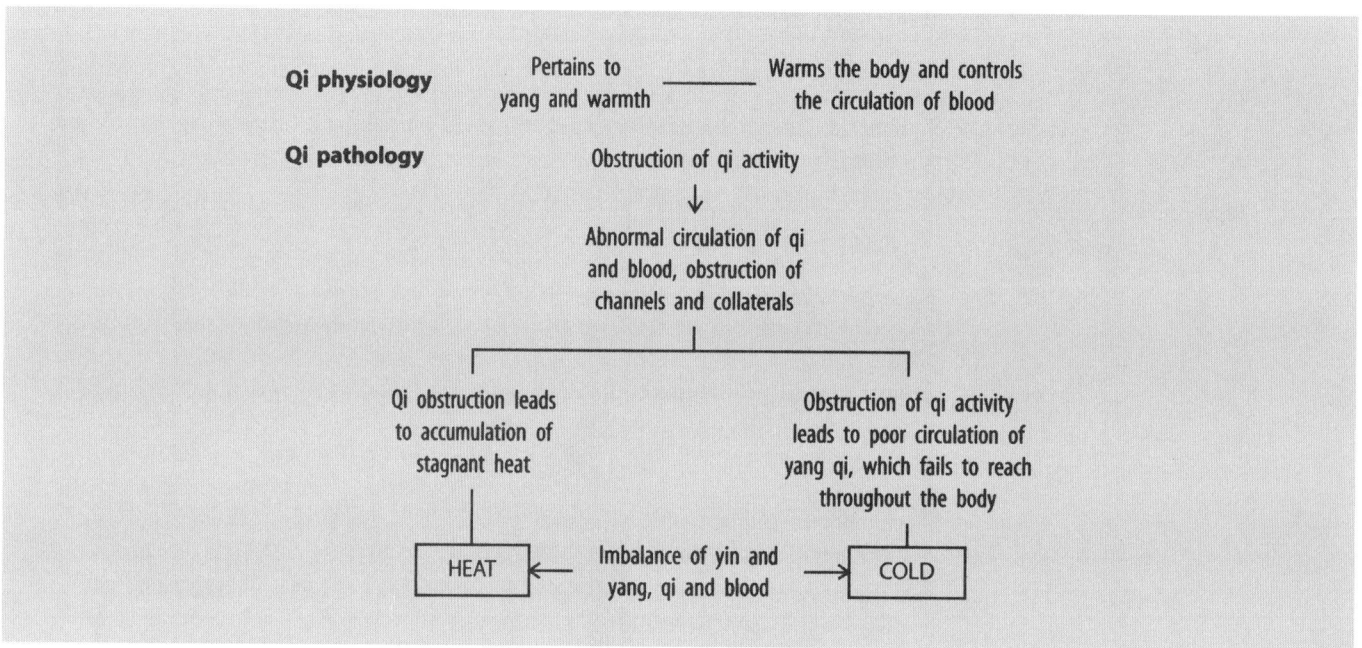

Cause of disease	Qi stagnation and insufficiency of antipathogenic factors
	The symptoms here are irregular and changeable, and are often associated with emotional upset or intense feelings, such as fright and anger; this is evidence of qi stagnation. Since the qi activity is obstructed, the circulation of qi and blood is sluggish.
	The patient also has symptoms that reflect deficiency of the antipathogenic factors: poor appetite, insomnia, dream-disturbed sleep, and a forceless pulse.
Site of disease	Channels, Heart, Spleen, and Kidney
	The patient has abnormal sensations of heat and cold in various parts of the body, which suggests that the site of disease is in the channels.
	Difficulty in falling asleep and the nightmares indicate a dysfunction of the Heart spirit.
	The poor appetite despite a feeling of hunger suggests a problem in the Spleen.
	The feeling of cold in the lower back and lower limbs, and the forceless pulse at both proximal positions, are evidence of a Kidney disorder.
Pathological change	The symptoms in this case are associated with disorders of various internal Organs. The characteristics of deficiency, excess, heat, and cold will therefore vary. When the problems are analyzed and diagnosed, it is necessary to group the symptoms, decide on the pathological characteristics in each group, and then examine the relationships among the various pathological changes.
	Intermittent and alternating sensations of heat and cold in the body is one of the main symptoms in this case. The hot sensation occurs in the forehead, lateral side of the arms, the upper back, the front of the thighs, and both knees; the cold sen-

sation in the lower back, calves, and soles of the feet. These sensations of heat and cold are in the superficial parts of the body, and are thus associated with the impaired circulation of qi in the channels.

The location of these sensations involve the arm and leg yang brightness, the arm lesser yang, the leg greater yang, and the leg greater yin channels. It is also noteworthy that the heat is found mainly in the yang aspects of the body, and the cold mostly in the yin. It can thus be concluded that there is disharmony of the yin and yang in the channels. The heat is attributable to qi constraint, and the cold to insufficiency of qi.

Qi itself is unformed and invisible, unlike the substantial pathogenic factors; and because the qi is active, symptoms of pathology are changeable and intermittent. The distending sensation is also characteristic of qi stagnation in the channels. Because emotional upset is closely related to qi activity, a change in one will affect the other; this is why the symptoms are aggravated by a strong emotional upset such as sadness, fright, or anger.

The Heart governs the spirit. The insomnia in this instance is characterized by difficulty in falling asleep and nightmares. This suggests that there is a deficiency of yin in the Heart, and that heat from deficiency has accumulated in the body. The spirit is badly disturbed, leading to this type of insomnia.

The appetite is closely related to the function of the Spleen. Spleen deficiency impairs the Organ's transportive and transformative functions, suppressing the appetite. In this case, the patient's appetite is poor despite the fact that she feels hungry: this is characteristic of Spleen yin deficiency. When the Spleen yin is deficient, heat from deficiency accumulates in the Spleen, limiting its ability to transport and transform food. This can suppress the appetite.

The reason for the foul breath is a disruption in the upward-moving action of Spleen qi, coupled with a disruption in the downward-moving action of Stomach qi. As a result, turbid qi reverses upward from the Stomach, causing bad breath. Because the normal upward and downward movements of the qi activity in the Spleen and Stomach are disrupted, the qi stagnates in and obstructs the middle burner, causing abdominal distention. But because of the patient's poor appetite, the amount of food she can consume is very limited, and the abdominal distention is therefore not significantly increased when she eats. The impairment of the Spleen's transportive and transformative functions has also interfered with its capacity for separating the food essence from the waste, so the clear and turbid parts (essence and waste) become mixed together. This mixture drains into the Large Intestine, and the feces are consequently greasy and unformed. The stagnation of qi in the middle burner also affects the Large Intestine, where the qi cannot move properly; thus, the bowel movements are reduced to once every three to four days.

The Kidneys are located in the lower burner and have the important function of warming and nourishing both the body in general, as well as the local area (the lower burner). It is the obstruction in the channels and collaterals, as well as the deficiency of Kidney yang, that reduces the warmth provided to the lower back and limbs, and thereby accounts for the feeling of cold.

Examining the relationships among the various pathological changes in this case, we can identify two main patterns: the first is qi stagnation, and the second is injury to the antipathogenic factors. Qi stagnation is a type of excess, and the injury to the antipathogenic factors is a type of deficiency. In this case, the excess has occurred in the channels and collaterals, which pertain to the superficial parts of the body. The problems in the Heart, Spleen, and Kidney are primarily due to deficiency.

Turning to the heat and cold aspects, the Heart and Spleen have a deficiency of yin, which pertains to heat, while the Kidney has a deficiency of yang, which pertains to cold, although it is not very severe. Regarding the location of the heat and

Fig. 7-8

cold, the heat has accumulated in the upper (yang) part of the body, while the cold symptoms appear in the lower (yin) part; there is thus a combination of heat and cold patterns in this case, which is known as heat above and cold below.

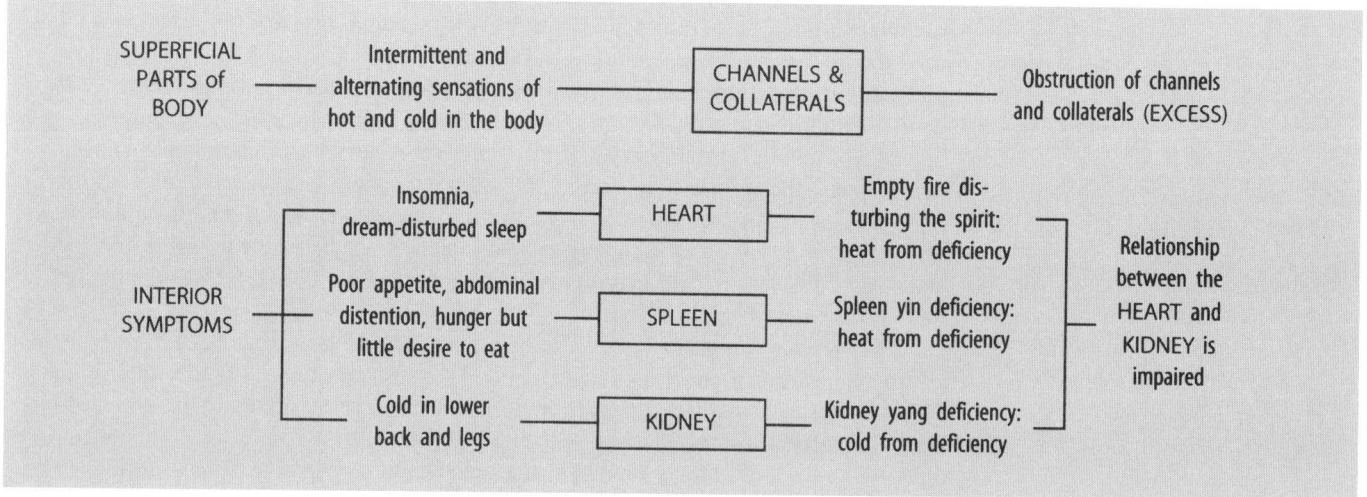

Among the relationships of the five yin Organs with the five phases, the Heart is located in the upper burner and is associated with fire, and the Kidney is located in the lower burner and is associated with water. In Chinese medicine the physiological relationship between these two Organs is described as one of harmony between Heart and Kidney, or of balance between fire and water. The Heart yang descends to help warm the Kidney water, and to support and increase the Kidney yang, ensuring that the Kidney water is not too cold. In this case, however, instead of descending, the Heart fire has risen upward. This has disrupted the normal relationship between the Heart and Kidney, and given rise to symptoms associated with Kidney yang deficiency. Thus, in this instance, the Kidney and Heart disorders are interrelated.

The red color of the tongue indicates the presence of heat, and the dark aspect indicates a dysfunction in the circulation of blood. Because qi is the "commander" of blood, when its circulation is disturbed, the circulation of blood will also be impaired. The white coating indicates cold, and the slightly yellow and dry coating indicates heat. The sunken, lax, and forceless pulse reflects interior deficiency. The pulse at the proximal position is associated with the Kidney; its forceless quality in this case reflects Kidney deficiency.

Pattern of disease

There is dysfunction of qi in the channels and collaterals, indicating a channel-collateral pattern. There are also disorders of the Heart, Spleen, and Kidney, indicating an interior pattern. Thus, there are both interior and channel-collateral patterns in this case.

There is also a combination of heat and cold patterns: heat from deficiency because of the yin deficiency of the Heart and Spleen; cold (loss of warmth) owing to the Kidney yang deficiency.

The obstruction of qi in the channels and collaterals is characterized as excess, and the injury to the antipathogenic factors as deficiency.

Thus, from all the complications in this case, three combinations of patterns can be identified: the interior and channel-collateral combination, of which the interior is the main pattern; the heat and cold combination (heat above and cold below), of which heat is the main pattern; and the deficiency and excess combination (excess within deficiency), of which deficiency is the main pattern.

Additional notes

1. What is the cause of the spontaneous sweating?

Spontaneous sweating is generally associated with yang deficiency. The pathogenesis is usually that the protective qi loses control over the opening and closing of the pores, and body fluids therefore drain out through the pores in the form of sweat. The Lung is the Organ that disperses protective qi to the surface of the body, and thus spontaneous sweating is found in patterns of Lung qi deficiency.

However, in this case there are no Lung disorders. Instead, the spontaneous sweating here is attributable to the qi disorder in the channels and collaterals; it is therefore related to the disharmony of yin and yang. Because the protective qi cannot reach the body surface through the channels and collaterals, the normal opening and closing of the pores is impaired, resulting in spontaneous sweating. Although the Lung qi is not deficient in this instance, regulating the Lung qi and promoting the Lung function will nonetheless be beneficial in the treatment of the spontaneous sweating.

2. In light of the fact that multiple Organs are affected, is the patient's condition very severe?

Although it is true that the disease has affected the Heart, Spleen, and Kidney, the injury or dysfunction in each Organ is not very severe. Moreover, the patient's general condition is not very weak. The deficiency in the Organs is not severe; rather, it is a dysfunction in qi activity that has disrupted the balance and harmony among the Organs. Thus, the patient's condition in this case is not very severe.

3. What is the cause of this patient's long history of being easily frightened, upset, and sad?

In Chinese medicine there are seven varieties of emotional upset: joy, anger, worry, over-thinking, grief, fear, and fright. Each of these emotions is associated with a different yin Organ. In general, qi stagnation in the five yin Organs is associated with hyperactive emotions such as irritability, anger, and anxiety. On the other hand, qi deficiency in the yin Organs is associated with hypoactive emotions such as timidity, fright, sadness, ponderousness, depression, and fear.

In this case, there is both qi stagnation and deficiency, but because qi deficiency in the yin Organs is predominant, the patient is susceptible to fright and sadness, and her other symptoms will often be aggravated after a fright.

Conclusion

1. According to the eight principles:
   Combination of interior and channel-collateral patterns, combination of heat and cold patterns (heat above and cold below), combination of deficiency and excess patterns (excess within deficiency)—interior, heat, and deficiency predominate.

2. According to yin-yang theory:
   Disharmony between yin and yang.

3. According to theory of qi, blood, and body fluids:
   Qi stagnation.

4. According to theory of channels and collaterals:
   Disharmony of yin and yang and qi and blood in the channels and collaterals.

5. According to Organ theory:
   Heart and Spleen yin deficiency, Kidney yang deficiency.

Treatment principle

1. Nourish the yin and strengthen the yang.

2. Harmonize the qi and blood.

3. Regulate qi and remove the qi obstruction.

Explanation of treatment principle

In order to nourish the yin, the cooling method is used; conversely, in order to tonify the yang, the warming method is used. If a case involves both yin and yang deficiency, it is important to determine which is predominant. In this case we must nourish the yin, although it is also necessary to strengthen the Kidney yang to some degree; care must be taken to avoid over-strengthening the Kidney yang, however, as this may increase the fire, and thereby further injure the yin.

Regulating and harmonizing the yin, yang, qi, and blood and removing the obstruction from the qi activity is essential in the treatment of this patient. In order to do this, we should promote the qi activity in the channels and collaterals to restore normal function to the channels, and remove the obstruction to the circulation of qi and blood in general in order to balance the yin and yang. Because the Lung and Liver are closely associated with the qi activity of the entire body, proper regulation of these Organs is also indicated.

Selection of points

BL-14 *(jue yin shu)*
BL-15 *(xin shu)*
BL-18 *(gan shu)*
BL-20 *(pi shu)*
BL-23 *(shen shu)*

Explanation of points

BL-14 *(jue yin shu)* is the back associated point of the pericardium, which is associated with the terminal yin channel. It calms the Heart spirit, stops vomiting, and harmonizes the middle burner. It is also used for pain associated with disorders of the chest, diaphragm, and Heart.

BL-15 *(xin shu)* is the back associated point of the Heart, and is located where the qi of the Heart (arm lesser yin) channel accumulates. It settles the emotions, calms the Heart spirit, and harmonizes the nutritive and protective qi. It can be used to nourish the Heart and treat emotional and psychological disorders with such symptoms as fright, palpitations, anxiety, depression, epilepsy, restlessness, insomnia, and poor memory, as well as manic disorders.

BL-18 *(gan shu)* is the back associated point of the Liver. It promotes the free-flow of Liver qi, nourishes the Liver, promotes the Gallbladder function, and can be used in treating eye disorders. It can also be used for blood disorders, emotional and psychological problems, and patterns involving pain.

BL-20 *(pi shu)* is the back associated point of the Spleen. It strengthens the Spleen, harmonizes the functions of the middle burner, and removes dampness. It is used to promote the transportation and transformation of food and the metabolism of water, and in treating such symptoms as abdominal distention, vomiting, diarrhea, jaundice, and dysentery.

BL-23 *(shen shu)* is the back associated point of the Kidney. It is an important point in the treatment of Kidney deficiency patterns, including Kidney yin, yang, essence, and qi deficiency. In clinical practice, symptoms like lower back pain caused by Kidney deficiency, impotence, involuntary seminal emissions, urinary incontinence, irregular menstruation, deafness, tinnitus, edema, and coughing and asthma associated with Kidney deficiency, can all be treated with this point.

Combination of points

A group of back associated points is used in the treatment of this case. The fact that all the points are on the Bladder channel does not mean that they all treat Bladder disorders. When there is disharmony of yin and yang, and a combination of heat and cold, gentle, superficial puncturing and tonification (but not moxibustion in the beginning) are indicated. The purpose is to regulate the yin and yang, gradually nourish the yin, gently promote the yang of the body, and remove the obstruction to the qi activity in order to solve the problem.

Follow-up

The patient was given acupuncture treatment once daily. After three weeks her sleep had become normal, her appetite was much better, the panic attacks had disappeared, and the abdominal distention was alleviated. However, she still felt cold in the lower limbs, and occasionally in the lower back as well. The treatment was therefore changed slightly: warm needle technique (moxa on top of the needle) was used at BL-23 *(shen shu)*. Treatment was administered twice weekly. Over a period of two months the symptoms gradually diminished, so treatment was terminated. The patient was very satisfied with the result, and stated that this was the first time that she felt her old self again after ten years of poor health. It was suggested that the patient herself use moxa sticks above BL-23 *(shen shu)* at least three times a week, and she was advised to continue this for at least a year.

In clinical practice, patterns that involve disharmony of yin and yang, and a combination of heat and cold, are complicated and difficult to treat. Treatment frequently lasts a rather long time, and treatment of yang deficiency often takes longer than yin deficiency. This should be explained to patients so that they may cooperate. In addition, self-treatment is important as a support for long-term stability.

CASE 33: **Male, age 27**

Main complaint

Paroxysmal fear and anxiety (panic attacks)

History

Over a year ago the patient, for no apparent reason, began to develop paroxysmal fear and anxiety. During the attacks he feels very nervous for no apparent reason, is unable to think clearly, and, because he is so anxious, cannot stand or sit still. Sometimes these symptoms can lead to depression and a lack of confidence. During the attacks he also feels cold over his entire body, experiences cold sweats and nausea, and is tense both in the nape and the shoulders. The symptoms can last anywhere from a few seconds to a few minutes, and the intervals between attacks are very irregular in duration.

At one stage the patient used conventional tranquilizers, antidepressants, and anti-anxiety medications, which had some effect, but did not last. He stopped taking the tablets on his own.

During the interval between attacks the patient has no physical or mental symptoms, and his appetite, sleep, bowel movements, and urination are all normal. Since the problem began, he has noticed that his memory has suffered considerably, and he always feels the presence of a foreign substance in his throat. A formal otolaryngological checkup and a barium meal for his esophagus showed no organic disorder in the throat or esophagus.

Tongue

Slightly red with a thin, white coating

Pulse

Wiry

Analysis of symptoms

1. Paroxysmal attacks of short duration, occurring at irregular intervals—disorder of qi.
2. Depression, lack of confidence, and a feeling of a foreign substance in the throat—stagnation of Liver qi.
3. Anxiety, nervousness, and stress—disturbance of Heart spirit.
4. General feeling of cold, cold sweats, tension in the nape and shoulders—impaired circulation of qi in the channels and collaterals.
5. Nausea—reversal of Stomach qi.
6. Slightly red tongue with a thin, white coating—absence of blood disorder and absence of pathogenic excess.
7. Wiry pulse—dysfunction of qi activity.

Basic theory of case

In this case, it has been noted that the patient feels as though his throat is blocked by some foreign substance, which he can neither swallow nor spit out, although the otolaryngological checkup and barium meal have shown no organic disorder. In conventional medical terms this is simply noted as a sensation of a foreign substance in the throat. In Chinese medicine it is termed "plum-pit qi" *(méi hé qì))*, as the sensation is similar to that of having the pit of a plum lodged in the throat. While there is, in fact, nothing substantial lodged in the throat, the sensation is nonetheless real. This condition is often reported by patients suffering from stagnation of Liver qi. Its pathogenesis is a combination of qi stagnation and phlegm in the throat.

If the problem was only Liver qi stagnation, the location of the disorder would not be fixed and the manifestations would be changeable; these are the general characteristics of a qi disorder. There would be no visible or definite form to the disorder because qi itself lacks form and is invisible. Phlegm, on the other hand, is a substantial and formed pathogenic factor; its location is usually fixed, and its manifestations change very little. Thus, for example, when there is an accumulation of phlegm in the skin or otherwise close to the body surface, lumps or swellings may appear, that is, it will be visible or palpable.

If there is a qi disorder with an accumulation of phlegm, this means that a combination of substantial and insubstantial pathogenic factors are involved; the disease will therefore have two characteristics. When this occurs on the right side of the throat, as in this case, the disorder will be relatively fixed, but the symptoms will be invisible and impalpable. This explains the patient's plum-pit qi symptom, which was described above.

Fig. 7-9

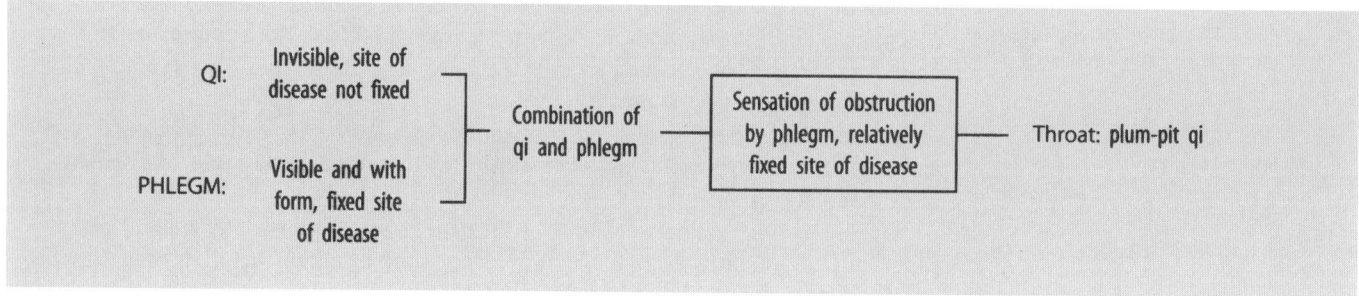

Cause of disease

Qi stagnation

There are no symptoms associated with an invasion of an external pathogenic factor. The main symptoms are connected with emotional upset and come and go on an irregular basis, which is evidence of qi stagnation.

Site of disease

Heart and Liver

The patient's anxiety, tension, and restlessness are associated with the Heart.

The symptoms related to emotional factors (depression, lack of confidence), and the sensation of a foreign substance lodged in the throat, are evidence of a Liver disorder.

Pathological change

In Chinese medicine, disorders resulting from emotional upset are most commonly associated with the Heart and Liver. The Liver regulates the qi activity throughout the body, ensuring that the qi and blood circulate smoothly and harmoniously; when this occurs, the emotions are normal. Normal emotions, such as calmness and happiness, reflect the health of the Liver in regulating the free-flow of qi. By contrast, this patient's paroxysmal or episodic bouts of fear and anxiety reflect the Liver's inability to regulate the free-flow of qi, owing to the obstruction of qi activity and consequently the impaired circulation of qi and blood.

There are two primary types of abnormal Liver qi activity. In the first, called transverse reversal of Liver qi *(gān qì héng nì),* the Liver qi is too active, leading to hyperactive and dramatically labile emotions such as irritability, poor temper, and anger. In the second pattern, called constrained or stagnant Liver qi *(gān qì yù jié),* the qi is not active enough, causing hypoactive or depressed emotions, such that the patient feels very anxious and depressed, lacks confidence, loses interest in work, and thinks negatively. The present case belongs in the latter category. In addition, this patient feels as if a foreign substance is lodged in his throat, which also suggests stagnation of Liver qi stagnation.

The Heart houses the spirit. Under normal circumstances, the Heart spirit is supported by the qi and blood. When the qi and blood circulate properly, the spirit is nourished and normal psychological functions can be sustained. However, if the circulation is impaired, the Heart spirit will be disturbed and the patient, for no particular reason, will experience tension, stress, anxiety, inability to think clearly, and a poor memory. All of these symptoms indicate malnourishment of the spirit owing to a deprivation of blood.

Fig. 7-10

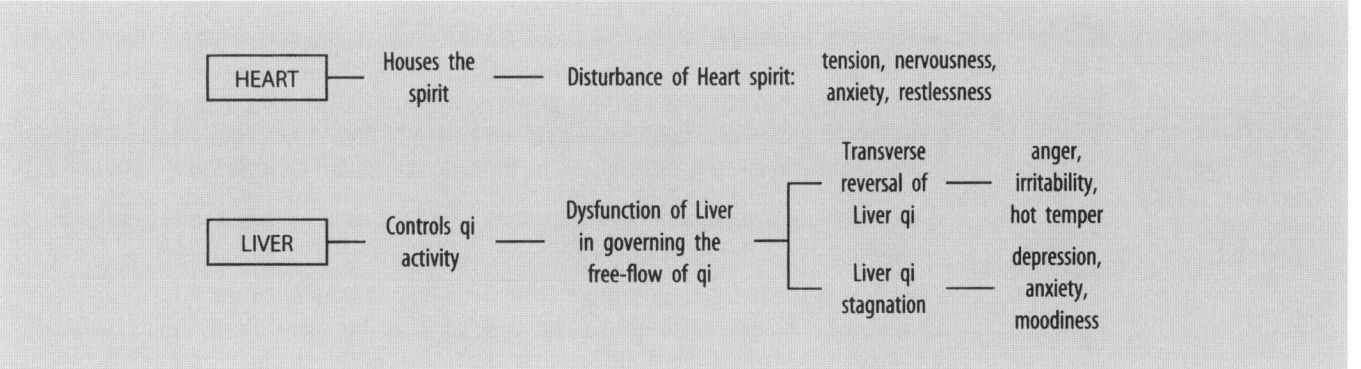

Disorders of qi activity not only give rise to emotional symptoms, but also to physical symptoms. The coldness felt over the body, as well as the cold sweats, indicate that the protective qi is unable to reach the body surface, which is thereby deprived of its normal warmth. The body will then feel cold, and, because the pores are not opening and closing properly, body fluids will flow out in the form of sweat. The tension in the nape and shoulders indicates an impediment to the circulation of qi in the channels and collaterals. It is the yang channels that pass through this area, and the tension is due to poor circulation of yang qi in the body. The upward and downward movement in the middle burner is closely associated with the Liver's regulation of the free-flow of qi. When this Liver function is impaired, the Stomach qi may not descend properly, but will reverse upward, causing nausea.

The color of the tongue body is closely associated with the circulation of blood, while the tongue coating generally reflects the condition of the Stomach qi and the existence of pathogenic factors. Because the disorder here is in the qi level, the blood has not been affected much. The absence of external pathogenic factors has likewise left the tongue proper unaffected. The wiry pulse suggests stagnation of qi, which reflects the qi disorder in the Liver.

Pattern of disease

The disorder is in the qi level, which pertains to an interior pattern.

During the intervals between attacks, the patient experiences no hot or cold sensations, and his appetite, bowel movements, urination, and tongue are all basically normal. This indicates that there is neither a pattern of heat nor cold. During attacks, although the patient experiences a cold feeling in general, the cause of this symptom is not deficiency of yang, and it is therefore not a pattern of cold. (For further discussion of this point, see note 2 below.)

Although the patient's condition has lasted for over a year, the antipathogenic factors have not been injured. This is, accordingly, a pattern of excess.

Additional notes

1. Is the fear associated with a disorder of the Kidney?

Among the relationships between the emotions and the five yin Organs, fear and fright are associated with the Kidney. This would suggest that severe fear or fright can overstimulate or injure the Kidney qi, leading to such symptoms as incontinence of urine and stool.

However, it must be noted that this is only a generalization, and that in the clinic it is not always the case that fear is associated only with the Kidney. On the other hand, the reverse can also happen: disorders of the internal Organs can lead to psychological or emotional problems. Fear can occur following a disorder of an internal Organ; it is not only associated with the Kidney. As a practical matter, fear is encountered much more often in patterns of Gallbladder qi stagnation or Gallbladder qi deficiency than in patterns of Kidney deficiency.

In this case it has been established that source of the disorder is Liver qi stagnation. The Liver and Gallbladder have an interior/exterior relationship; a disorder in one will often affect the other. Also, apart from the symptom of fear, there is no other evidence to suggest Kidney deficiency or an injury to the Kidney qi in this case. We may therefore conclude that the patient's fear is not associated with the Kidney, but is caused by stagnation of qi in the Liver and Gallbladder.

2. Is there any yang deficiency in this case? And if there is, could a cold pattern be diagnosed?

During attacks, the patient suffers from a feeling of generalized cold, as well as cold sweats. As explained above, the yang qi is unable to reach the body surface because of the impediment to the circulation of qi in the channels and collaterals. Yet why can it not be said that this is caused by yang deficiency?

If the cold symptoms were to be viewed in isolation, it could be said that they are common symptoms of yang deficiency, either Heart or Kidney yang deficiency, but in both cases the symptoms would be continuous. Here, the symptoms only occur during the attacks, which are paroxysmal and last for only a few seconds or minutes; we must therefore rule out yang qi deficiency, which is a chronic, ongoing condition. The paroxysmal feeling of cold and cold sweats in this case is the result of the disorder in the qi activity in the channels and collaterals, and is an indication that the protective qi cannot reach the body surface. In the absence of yang qi deficiency, there is no retention of pathogenic cold, and thus no cold pattern.

3. Since plum-pit qi is one of the symptoms, why is phlegm not mentioned as one of the causes of this disorder?

Earlier it was mentioned that qi stagnation and retention of phlegm are the cause of the symptom called plum-pit qi. It was established that this patient is suffering from symptoms typical of this problem, that his condition has lasted for over a year, and that the source of the disorder is qi stagnation. Liver qi stagnation can interfere with the upward and downward movements of the Stomach and Spleen qi, which can thereby affect water metabolism. The patient may therefore have symptoms associated with phlegm and dampness, as well as reversal of Stomach qi, such as nausea and plum-pit qi. However, based on the general symptoms and the tongue and pulse signs, the damp-phlegm in this case is not very severe. Moreover, as plum-pit qi is but one symptom, there is not enough other evidence to support an independent diagnosis of phlegm accumulation. The mild phlegm in this case is simply a result of the Liver qi stagnation. When the Liver qi stagnation is relieved, the phlegm and plum-pit qi will disappear by themselves.

Conclusion

1. According to the eight principles:
   Interior, neither heat nor cold, excess.

2. According to etiology:
   Qi stagnation.

3. According to Organ theory:
   Liver qi stagnation, and disturbance of the Heart spirit.

Treatment principle

1. Regulate qi and remove the stagnation of qi.
2. Calm the spirit.

Explanation of treatment principle

In Chinese medicine there are two general aspects to any treatment principle: the manifestation or symptoms of the disorder *(biāo)* and the root or cause of the disorder *(běn)*. An important principle of treatment is to search for the root in order to treat the disease: if the cause of the illness *(běn)* is removed, the manifestations or symptoms *(biāo)* will disappear by themselves.

In clinical practice both the root and the manifestations can often be treated together. Here, there are disorders involving the Liver and Heart. These Organs can be treated together. By calming the Heart spirit, we are treating the manifestations to alleviate the symptoms. And by regulating the qi, promoting the Liver function in regulating the free-flow of qi, and removing the stagnation, we are treating the root of the disorder. If both the manifestations and root are treated together, good results can be expected.

Selection of points

GB-13 *(ben shen)*   LI-4 *(he gu)* [left side]
CV-24 *(cheng jiang)*   CV-12 *(zhong wan)*
GB-20 *(feng chi)*   LR-3 *(tai chong)*
HT-7 *(shen men)* [right side]

Explanation of points

GB-13 *(ben shen)*. The name of this point means "rooted in spirit." It is located 3 units lateral to GV-24 *(shen ting)* and is responsible for the spirit, which is the "root" of the human being. The point is used to remove obstruction from the channels and collaterals, alleviate pain, calm the spirit, relieve muscular spasms, and expel pathogenic wind. As a Gallbladder channel point on the head, it is very suitable for calming the spirit and strengthening the brain functions; thus the expression that this point can "reach the spirit and recapture the consciousness." It also accounts for the point's name.

Because of the interior/exterior relationship between the Liver and Gallbladder, if the Liver qi becomes stagnant, it will interfere with the Gallbladder function, especially since qi stagnation is a yang disorder. The function of the Gallbladder channel, exteriorly, is to promote and regulate the yang qi, remove qi stagnation, and calm the spirit. This point has both a local as well as a channel-wide function. By this is meant that it can be used to treat disorders along the Gallbladder channel. It can remove qi stagnation from the channels and vessels, and treat disorders such as hemiplegia, as well as stiffness and pain in the nape and shoulders.

CV-24 *(cheng jiang)* is the terminal point of the conception vessel. Its name in Chinese means "to receive saliva." It is a meeting point of the arm and leg yang brightness channels, conception vessel, and governing vessel. Typically, this point is used in treating local disorders, such as those affecting the gums or face. It can also be used, to some degree, as a systemic point for calming the spirit, settling the emotions, and relieving convulsions. As a meeting point of four channels, it can regulate the qi in the yang brightness and conception channels. Here it is used to remove the qi stagnation, soothe the throat, and regulate the qi. It serves an important function in helping to remove plum-pit qi.

GB-20 *(feng chi)* is very commonly used to remove both internal and external wind. It can be used to treat symptoms in the head and neck, such as eye problems and stiffness and pain in the nape. Here, the point is used to extinguish Liver wind and remove the qi stagnation, which, in this case, come and go, just like wind.

The puncturing method in this instance is very important. The reducing method is used, then the needle is withdrawn so that the tip is just below the skin. The angle of the needle is then changed, and the tip is threaded in the direction of N-HN-54 *(an mian)*. The idea is that by puncturing just one point, we can both remove the qi stagnation, and also calm the spirit to relieve the patient's disorientation.

HT-7 *(shen men)* is the source point of the Heart channel. The name of this point means "gate of the spirit." The point serves to calm the Heart and spirit. In this case, it is used to relieve the anxiety and restlessness caused by the disturbance of the Heart spirit.

LI-4 *(he gu)* is the source point of the arm yang brightness channel. It is an important point for removing qi obstruction and alleviating pain. It is potent both as a local and systemic point, and can be used in treating a wide variety of disorders and patterns. In this case it is used to regulate the qi and remove the obstruction. There are certain symptoms in this case that involve yang brightness disorders. One example is the nausea associated with the reversal of Stomach qi. This point is very effective in removing qi stagnation and promoting the circulation of qi in the yang brightness channels.

CV-12 *(zhong wan)* is a meeting point of several channels: the arm greater and lesser yang, the leg yang brightness, and the conception vessel. It is also one of the eight meeting points for the yang Organs, as well as the alarm point of the Stomach channel. This point can be used to treat a wide range of illnesses that affect different channels, as well as the Stomach, Triple Burner, and Small Intestine. It is an important point for the treatment of deficiency patterns and for tonifying the body. It can also be used in treating patterns of excess. In this case it is used to treat the local abdominal symptoms, and also to promote the upward and downward movements of the middle burner qi in order to help remove the qi stagnation.

LR-3 *(tai chong)* is the source point of the Liver channel. It can be used to spread the Liver qi as a means of treating Liver qi stagnation or Liver qi rising. It can also control spasms, convulsions, and feelings of panic. Patterns of excess can be treated using the reducing method of needle manipulation, for example, in removing obstruction and qi stagnation not only in the Liver channel, but also in the qi activity in general. It is a very important point in the treatment of qi stagnation patterns.

Combination of points

HT-7 *(shen men)*, LI-4 *(he gu),* and LR-3 *(tai chong)* are all source points. The idea here is to use the four gate *(sì guān)* points, that is, LI-4 *(he gu)* and LR-3 *(tai chong)*, to remove the constraint, and HT-7 *(shen men)* to calm the spirit. This is an example of using slight tonification as part of treating an excessive disorder, thereby relieving the excess while nourishing the spirit. In this case, apart from the depression which is attributable to qi stagnation, there is also poor circulation of qi and blood. The spirit is deprived of the nourishment from blood, which contributes to the poor memory and inability to concentrate. Thus, it is important that treatment not only focus on relieving the obstruction of qi, but that is also address calming the spirit.

In this combination of points, LI-4 *(he gu)* is needled on the left side, and HT-7 *(shen men)* on the right. LR-3 *(tai chong)* is needled bilaterally. LI-4 *(he gu)* is a point on the Large Intestine channel, which is one of the yang channels. When focusing on the yang in men, the left side is needled. In this way the point is used to remove the obstruction, and can also draw on the yang qi from the yang channels for this purpose. HT-7 *(shen men)* is located on the Heart channel, which is one of the yin channels. For male patients, the right side is needled to nourish the spirit.

GB-20 *(feng chi)* and GB-13 *(ben shen)* are both on the Gallbladder channel. The disorder in this case is caused by Liver qi stagnation. Both points, one of which is close to the forehead and the other in the occipital region, are used to remove qi stagnation and relieve the constraint. This combination can be used in treating symptoms involving disorders of the head, and also for emotional problems such as headache, dizziness, depression, and stress, especially if they are caused by Liver qi stagnation. The effectiveness of these two local points can be attributed to the interior/exterior relationship between the Liver and Gallbladder channels.

Follow-up

The patient's work did not permit him enough time for regular treatments, and he was therefore treated only once a week. After the first two treatments there was a noticeable decline in the anxiety attacks, but there was little change in the other symptoms. Treatment was continued for another month, at the end of which there was obvious improvement. He only occasionally felt anxious, his depression was relieved, and the sensation of a foreign substance lodged in the throat became intermittent; yet his memory was still very poor. After another three weeks of treatment the patient's condition continued to improve, but he now complained of a feeling that something had lodged in his stomach, and there was also tension in the shoulders.

At this stage in the treatment, HT-7 *(shen men)* was removed from the prescription, LI-4 *(he gu)* was punctured bilaterally, and GB-21 *(jian jing)* was substituted for GB-20 *(feng chi)*. The purpose of these changes was to regulate qi, remove the obstruction from the channels locally, and relieve the depression. For patients with Liver qi stagnation, symptoms like shoulder tension are usually associated with qi stagnation or poor circulation in the Gallbladder channel; points on these channels were therefore used.

After five more treatments the stomach symptom disappeared. Thereafter, treatment was reduced to once every two weeks. Four months later all the symptoms were more or less resolved. The patient's memory was restored, and there were no further attacks of anxiety. The treatment was again reduced to once every month, for two months. After this, treatment was terminated. At a checkup six months later, no further symptoms were reported.

When patients suffering from anxiety come to the clinic for treatment, the condition frequently has lasted for over a year, and so has become quite fixed. Both patient and practitioner must therefore be prepared for long-term treatment. The probability of prolonged treatment should be explained to the patient so that he or she is able to cope with the situation.

CASE 34: **Male, age 56**

Main complaint

Severe depression

History

The patient had a bad car accident four years ago, and suffered a very severe cerebral concussion. There was no fracture of the cranium, but after the accident he developed severe headaches, dizziness, poor memory, and severe depression. He received conventional medical treatment for quite a long time, and was given anti-anxiety medication and antidepressants, as well as several courses of electrostimulation therapy. The latter was administered three years after the accident over the course of seven weeks, which was about ten months prior to his coming for acupuncture treatment.

The headaches are now gone, but the patient still feels depressed, especially in the mornings. He shows no interest in daily life and can sit inanimately for a long time, feeling very sad and often weeping. These symptoms usually last from morning until about 10a.m. or noon. In the afternoon his mood may improve a little, but he is unable to really concentrate on anything, and both his physical and mental energy are very poor. He is unable to work. His sleep is unsound. He wakes three to four times during the night and needs to urinate frequently. His appetite is good and he does not need to drink much. His bowel movements are normal.

Tongue	Pale and lusterless, swollen and soft, with a thick, slightly yellow, and not very dry coating
Pulse	Sunken and thin

Analysis of symptoms

1. Dizziness and headaches after car accident—stagnation of qi and blood in the head (the clear or pure orifices: the brain.)
2. Depression, sadness, inanimate state—disorder of spirit activity caused by a dysfunction of yang qi.
3. Poor memory and concentration—malnourishment of the spirit.
4. Fatigue and tiredness—Spleen qi deficiency.
5. Unsound sleep, often waking at night—disturbance of the Heart spirit.
6. Pale, swollen, soft tongue and sunken, thin pulse—yang qi deficiency.
7. Lusterless tongue—poor circulation of blood.
8. Thick tongue coating—interior disorder.

Basic theory of case

In Chinese medicine both the Heart and the brain have important functions in relation to the spirit. As noted in chapter 8 of *Basic Questions*, "The Heart stores the spirit," and in chapter 17, "The brain is the residence of the basal *(yuán)* spirit." The Heart and brain are both closely associated with emotional and psychological activities, and both depend upon the nutrition from the clear yang qi and blood to perform their physiological functions. Activation of the spirit relies on the activity of the yang qi. When this excitation is at its normal level, it manifests itself as clear thinking, calm emotions, and ease of mind.

The Spleen is responsible for the transportation and transformation of food, by means of which the food essence is produced; this in turn becomes the clear yang. The nutrient-bearing clear yang is dispersed by the action of the Lung throughout the entire body, including the brain and Heart. This, then, is the Spleen's upward-moving (ascending) function. If this function is impaired, the clear yang will fail to rise, the Heart and brain will be deprived of nourishment, and the activity of the spirit—which is supported by the yang qi—will weaken. As a result, patients may become very depressed, will be slow to respond to stimulation from their environment, and will show little interest in life and work.

In Chinese medicine the morning pertains to yang. On waking and after some initial activity, the normal yang, which is characteristically light of weight and upward-rising, gradually ascends to the upper part of the body and the brain. The level of activation increases until it reaches its normal level, quickly dispelling drowsiness and tiredness. However, if, because of injury or dysfunction, the yang qi fails to rise during the morning, this normal sequence will be delayed, and various symptoms will develop *(See Fig. 7-11)*.

Fig. 7-11

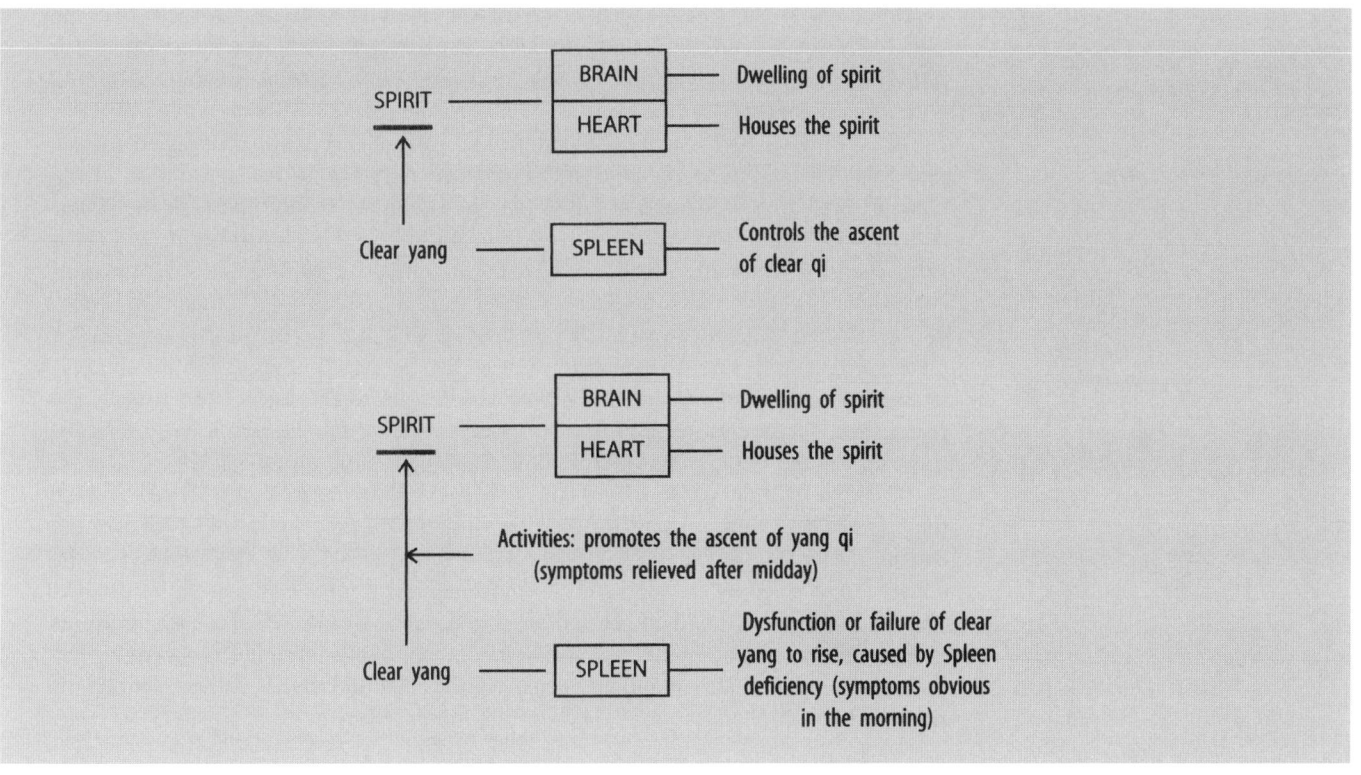

Cause of disease	Blood stasis
	The patient suffered trauma from a car accident. After the accident, he began to develop headaches and dizziness, suggesting blood stasis resulting from an injury to the vessels, channels, and collaterals in the head. Thus, the cause of disease is blood stasis.
Site of disease	Head, Heart, and Spleen
	The patient's history of head injury has left him with headaches and dizziness. The site of the disorder is obviously the head.
	The depression, poor memory, weak concentration, and unsound sleep suggest a disorder of the Heart and spirit.
	The poor energy and episodic symptoms in the morning indicate a disorder of the Spleen.
Pathological change	In the relationship between qi and blood, qi is the commander of blood, and blood is the mother of qi. The meaning of this well-known maxim is that the qi provides energy for the circulation of blood, but the blood provides substantial support and nourishment to the qi; thus blood is the substantial source of qi. In clinical practice, blood stasis caused by qi deficiency is a common occurrence: the qi lacks the necessary energy to circulate the blood. Conversely, blood stasis may occur first and cause qi deficiency, because it is unable to replenish the qi. That is, owing to its stasis, the blood cannot provide enough substantial support and nourishment for the qi, which becomes deficient. This is what occurred in the present case.
	The trauma here is the direct cause of the illness and is responsible for the blood stasis. Because of the stagnation and obstruction in the channels and vessels attributable to the poor circulation of blood, the clear yang qi was unable to rise properly to the brain, depriving it of nourishment. This accounts for the patient's headaches and dizziness during the early stage of the illness, and later his poor

memory, low emotions, and severe depression. After the patient's treatment by conventional medicine, the headaches disappeared, which would indicate that the blood stasis had been alleviated. However, because his emotional symptoms have remained unchanged, we must search for another explanation for the continuing emotional disorder.

According to the history, the patient has suffered from this condition for the past four years. The early stage of blood stasis resulted in the obstruction of the channels and vessels, which affected the circulation of blood, and thus the provision of nourishment to the various parts of the body. The Heart, brain, and spirit were thereby deprived of sufficient nourishment. The qi was also deprived of replenishment from the blood, and itself gradually became deficient. This especially affected the Spleen qi, which is responsible for the upward movement of clear yang. The failure of the clear yang to rise properly, aggravated the already-weakened activity of the spirit. This is why, in the later stage of the illness, the patient has become more sad and depressed, sits motionless, is unable to concentrate, and shows little or no interest in what is happening around him.

The development of this illness has thus moved into a secondary stage in which the spirit is deprived not only of the nourishment from blood, but also that of the qi—in particular, the clear yang. This has resulted in a severe dysfunction of the spirit. The symptoms are worse in the morning and improve during the afternoon. The patient feels fatigued and experiences general lassitude. All of these symptoms reflect Spleen qi deficiency, even though the patient's appetite is normal. The patient's sleep is unsound and he is easily awakened due to the malnourishment of the Heart spirit.

Fig. 7-12

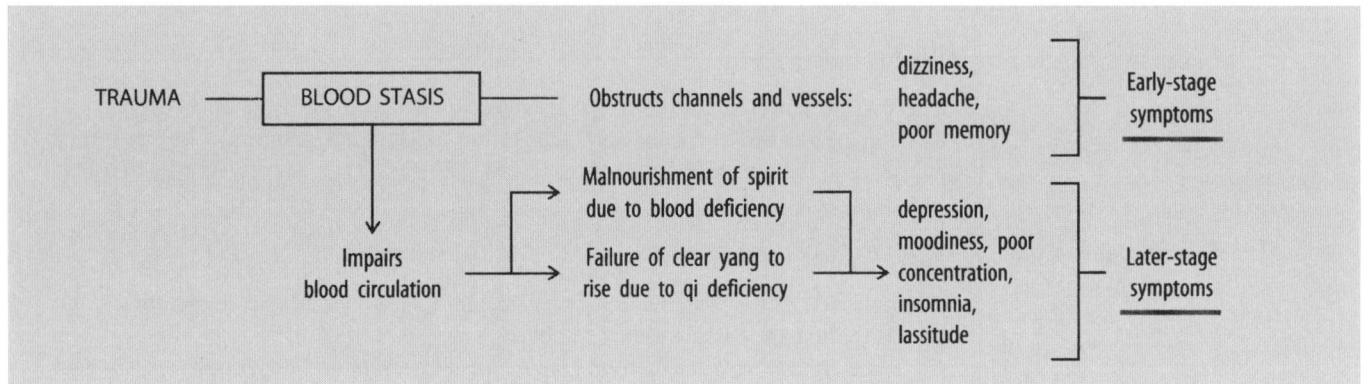

The lusterless quality of the tongue indicates a pattern of interior blood stasis, and the pale, swollen, and soft tongue, as well as the sunken, thin pulse, suggest yang qi deficiency.

Pattern of disease

The blood stasis and inability of Spleen qi to rise are both interior disorders.

The absence of heat or thirst, the pale, swollen tongue, and unrapid pulse indicate a pattern of cold.

The patient's general lassitude, fatigue, poor memory, and weak concentration suggest a pattern of deficiency. However, the blood stasis in the channels and collaterals is evidence of stagnation, which is excessive in nature. Thus, there is a combination of deficiency and excess in this case.

Additional notes

1. What is the explanation for the tongue signs?

When the tongue body is pale, swollen, and soft and the coating is white, thick, and moist there is yang deficiency of the Spleen and Kidney, as well as an internal accumulation of dampness and cold.

In this case, the condition of the tongue proper suggests yang deficiency, which can be attributed to the chronic Spleen qi deficiency gradually evolving into Spleen yang insufficiency. However, the tongue coating, which is yellow but not dry, is not evidence of heat. The yellowish coating is associated with a disruption in the upward and downward movements of the Spleen and Stomach qi. Because the clear qi is unable to rise and the turbid yin is unable to descend, the turbid qi in the Stomach reverses upward, which is reflected in the thick, slightly yellow coating. The fact that it is not dry suggests that the body fluids have not been affected by the illness. Taking into account all of the tongue signs, we find an early stage of yang deficiency and interior cold, but the illness is not very severe.

2. Is there Kidney qi deficiency in this case?

Urinary frequency at night is often associated with Kidney disorders, specifically Kidney qi deficiency leading to a loss of control over the Bladder. The patient in this case urinates three to four times nightly, but there are no other symptoms suggesting Kidney qi deficiency. A better explanation is that the body's general qi deficiency has led to a loss of Bladder control to some degree.

3. Is it more accurate to characterize this case as one of deficiency, or as a combination of deficiency and excess?

Blood stasis leading to qi deficiency combines deficiency with excess, and these two aspects are combined in this case.

The general lassitude is so severe that the patient is unable to work, but he has no headaches. This factor, together with the lusterless tongue, suggest that the predominant pattern is not blood stasis, but qi deficiency. However, because there is a certain degree of blood stasis, we must conclude that the overall pattern is a combination of deficiency and excess (excess within deficiency), rather than pure deficiency.

4. Depression is a common feature in both this and the previous case. What is the difference between the two cases?

In general, depression can be described as a very low response or reaction to the stimuli in one's environment. The cause of the depression in each of these cases is different. In the previous case it was Liver qi stagnation, and in this case, inability of the yang qi to rise, leading to a severe dysfunction of the spirit.

The general symptoms in these two cases are also different. In the previous case there was qi stagnation, while here there is qi deficiency. The nature of the depression is also different. In this case the depression is worse in the morning and improves in the afternoon. The patient suffers general lassitude related to Spleen qi deficiency and the inability of the clear yang to rise, which severely impairs the spirit and thereby causes depression. In the previous case, there was general depression.

Conclusion

1. According to the eight principles:
   Interior, cold, and a combination of deficiency and excess (excess within deficiency).
2. According to etiology:
   Blood stasis.
3. According to theory of qi, blood, and body fluids:
   Qi deficiency, blood stasis.
4. According to Organ theory:
   Deficiency of Spleen and Heart, and malnourishment of the spirit.

Treatment principle

1. Tonify the qi and promote the rising of the yang.
2. Nourish the blood and remove the obstruction from the channels and collaterals.

Explanation of treatment principle

There is no obvious blood deficiency in this case, but the poor circulation of blood has deprived the spirit of nourishment. Thus, in order to calm and nourish the spirit, we must both tonify the qi and nourish the blood. Two points should be kept in mind:

1. Because qi deficiency has prevented the clear yang from rising, we must promote the rising of the yang at the same time as we tonify the qi.

2. Blood stasis is the underlying cause of the symptoms. Although deficiency is the main problem at the moment, it is important that the blood stasis also be removed, otherwise normal blood cannot be produced. If all we do is tonify the qi and blood, the blood will still be unable to circulate and nourish the body, as the stasis will continue to obstruct circulation. We must therefore nourish the blood, but also remove the obstruction from the channels and collaterals.

If we keep these two points in mind and treat accordingly, we can improve the blood circulation, provide nourishment to the Heart spirit, and enable the clear yang to rise. The key to treatment is in pinpointing the cause.

Selection of points

GV-20 *(bai hui)*   BL-44 *(shen tang)*
GV-16 *(feng fu)*   BL-49 *(yi she)*
BL-15 *(xin shu)*   BL-50 *(wei cang)*
BL-20 *(pi shu)*   GV-4 *(ming men)*
BL-21 *(wei shu)*

Explanation of points

GV-20 *(bai hui)* is the meeting point of the yang channels in the head, thus its Chinese name , which means "hundred meetings." It is located in the middle of the top of the head, where the three leg and three arm yang channels, as well as the governing vessel, meet. This point is used to revive the spirit, settle the emotions, and restore the yang. It is a very important point in treating such disorders and symptoms of the head as headache, dizziness, tinnitus, nasal obstruction, and aphasia in windstroke. It also promotes the yang in general, and is used in treating the failure of clear yang to rise. Here, the point was used to enable the yang qi to rise, thereby calming the spirit and relieving the depression and anxiety. The tonification method was used at this point.

GV-16 *(feng fu)*. *Fēng* means wind or pathogenic wind, and *fǔ* means palace or meeting place. As its name suggests, this is an important point in treating disorders that involve wind. It is used to expel pathogenic wind and to remove obstruction (including blood stasis) from the head. It is especially useful in treating internal wind, with such symptoms as dizziness, stiff neck, dysphasia, hemiplegia, mania, and epilepsy. In the present case, the depresssion, which is worse in the morning, can be attributed to blood stasis, qi deficiency, and malnourishment of the spirit. This point not only helps remove the obstruction due to the blood stasis, but also assists GV-20 *(bai hui)* in promoting the yang.

BL-15 *(xin shu)* is the back associated point of the Heart. It soothes the Heart, promotes the Heart function, and calms the spirit. It harmonizes the nutritive and protective qi. It is used in treating many disorders associated with the Heart and Heart channel, psychological problems like panic attacks, precordial pain, palpitations, insomnia, poor memory, restlessness, night sweats, and especially deficiency patterns.

BL-20 *(pi shu)* is the back associated point of the Spleen. It strengthens the Spleen, harmonizes the functions of the middle burner, and resolves dampness. This point is used to treat disorders of the middle burner, including disharmony between the Spleen and Stomach. It is an important point in the treatment of such problems as poor appetite, abdominal distention, nausea, vomiting, diarrhea, poor digestion, stools containing undigested food, jaundice, edema, and dysentery. In this case, it is one of the main points used for treating the Spleen deficiency.

BL-21 *(wei shu)* is the back associated point of the Stomach. It is used to strengthen the Spleen and Stomach, harmonize the functions of the middle burner, and promote the downward movement of the Stomach qi, thus treating reversal of Stomach qi. This is another useful point in treating disorders of the middle burner. It is used to treat diseases involving the Stomach, as well as symptoms of the yang Organs associated with the yang brightness channels (Stomach and Large Intestine) such as epigastric pain, regurgitation, borborygmus, chest and hypochondrial pain, nausea, vomiting, and abdominal distention. In this case, the point serves as an assistant: the main pattern involves Spleen and Heart deficiency, and this point is used to promote the functions of the middle burner in order to help treat the deficiency in the Spleen.

BL-44 *(shen tang)*. The name of this point means "dwelling place of the spirit." It is used for releasing qi stagnation in the chest, promoting the Heart functions, and calming the Heart spirit. The point is not only useful in treating such physical disorders as cough, wheezing, asthma, shortness of breath, fullness in the chest, and shoulder pain, but is also important in the treatment of psychological symptoms. In the clinic it is used in accordance with the theory of the Organs, and is especially suitable for Heart disorders leading to malnourishment of the spirit, or a disturbance of the Heart spirit. The point is useful in treating symptoms associated with these disorders, such as anxiety, palpitations, insomnia, and depression.

BL-49 *(yi she)*. The psychological aspect associated with the Spleen is intention *(yi)*, which is also translated as intelligence or reflection. The Chinese name for this point means "dwelling of the intention." It strengthens the Spleen and promotes both digestion and appetite. It treats disorders involving the Spleen, Stomach, and Large Intestine such as abdominal distention, borborygmus, diarrhea, vomiting, nausea, and poor appetite. It can also treat emotional problems such as obsessive thinking, which can lead to Spleen deficiency with such symptoms as poor appetite and digestion, abdominal distention, and nausea.

BL-50 *(wei cang)*. The Chinese name for this point means "storehouse [granary] of the Stomach." This point regulates the qi, harmonizes the middle burner functions, and treats disorders like stomachache, poor appetite, and abdominal distention. It is an assistant point in this case, used in treating Heart and Spleen deficiency.

GV-4 *(ming men)* is located midway between the back associated points of the Kidney, BL-23 *(shen shu)*. Kidney qi is the root of the qi for the entire body, thus the Chinese name for this point, which means "gate of vitality." The function of this point is to strengthen source qi, promote vitality, and to improve the functioning of the lower back and knees. It is used in treating such disorders as back pain, abdominal pain, and chronic diarrhea. In women it is used for such problems as menstrual disorders and excessive leukorrhea. In men it is used for impotence and seminal emissions. It can also be used in treating such emotional disorders as insomnia, depression, panic attacks, and fright. In this case it serves as an assistant point: in view of the Heart and Spleen deficiency, it is used to tonify the Kidney in order to treat the Heart deficiency, and to harmonize the Heart and Kidney in order to treat the emotional disorder—the depression in this case.

Combination of points

GV-16 *(feng fu)* and GV-20 *(bai hui)* is one of the classical combinations from *Songs of the Essentials of Practicing Acupuncture (Xing zhen zhi yao ge)*. It is an important combination for treating disorders involving wind, especially internal wind. In patterns caused by wind, the attacks are sudden and the symptoms are changeable. When wind attacks the head, it frequently obstructs the channels there, disrupting the functions associated with the head. These two points on the governing vessel are used since this channel governs the general yang qi of the body; the points are helpful in removing wind from the head. Also, because a portion of the channel goes around the middle of the center line of the head, it is very useful in treating psychological and emotional disorders. These two points are effective in calming the spirit and removing obstruction from the head.

Combination of back associated points and "spirit" points

The back associated points are located along the first line of the Bladder channel on the back; they draw on the qi from the channels of each yin or yang Organ in treating disorders (especially deficiency patterns) of the yin or yang Organs. The back associated points of the yin and yang Organs are as follows:

BL-13 *(fei shu)* . . . . Lung
BL-14 *(jue yin shu)* . . . . Pericardium
BL-15 *(xin shu)* . . . . Heart
BL-19 *(dan shu)* . . . . Gallbladder
BL-18 *(gan shu)* . . . . Liver
BL-21 *(wei shu)* . . . . Stomach
BL-20 *(pi shu)* . . . . Spleen
BL-25 *(da chang shu)* . . . . Large Intestine
BL-23 *(shen shu)* . . . . Kidney
BL-27 *(xiao chang shu)* . . . . Small Intestine
BL-28 *(pang guang shu)* . . . . Bladder

As this list shows, there are 11 back associated points in all: five for the yin Organs and six for the yang. Among them, it is the back associated points of the yin Organs that are mainly used in treating psychological and emotional disorders.

The five "spirit" points are also located on the back, on the second line of the Bladder channel:

BL-42 *(po hu)*, 3 units lateral to BL-13 *(fei shu)*, the back associated point of the Lung

BL-44 *(shen tang)*, 3 units lateral to BL-15 *(xin shu)*, the back associated point of the Heart

BL-47 *(hun men)*, 3 units lateral to BL-18 *(gan shu)*, the back associated point of the Liver

BL-49 *(yi she)*, 3 units lateral to BL-20 *(pi shu)*, the back associated point of the Spleen

BL-52 *(zhi shi)*, 3 units lateral to BL-23 *(shen shu)*, the back associated point of the Kidney

When each of the first characters in the Chinese names for these points are arranged according to the order of the five elements, we can clearly see their correspondences to the five psychological aspects, which in turn are associated with the five yin Organs:

shén (spirit) . . . . Heart
hún (ethereal soul) . . . . Liver
yì (intention or reflection) . . . . Spleen
pò (corporeal soul, courage, or daring) . . . . . . Lung
zhì (purpose, will) . . . . Kidney

The second character in each of the Chinese names for these points refers to parts of a dwelling: *táng* means hall or dwelling place, *mén* means a gate or door, *shè* means abode, *hù* means a door, and *shì* means a room or chamber. These points are used in treating the psychological and emotional problems caused by physical illness, as well as the physical illnesses caused by psychological and emotional disorders. The points are frequently used, since in Chinese medicine, psychological and emotional disorders are directly related to the various internal Organs. In clinical practice the combination of back associated points and spirit points is very useful. If the diagnosis is correct, the results will be excellent. In this case, although the disorder has lasted a long time, once the cause of the disease is corrected, the symptoms of depression will be relieved rather quickly.

Follow-up

The patient was treated twice a week. After the very first treatment he felt as if a door had suddenly opened and fresh air had entered his head. He also noted that the morning depression was largely alleviated, and did not last as long. Because he had been taking antidepression and anti-anxiety medication for four years, his physical and mental energy were still poor, and the urinary frequency was basically unchanged. Treatment was continued for two weeks, during which the patient's energy and emotions were much improved, and the morning depression occurred for only a very short time. He slept much better, and only had to get up once during the night to urinate. His appetite returned to normal and he fully enjoyed his food.

The treatment was continued, this time once a week, for another three weeks, after which all the symptoms were alleviated.

The patient returned a year later for a checkup and reported that there was no further depression and that he was working once again on a daily basis.

It is important to note that while the patient was diagnosed as having blood stasis four years ago, at the time of treatment the blood stasis was no longer a major problem, and there were few related symptoms. By the time he came to the clinic, qi deficiency was the main problem, with only a little residual blood stasis (as evidenced by the history and lusterless tongue). Treatment, therefore, did not focus on the blood stasis, although a small part of the treatment was used to remove the residual blood stasis from the channels and collaterals, to improve the blood circulation and thereby help the qi deficiency. Still, an understanding of blood stasis and its ramifications is crucial to understanding the dynamic of the problem in this case, and in arriving at an appropriate treatment plan.

CASE 35: **Male, age 34**

Main complaint

Recurrent stress and anxiety

History

The patient has been engaged in very intense and stressful mental work at his office for a long period of time. During the past ten years he has developed severe episodic stress and anxiety. When stressed and anxious, he feels hot all over his body, sweats, has palpitations, and becomes very restless. Sometimes he suffers from depression. His memory is poor, he cannot concentrate or control himself properly, and the symptoms worsen after he has been thinking for a long time. He is often angry and irritable. At one point he was given conventional medical treatment and took tranquilizers, antidepressants, and anti-anxiety medication. However, because he disliked taking them, their use was soon discontinued.

The patient has developed a large appetite, and he tends to eat in order to help relieve the tension and stress; his body weight has consequently increased. His general energy is normal, although his sleep is not very sound; he finds it difficult to fall asleep, and wakes early in the morning. Skin flakes from his scalp, which has become dry, and he is losing his hair. He often develops rashes on his chest and back, and his skin can be red, dry, and itchy. When the tension and anxiety is at its worst, he tends to scratch himself all over. His urine is yellow and his stools tend to be dry.

Tongue

Deep red with a thin, yellow coating

Pulse

Sunken and wiry, slightly forceless in the left distal position

Analysis of symptoms

1. Episodic stress, tension, anxiety, restlessness, and palpitations—disturbance of Heart spirit.
2. Diminished ability to think, poor memory and concentration—malnourishment of the spirit.
3. Reduced self-control, irritability, and occasional depression—disruption in the free-flow of Liver qi.
4. Unsound sleep, difficulty in falling asleep, and waking early in the morning—disturbance of the Heart spirit by pathogenic heat.
5. Increased appetite—Stomach fire.
6. Feeling hot, sweating, yellow urine, and dry stools—heat pattern.
7. Dry scalp, dandruff, hair loss, and skin rash—heat in the blood.
8. Deep red tongue with yellow coating—heat in the blood.
9. Sunken pulse, forceless in the left distal position—interior deficiency pattern.

Basic theory of case

A pattern of blood heat can emerge when pathogenic heat affects the blood. Symptoms that are characteristic of this pattern can be divided into three groups: those that involve heat, bleeding, and injury to the yin.

1. *Heat symptoms:* red face, hot sensation over the entire body, restlessness, "butterflies" in the chest, insomnia, deep red tongue, rapid pulse. Severe cases can include unconsciousness and delirium.

2. *Bleeding symptoms:* hemorrhage and bleeding in various parts of the body such as hemoptysis, hematemesis, epistaxis, subcutaneous bleeding, blood in the urine and stools.

3. *Injury to the yin:* restlessness, hot sensation in the palms, soles, and chest, night sweats, dry mouth, deep red tongue with very little coating, a thin and forceless pulse.

Blood heat patterns can be of either external or internal origin.

External pathogenic heat can invade deeply to the nutritive or blood level, is excessive in nature, and is characterized by an acute onset and severe symptoms. A severe hemorrhage caused by excessive heat pushing the blood out of the vessels is often encountered.

Blood heat patterns of internal origin can be either excessive or deficient in nature. A strong emotional upset or disturbance can cause hyperactivity, which leads to excessive internal heat. By contrast, long-term stress can consume the yin and blood, especially the Heart and Kidney yin, leading to heat and fire from deficiency, which can affect the blood. Thus, while blood heat patterns of internal origin may be either excessive or deficient, attacks are usually chronic, and the duration of the illness is relatively long.

The deep red (*jiàng*) tongue is a very important diagnostic indicator for patterns of blood heat. If the heat becomes stronger, the tongue can turn purplish. This pathological change occurs because the pathogenic heat accelerates the circulation of blood. As the fire and heat rise, the circulation of blood in the tongue becomes excessive and the color turns purplish.

Fig. 7-13

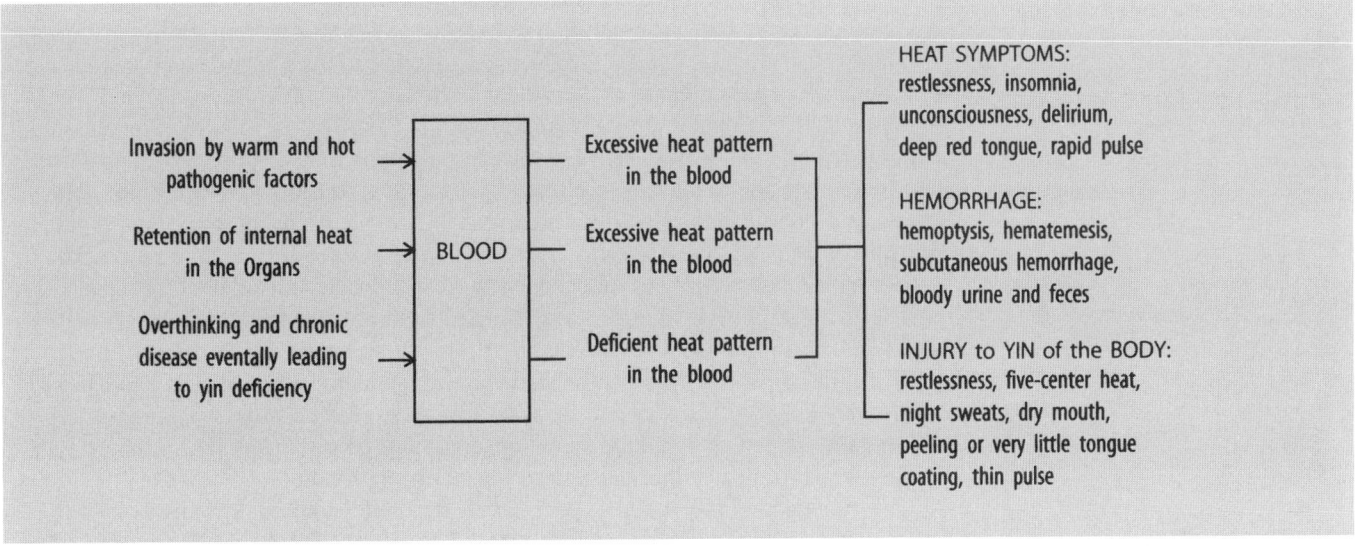

Cause of disease	Emotional upset and pathogenic fire

Over the years, the patient's high-powered job has resulted in psychological stress, which has led to stagnation of qi. This has then transformed into heat, which has injured the yin, resulting in Heart fire. Thus, both the emotional stress and the interior fire are pathogenic factors in this case.

Site of disease	Heart and Kidneys

The patient is restless and suffers from palpitations, stress, anxiety, and a poor memory, all of which are evidence of a Heart disorder.

    The long-term nature of the disorder, hair loss, symptoms associated with heat from yin deficiency, and the sunken pulse indicate a disorder of the Kidneys.

Pathological change	As we saw in previous cases, emotional disturbance or upset that causes qi stagnation, which then transforms into fire, is commonly seen in the clinic. This patient has no history of anger or chronic depression caused by Liver qi stagnation, but for a long time he has experienced a great deal of pressure at his job, which can be very stressful psychologically. If this persists too long, it can affect the free-flow of qi, and the ensuing obstruction can lead to heat. Over the long term, the desk-bound, mental nature of the patient's work can also injure the Heart yin and blood, leading to an imbalance of yin and yang, and gradually giving rise to Heart heat and fire. The qi stagnation in this case also contributes to the production of heat. Because the Heart governs the circulation of blood and the functioning of the vessels, when Heart fire is strong, it can directly affect the blood, leading to blood heat.

    The Heart spirit is normally housed in, supported, and nourished by the Heart blood. When heat disturbs the blood, however, the Heart spirit cannot remain calm, and the patient will suffer from anxiety, palpitations, restlessness, and insomnia. The injury to the yin and blood caused by the patient's stressful work can aggravate the imbalance between yin and yang, which in turn may increase the blood heat, which further injures the yin and blood. Thus, the Heart becomes more deficient in yin and blood.

    Malnourishment of the Heart spirit impairs the memory. The decline in one's ability to think and concentrate is also a manifestation of the malnourishment of the Heart spirit. This is because thinking, as a function or action of the body, is a yang activity; as such, it can consume the substance of the body, that is, the yin and blood. Thus, the patient's strenuous mental work over a long period of time can aggravate the deficiency of Heart blood, and the physical symptoms will worsen.

The Liver is regarded as the "sea of blood." Injury to the yin and blood can lead to deficiency of Liver blood. When there is deficiency or insufficiency of Liver blood, the Liver is unable to maintain the normal free-flow of qi, which results in irritability, poor self-control, and symptoms associated with depression. In this case, the symptoms related to the interruption in the free-flow of qi are not very severe, and are secondary to the injury to the Heart yin and blood. Thus, if the Heart disorder is resolved, these symptoms should disappear of their own accord. It is therefore unnecessary to independently treat the Liver disorder in this case.

The yang brightness channels and yang Organs are very rich in qi and blood. When heat in the blood level affects the Stomach and yang brightness channels, impeding the Stomach's ability to warm and digest food, the digestive function itself will become overactive, and the patient will develop an excessive appetite. At present, the patient in this case does not complain of poor energy, tiredness, or fatigue, which indicates that the Spleen has not been affected.

The function of the blood is to nourish the body, that is, the yin and yang Organs, various tissues, and sensory organs. The adage "The hair is the surplus of the blood" means that the hair relies on the nourishment from blood to maintain its luster, color, thickness, strength, flexibility, and softness. The skin of the scalp also relies on the nourishment from blood. The health of the Kidney is manifested in the hair (glossiness), thus the qi and essence of the Kidney play a very important part in the normal growth of hair. Heat in the blood will affect its ability to provide nourishment, and can reduce the fluid in the blood. Heat or fire can also descend from the Heart and consume the Kidney yin. Kidney yin deficiency can then lead to, or aggravate, heat or fire from deficiency. The deficiency deprives the hair of nourishment, causing it to become dry, brittle, and easy to fall out. Dryness of the scalp and dandruff can also result.

Pathogenic heat in the blood can be reflected in the skin as a rash. When fire and heat accumulate in the body, the body fluids are injured and pushed out of the body. The patient accordingly feels hot and sweats, his urine becomes yellow, and his stools are dry.

The deep red tongue and yellow coating in this case are evidence of heat in the blood. The pulse, which is sunken and forceless in the left distal position, suggests deficiency of yin and blood in both the Heart and Kidney, and especially injury to the Heart yin, which has become very obvious.

Pattern of disease

The fire has deeply affected the blood and vessels, indicating an interior pattern.

The patient's restlessness, sensation of heat, deep red tongue, and yellow coating suggest a pattern of heat.

The yin and blood deficiency, and the malnourishment of the spirit, are evidence of deficiency. The presence of excessive pathogenic heat is an element of excess.

Additional notes

1. Is the heat in this case deficient or excessive in nature?

Pathogenic heat or fire as an independent factor can be deficient or excessive, depending on the cause.

The main symptoms in the pattern of excessive Stomach heat are a big appetite, frequent hunger, a hot, burning sensation and pain in the area of the Stomach, regurgitation, indeterminant gnawing hunger (*cáo zá*), swollen and painful gums, foul-smelling breath, constipation, red tongue with a yellow coating, and a rapid and forceful pulse. The main symptoms of Stomach yin deficiency include hunger, but with little appetite, a dull, mild pain in the Stomach area, dryness in the mouth, dry stools, red tongue, dry tongue coating, and a thin and rapid pulse.

In this case, the patient has a big appetite and has also been gaining weight. Based on these symptoms alone, one would expect the nature of the Stomach heat to be excessive. However, when viewing the condition in its entirety, there are more symptoms of heat from deficiency, such as restlessness, insomnia, waking early, poor memory and concentration, dryness in the scalp, and loss of hair. Once a combination of deficiency and excess has been diagnosed, we must then decide which of the two is the main problem. Here, having analyzed the entire case, we can conclude that there is excess within a larger pattern of deficiency, that is, deficiency is the main problem.

The pulse is also of interest here. If there is only excessive heat, the pulse is usually rapid and forceful; if the heat is only from deficiency, the pulse is rapid but forceless. Because the pulse here is sunken and forceless, we have determined that fire from deficiency is the main problem. The lack of a rapid pulse runs counter to the diagnosis of heat, but, in light of the remainder of the presentation, this can be disregarded for the moment.

Heart fire was diagnosed in both this case and case 30, but the fire in the earlier case was excessive and therefore associated with a pattern of excess; the patient's restlessness and sensation of heat were quite severe. In this case, the deficiency of yin and body fluids in the Heart and Kidney has resulted in the rising of fire from deficiency. In contrast to the earlier case, the restlessness and sensation of heat are relatively mild here, but the patient's anxiety is very obvious. This explains why the two cases are treated differently.

2. How does one distinguish between patterns of the qi system and patterns of the blood system?

When diagnosing according to the theory of qi, blood, and body fluids, problems of the qi are said to reflect a disruption in the body's inner defensive system, while problems of the blood indicate that there is trouble with the flow of blood, or within the blood vessels. Other distinguishing points include the following:

- *Site of disease*: Disorders of the qi mainly occur in the Lung, Spleen, Stomach, and, to a certain degree, the Liver (Liver qi stagnation, Liver fire rising); this would not include disorders involving Liver blood or yin. Disorders of the blood occur in the Heart, Kidney, and Liver blood and yin.

- *Symptoms:* Heat patterns affecting the qi are excessive in nature. If the heat is very strong, the patient generally sweats excessively, is very thirsty, and is inclined to drink a lot of cold beverage. In some cases there may be symptoms associated with stagnation of qi, such as irritability, poor temper, and a full or distending sensation in the intercostal and hypochondrial regions. However, with patterns affecting the blood, the heat is generally from deficiency. There may sometimes be excessive heat in the blood, but the heat and thirst are not as strong as the heat affecting the qi. Also, such symptoms as restlessness, dry and hot sensation over the entire body, insomnia, anxiety, and poor memory are associated with a disturbance of the Heart spirit by heat, or malnourishment of the Heart spirit. These symptoms often occur in blood patterns.

- *Tongue and pulse:* With patterns of excess affecting the qi, there is a red tongue with a thick, yellow, and dry coating, and the pulse is flooding, rapid, and forceful. If a qi pattern involves stagnation of qi activity, the tongue generally does not change very much, and the pulse will be wiry. With heat patterns of the blood, the tongue is deep red with a yellow coating, and in patterns of heat from deficiency, the tongue coating is very slight and dry. The pulse is usually rapid, or thin, rapid, and forceless.

The main complaint in both this case and case 33 is anxiety, but in the earlier case the disorder was associated with a pattern that mainly involved Liver qi stagnation.

Fig. 7-14

The symptoms there were due to impaired qi activity affecting the Heart qi and Heart blood. By contrast, here the disorder is associated with a pattern involving the blood, as it was caused by deficiency of yin and blood in the Heart and Kidney, and by fire in the Heart. The symptom of anxiety is caused by a dysfunction of the Heart itself, while the symptoms associated with Liver qi stagnation are not severe in this case.

	HEAT PATTERN in QI SYSTEM	HEAT PATTERN in BLOOD SYSTEM	PATHOLOGICAL CHANGE in BLOOD SYSTEM
SITE of DISEASE	Lung, Spleen, Stomach, Liver (Liver qi)	Heart, Kidney, Liver (Liver blood, Liver yin)	
SYMPTOMS	High fever, excessive sweating	Hot sensation all over, worse during the night, or hot sensation in the chest, palms, and soles; night sweats	Yin system of body deeply invaded by pathogenic factors, or heat from deficiency
	Thirst, preference for cold drinks	Slight thirst	Pathogenic heat injures the nutritive system
	Irritability and hot temper	Restlessness, insomnia	Heart spirit disturbed by heat
TONGUE and PULSE	Red tongue	Deep red tongue	Nutritive and blood systems deeply invaded by pathogenic heat; Stomach yin already badly injured; deficiency of yin and blood
	Yellow, thick, dry and cracked tongue coating	Very little tongue coating, partially or completely peeled coating, or no coating	
	Flooding and rapid pulse	Rapid or thin and rapid pulse	

Conclusion

1. According to the eight principles:
   Interior, heat, combination of deficiency and excess (excess within deficiency).

2. According to etiology:
   Emotional factor (stress) is the cause of the illness.

3. According to theory of qi, blood, and body fluids:
   Blood heat pattern.

4. According to Organ theory:
   Disharmony of the Heart and Kidney, rising of heat from deficiency, and heat pattern in the Stomach.

Treatment principle

1. Nourish the yin and clear the heat.

2. Harmonize the Heart and Kidney.

3. Cool the blood and calm the spirit.

Explanation of treatment principle

Blood heat can be either deficient or excessive in nature, and each is treated differently.

For excessive heat, the blood must be cooled and the heat cleared; the reducing method is therefore used. However, it is heat from deficiency that is the main problem in this case. It was caused by yin deficiency, which led to a preponderance of yang, resulting in the rise of heat or fire from deficiency. Thus, if we use only the cooling method to reduce the heat, we risk aggravating the yin deficiency and making the symptoms worse. We must therefore also nourish the yin.

The main method in this case is to nourish the Heart and Kidney yin. As the yin becomes stronger, the imbalance of yang and Heart fire will be brought under control. At the same time, we must clear the heat so that it stops injuring the yin and body fluids.

Selection of points

First prescription:

LI-11 *(qu chi)*
LI-4 *(he gu)*
KI-6 *(zhao hai)*
N-HN-54 *(an mian)*

Second prescription:

BL-13 *(fei shu)*
BL-15 *(xin shu)*
BL-17 *(ge shu)*
SP-10 *(xue hai)*

Explanation of points

First prescription:

LI-11 *(qu chi)* is the sea point of the arm yang brightness channel. It soothes wind, clears heat, and regulates the nutritive and protective qi of the body. It is very effective in treating febrile diseases involving the entire body, skin rashes, and fungal infections. This point is very useful for clearing heat, especially from the qi level, and from the yang Organs, especially those associated with the yang brightness channels. Clearing the heat from the qi level also assists in cooling the blood.

In this case, the point is used to clear the Stomach heat, and also the dry, itchy skin and skin rash.

LI-4 *(he gu)* is the source point of the arm yang brightness channel. It is very effective in clearing heat and alleviating pain. It is one of the most important points used in the clinic. It is also excellent for regulating qi in order to remove obstruction from the channels and collaterals, expelling pathogenic wind, and removing external diorders. It is used in treating patterns of heat, spontaneous sweating, and depression. It is one of the four gate points.

In this case, the point is used to clear the heat, settle the emotional and psychological symptoms, and treat the restlessness and skin disorders.

KI-6 *(zhao hai)* nourishes the yin, tonifies the Kidney, and soothes the spirit. In this case, it treats the heat from yin deficiency, which underlies the disharmony between the Heart and Kidney.

N-HN-54 *(an mian)* calms the spirit and improves sleep. In this case, the point is used for the insomnia (as the patient's Heart spirit is obviously disturbed), unsound sleep, early wakening, and irritability.

Second prescription:

BL-13 *(fei shu)* is the back associated point of the Lung. It promotes the dispersing function of the Lung, regulates the qi in the upper burner, and treats cough, asthma, and a stifling sensation in the chest. It is also used in promoting the yin of the body, and in clearing heat. It can be used for treating tidal fever, night sweats, and "steaming bone disorder"*(gǔ zhēng)*, the term used to describe heat coming from deep inside the body—patients feel that the internal heat is so intense that it is "steaming" the bones.

In this case, it serves as a secondary point to promote the yin of the body, clear the heat from the upper burner, calm the spirit in order to remove the anxiety, and promote the pectoral qi in the upper burner in order to support the Heart spirit.

BL-15 *(xin shu)* is the back associated point of the Heart. It calms the Heart, soothes the emotions, and regulates the nutritive and defensive qi. In the clinic, this point is often used for such symptoms as palpitations, anxiety, restlessness, and frightfulness.

In this case, the point is used to nourish the Heart blood and spirit in order to treat the patient's poor memory and concentration.

BL-17 *(ge shu)* is the influential point for the blood. It regulates the blood, treats blood deficiency, harmonizes the functions of the Spleen and Stomach, and removes qi stagnation from the middle burner.

In this case, the patient's excessive mental work and exhaustion have consumed the yin and blood, which has led to the blood deficiency in the Heart and the disharmony between the Heart and Kidney. In view of the skin problem caused by the heat in the blood, as well as the Stomach heat, this point is used to harmonize the middle burner and nourish the blood.

SP-10 *(xue hai)* regulates and cools the blood, and regulates the qi in the channels and collaterals. This is a very important point in treating blood disorders.

In this case, the point is mainly used in treating the consumption of yin and blood caused by the heat in the blood. It can also help in treating the skin disorders.

The first prescription is mainly used to clear the heat from the qi aspect, and the second to clear the blood heat, nourish the yin, and calm the Heart spirit. The back associated points serve as the main points in the second prescription; they are used to clear the blood heat, nourish the blood, and calm the spirit. Thus, each prescription has its own characteristics. Here, they are used alternately.

Combination of points

LI-11 *(qu chi)* and LI-4 *(he gu)* are both located on the yang brightness channel. Both points clear heat, regulate qi, remove exterior patterns, and treat similar skin disorders as rashes. LI-11 *(qu chi)* is more effective in clearing heat from the yang Organs than is LI-4 *(he gu)*. It is also good for eliminating stagnation and depression. Together, both points strengthen the function of clearing the heat and removing the symptoms from the body surface. They can also treat the anxiety, irritability, and heat in the yang Organs.

BL-17 *(ge shu)* and SP-10 *(xue hai)*. The former is the influential point for the blood, and the latter's Chinese name means "sea of blood"; thus, both of these points are important for treating blood disorders. BL-17 *(ge shu)* is more effective in treating blood deficiency, while SP-10 *(xue hai)* is better for regulating the blood and clearing blood heat. Together, the two points form an important combination for treating heat from blood deficiency, which disturbs the spirit. In this case, the combination was used to calm the spirit.

Follow-up

Because of the patient's intense work, responsibility, and long hours, he could not spare much time for treatment. It was therefore decided to give him short courses of treatment, each lasting four weeks, during which he would be given acupuncture once a week, alternating the two groups of points. There was a three-week interval between each of the courses of treatment.

After just two courses, there was an obvious improvement in his condition. The dry skin had more or less disappeared, there was very little spontaneous sweating, his self-control was much better, he slept longer at night, and his concentration and memory were slightly improved. It was suggested that he modify his lifestyle a little, and reduce his hours of work.

Subsequently, treatment was reduced to twice a month, in the first and second weeks of the month. Treatment was continued in this manner for another three months, after which the symptoms had more or less disappeared. Three years later there had been no recurrence of any of the symptoms mentioned in the history. The patient's emotions had become quite stable, and his memory and concentration were both good.

CASE 36: **Female, age 61**

Main complaint

Paroxysmal fear and panic attacks

History

When the patient was young, she developed into a very sensitive person whose emotions and mental state were easily affected by changes in her environment. She became nervous or tense quite easily, and would then need to visit the bathroom to move her bowels. Her stools were often unformed, but she never suffered any abdominal pain.

Over the past couple years the symptoms have worsened and her attacks are now accompanied by fear, anxiety, and depression; such episodes occur on an irregular basis and are paroxysmal in nature. She sometimes wakes during the night with a feeling of panic, and often has palpitations and shortness of breath. These attacks can occur while she is driving, or when she is in other situations. The symptoms only last a few seconds and then disappear. They are accompanied by general dizziness and nausea during the attacks, but there is no sensation of heat. She has tried conventional medication (tranquilizers and anti-anxiety tablets), but without much success.

Generally speaking, the patient's energy is poor, and she tires easily. Although she is not a very big eater, her appetite has remained the same for many years, and so can be considered normal. She sleeps soundly, apart from the panic attacks. Her urination is normal, but her stools are not properly formed. A conventional medical checkup revealed no abnormality.

Tongue

Dark and red, with a thick, white, greasy, and moist coating

Pulse

Sunken and wiry

Analysis of symptoms

1. Long-term emotional sensitivity, easily affected by changes in her environment—Heart qi deficiency.
2. Bowel movements and unformed stools caused by mental stress—controlling function of Kidney qi is impaired.
3. Paroxysmal panic attacks, depression, and anxiety—Heart qi deficiency.
4. Palpitations and shortness of breath during attacks—impaired qi activity in the chest.
5. Chronic dizziness and poor energy—qi deficiency.
6. Dark red tongue—impaired blood circulation.
7. Thick, white, greasy, and moist tongue coating—internal cold and retention of dampness.
8. Sunken and wiry pulse—impaired qi activity.

Basic theory of case

There is an adage in Chinese medicine, "The Kidney controls urination and defecation *(shèn sī èr biàn)*". That is to say, the Kidney's functions, which include the warming function of Kidney yang and the controlling function of Kidney qi, are closely related to the removal of waste from the body.

The warming function of Kidney yang acts to replenish the Spleen and Stomach yang, which is responsible for the transportation and transformation of food, to meet the body's need for food essence and body fluids. After the middle burner absorbs the essence from the food and water, waste is discharged from the body in the form of urine and feces.

Kidney qi plays an important role in both urination and defecation by providing the energy for two related functions. One is the expulsion of urine and stool at the appropriate times, and under conscious control; the other is the retention of urine and stool at other times, thereby preventing incontinence. These functions must be coordinated to facilitate the removal of urine and stool at the proper times.

In Chinese medicine these twin functions are referred to as "opening and closing *(kāi hé)*."

Deficiency of the Kidney yang will affect the transportive and transformative functions of the Spleen and Stomach, causing poor digestion and poor metabolism of water. This will produce cold, retention of dampness, and diarrhea. Impairment of the controlling function of the Kidney qi will cause abnormal urination and defecation. In mild cases, the patient will have urinary frequency, or drip urine after urinating, or there may be desire to defecate frequently, and difficulty in controlling urination and defecation. In severe cases, there will be incontinence of urine or stool.

Fig. 7-15

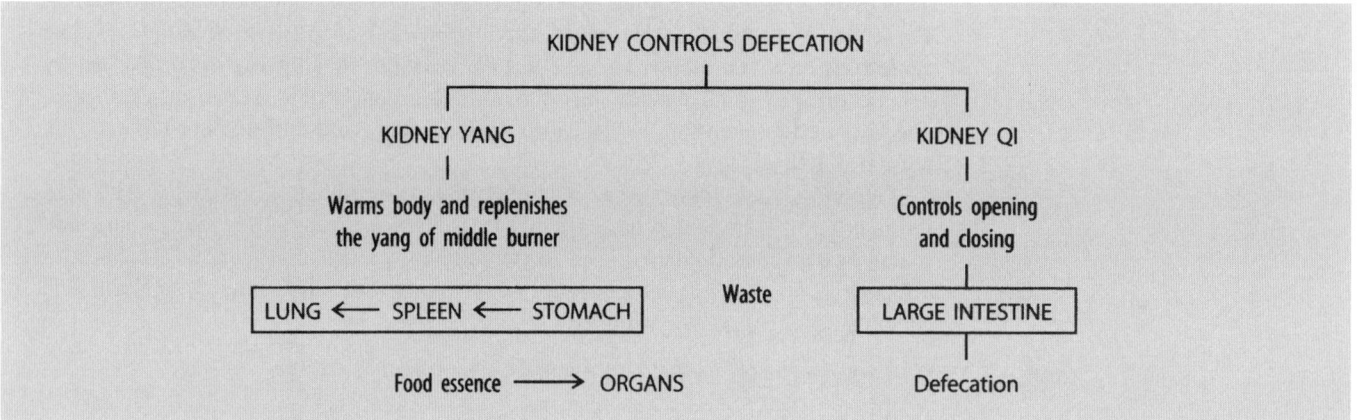

Cause of disease

Deficiency of antipathogenic factors

In this case there is no history of an invasion by external pathogenic factors, but the disorder has lasted a long time. The symptoms represent physiological dysfunctions that have gradually worsened. Thus, the antipathogenic factors have become deficient.

Site of disease

Heart and Kidney

The patient is very sensitive emotionally, and is easily affected by her immediate environment. She has paroxysmal panic attacks, anxiety, depression, and palpitations, all of which are evidence of a Heart disorder.

The nervousness or emotional stress that causes her to have bowel movements indicates a disorder of the Kidney.

Pathological change

The condition of one's spirit, the ability to think, the clarity of consciousness, and the capacity to adapt to one's environment are associated with the activities of various Organs. The Heart is responsible for these functions in general. There is a reference to this in chapter 8 of the *Divine Pivot:* "That which is responsible for things *(rèn wù)* is called the Heart." Commentators have interpreted this passage to mean that the Heart reacts to, and bears the effect of, all factors outside the body. In the *Classified Classic,* Zhang Jie-Bing observed that "The Heart is the ruler of the yin and yang Organs. It assembles and controls *(zǒng tǒng)* the ethereal soul and corporeal soul [courage], and also links together *(gāi)* intention and will." He also stated, "As for emotional injuries, each of the five yin Organs has those for which it is responsible. However, if you want to search for their origin, there is none that does not emanate from the Heart." The external environment (including both the social and physical environments) can influence human emotions and the physiological functions of the Organs. Yet the Heart plays a very important role in one's sensitivity to the environment. Those with sufficient Heart qi will be adaptable, but not unduly influenced by their surroundings.

In this particular case, the patient, from a very young age, has been over-sensitive to her environment, and her emotions are very easily affected by it. This indicates a congenital insufficiency of Heart qi. This condition deprives the Heart spirit of sufficient support from the yang qi, which explains why the patient is so intolerant of change in her environment.

Compared with the norm, those who suffer from deficiency are less able to cope with attacks from various pathogenic factors, and their antipathogenic factors are more easily injured. The patient here belongs to this category. Any change in the social and physical environment, no matter how benign, can still add an additional burden to the Heart qi, which is already congenitally deficient. This is the reason that the symptoms have gradually worsened. The Heart spirit governs psychological activity, and when the Heart qi is deficient, the Heart spirit is unable to control this activity. The patient will then manifest irregular and paroxysmal attacks of abnormal emotions. Anxiety, or the sudden onset of a panic attack, accompanied by palpitations and shortness of breath—regardless of whether it occurs while sleeping or awake—indicates a disturbance of the Heart spirit and its inability to control the emotions and psychological activity. Depression indicates that the deficiency of qi is such that the Heart spirit has been deprived of its stimulation and support from the yang.

Heart qi is part of the body's qi. Chronic Heart qi deficiency will eventually affect the qi in the body, resulting in general qi deficiency. This explains why the patient suffers from such general symptoms as dizziness and poor mental and physical energy.

When the patient is nervous, she suffers from diarrhea. This indicates a chronic insufficiency of Kidney qi. When there is no change in the environment, the qi and blood circulation is normal, and the Kidney qi is able to control the Large Intestine. But when her emotions are stimulated by the environment and she becomes nervous, the circulation of qi and blood are disturbed. The insufficiency of Kidney qi makes it harder to control the Large Intestine, which in turn makes the patient feel as if she must have a bowel movement, or that she is about to have diarrhea. Others can also suffer from abnormal urination.

Fig. 7-16

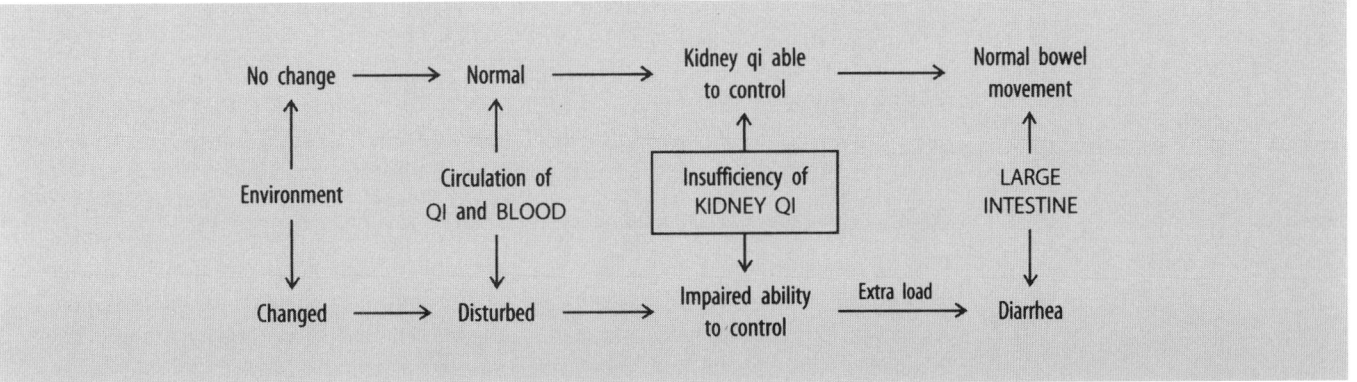

Heart qi deficiency impedes the circulation of blood. This accounts for the patient's dark tongue. The thick, white coating reflects the absence of pathogenic heat. The sunken and wiry pulse suggests that the qi activity is impaired, which, in this case, is caused by poor circulation of qi and blood.

Pattern of disease

The site of the disease is the Heart and Kidney, and there is no evidence of invasion by an external pathogenic factor. It is therefore an interior pattern.

The presence of cold is evidenced by the lack of heat, and by the dark quality of the tongue with its thick, white, greasy, and moist coating.

Organ function has declined, the patient suffers from dizziness, palpitations, and shortness of breath, and has poor physical and mental energy. All of these symptoms suggest a pattern of deficiency.

Additional notes

1. Why are the antipathogenic factors deficient?

Deficiency of the antipathogenic factors has been identified as the primary cause of this illness, but what has caused the deficiency?

The patient's history reveals that the symptoms associated with insufficiency of Heart and Kidney qi began when she was very young. We must therefore consider the possibility that congenital Heart and Kidney deficiency is the basis of this disorder. By the time she came for treatment she was 61 years of age, and her qi deficiency had become more marked, with a corresponding worsening of the symptoms. Generally speaking, problems associated with deficiency become aggravated as one gets older, as aging is a degenerative process. Thus, we can identify two reasons for the deficiency of antipathogenic factors in this case: a congenital disorder and aging.

2. Is there any disorder of the Spleen and Stomach?

The patient's fear and panic attacks are often accompanied by such symptoms as nausea, which indicates a reversal of Stomach qi. In general, the stools are unformed, which is often found in patterns of Spleen qi deficiency. The tongue coating is white, thick, greasy, and moist, which is indicative of damp-cold retention in the body. This is often caused when the transportation and transformation of water by the Spleen is impaired. Would it then be correct to diagnose a disorder of the Spleen and Stomach?

Nausea only occurs during the patient's fear and panic attacks. It is caused by an emotional upset, which affects the upward and downward movement of the qi activity in the middle burner, resulting in a reversal of Stomach qi, and thus the nausea. When the psychological and emotional symptoms are relieved, the qi activity is restored to normal, and the nausea spontaneously disappears. This confirms that there is no disorder of the Stomach itself.

Based on the characteristics of the bowel movements, the nature of the tongue coating, and the Kidney deficiency, we might consider a tendency toward deficiency of Kidney yang qi in this case. In this pattern there is retention of dampness and harmful water in the body—which accounts for the moist, greasy tongue coating—which drains downward to the Large Intestine, causing diarrhea. A Spleen disorder can be ruled out, since the patient has a normal appetite.

3. Why does tension cause diarrhea or the need for a bowel movement?

The relationship between diarrhea or bowel movements and an emotional disorder is a common one. In this respect, the most common emotions are anxiety, nervousness, irritability, fear, and panic attacks. The affected Organs include the Kidney, Liver, Spleen, and Large Intestine, but especially the Kidney and Liver. The most common pathogenesis is as follows. The Kidney controls defecation by regulating the opening and closing of the Large Intestine. Deficiency of either Kidney qi or Kidney yang can lead to this type of abnormal bowel movement. The emotions involved are usually panic, nervousness, or fear. Symptoms accompanying Kidney yang deficiency are of a cold nature, such as feeling cold, cold extremities, pale complexion, watery stools, pale and flabby tongue with a white, moist coating, and a sunken, slow pulse. There are no such cold symptoms associated with Kidney qi deficiency.

With respect to the Liver, when its function in regulating the free-flow of qi is impaired, there may be a transverse attack against the Spleen (disharmony between the Liver and Spleen) which interferes with its transportive and transformative functions. This can lead to diarrhea or abnormal bowel movements. The emotions most often implicated in this Liver pattern are anxiety, irritability, anger, or nervousness. After experiencing such emotions, the patient will have abdominal pain, followed by a bowel movement or diarrhea. The pain is relieved after defecation, and the patient feels comfortable. Other symptoms include pain and distention in the hypochondria, frequent sighing, and poor appetite.

In this case, there are no cold symptoms that would suggest deficiency of Kidney yang, and no symptoms suggesting disharmony between the Liver and Spleen. Thus, the diagnosis is very clearly deficiency of Kidney qi.

Conclusion

1. According to the eight principles:
   Interior, cold, and deficiency.

2. According to etiology:
   Qi deficiency.

3. According to Organ theory:
   Heart and Kidney qi deficiency.

Treatment principle

1. Warm and tonify the Heart and Kidney.

2. Calm the spirit.

Explanation of treatment principle

Qi and yang both pertain to yang in a general sense, but in terms of their physiological functions, qi and yang have different characteristics. The function of qi is to circulate, move, and promote normal functioning, whereas the function of yang is to warm. Symptoms associated with Heart and Kidney qi deficiency are therefore different from those involving Heart and Kidney yang deficiency. The former is characterized mainly by hypofunction, but there are no cold symptoms. By contrast, the latter is associated with cold symptoms.

In theory, just tonifying the qi should be sufficient for treating Heart and Kidney qi deficiency—it is not particularly necessary to also warm the yang. However, in view of the fact that qi and yang both pertain to yang, we can use the yang, especially Kidney yang, to warm the body. In clinical practice, tonifying the qi and warming the yang are often used in treating qi deficiency, and this practice clearly increases the efficacy of treatment. Warming the yang is very important to the production of qi and blood, since both need warmth to circulate, and cold causes constriction and congealing. Thus, when treating a patient with qi deficiency, the tonification of qi will be improved if accompanied by warming the yang.

Selection of points

GV-20 *(bai hui)*
BL-42 *(po hu)*
Bl-44 *(shen tang)*
KI-3 *(tai xi)* [right side]
BL-60 *(kun lun)* [left side]

Explanation of points

GV-20 *(bai hui)* promotes the function of the brain, restores the yang, and is very potent in tonifying the yang qi of the body. It is very effective in treating patterns involving sinking of the yang, and is good for extinguishing wind in the head.

In this case, because the patient's irregular, episodic, and paroxysmal panic attacks are akin to the changeable characteristics of wind, the point is used to settle the spirit and extinguish the wind and thereby relieve the panic.

BL-42 *(po hu)*. The word *pò* means courage or daring, and *hù* means door. *Pò* is often translated as corporeal soul, but in medicine, we believe that it refers more to a person's courage or emotional strength (see also case 34 above, and case 16 in

Acupuncture Patterns and Practice). This point is located 1.5 units lateral to BL-13 *(fei shu),* the associated point of the Lung. Each of the five yin Organs is associated with different psychological qualities, and emotional strength *(pò)* is associated with the Lung. The health of the Lung may thus affect emotional strength (that is, courage or daring), and this point, which promotes the Lung qi, can thereby also support emotional strength. BL-42 *(po hu)* promotes the Lung qi in treating disorders of the upper burner, such as cough and asthma, and can also be used in treating qi deficiency in the upper burner, which leads to a lack of courage and daring. It is this function for which the point has been selected here.

Bl-44 *(shen tang).* The name of this point means "spirit hall," which we know is the Heart. This point is 1.5 units lateral to BL-15 *(xin shu),* the associated point of the Heart. It removes stagnation from the chest, regulates the qi in the upper burner, and calms the spirit. It can also be used in treating Heart and Lung disorders, such as a stifling sensation in the chest, cough, and asthma. Here, the point is used to calm the spirit and treat the anxiety and palpitations.

KI-3 *(tai xi)* is the source point of the Kidney. It nourishes Kidney yin, tonifies the Kidney, and regulates both the penetrating and conception vessels. It can be used in treating both Kidney yin and Kidney yang deficiency. In this case, the point is used to strengthen the qi and yang of the lower burner. The tonification method is utilized.

BL-60 *(kun lun),* in this case, was threaded to KI-3 *(tai xi),* which was difficult to puncture on the right side because the patient preferred to lie on that side. The Bladder channel is both interiorly and exteriorly related to the Kidney channel, and these two points are very close to each other: KI-3 *(tai xi)* is on the medial side of the ankle, whereas BL-60 *(kun lun)* is on the lateral side, and therefore more accessible.

Combination of points

BL-42 *(po hu)* and Bl-44 *(shen tang)* are associated with the Lung and Heart, and both are located on the second line of the Bladder channel. Both points can be used in treating qi deficiency in the upper burner, and disturbance of the spirit. Deficiency of pectoral qi, or Lung/Heart qi insufficiency can result in a disorder of the spirit with such symptoms as palpitations, anxiety, and panic attacks. The combination of these points promotes the yang qi in the chest, settles the emotions, calms the spirit, and treats the disturbance of spirit caused by the disorder in the upper burner.

Follow-up

The patient was treated four times altogether, once a week. After the second treatment the panic attacks disappeared. Emotionally, she was much calmer. She was very pleased with the result, and continued with the treatments for another two weeks. After her fourth visit to the clinic, all the symptoms were alleviated and the treatment was concluded. At a checkup ten months later the patient reported no further panic attacks.

Diagnostic Principles for Constraint Disorders

Constraint disorders *(yù zhèng)* is a term used for a group of disorders that are characterized primarily by abnormal emotional states, or in which such emotions lead to Organ disorders.

I. The relationship between constraint disorders in Chinese medicine and psychological disorders in conventional biomedicine

Psychological disorders are now a common occurrence, as many people have difficulty in adapting to modern life. The causes of these disorders can be either social or personal.

With the development of science and technology, the speed and intensity of work has increased dramatically when compared to the past. While physical labor decreases, mental work increases. And because of the responsibility placed on each individual and the intensive competition among the professions, every single worker now carries a greater psychological load. Advanced communications and modern information systems have shortened the geographical distance between people, yet widened the emotional distance between them. In many ways, it is now more difficult than ever for people to communicate on an emotional level.

For various reasons, the psychological health of each individual is different, and each of us has a different way of expressing our emotions. If someone cannot tolerate the psychological pressures that life imposes on us, or is unable to express his or her emotions, eventually an imbalance will result, leading to psychological disorders or psychosomatic illness.

At the same time, it is important to remember that psychological disorders are not just the product of modern society, but have occurred throughout history. Despite the lack of high technology in ancient China, there are numerous reports of psychosomatic illness. One such account will serve as an example.

The patient was very wealthy, enjoyed a high position in society, and was well educated. He was regarded as a typical gentleman and something of a snob, but in fact deep inside he was a very tense person. His family noticed that he had developed a very poor appetite, that his sleep had become very poor, and that he had little energy; mental fatigue ensued, and became more obvious as time went on. Eventually he became so weak that he could no longer rise from his sickbed. Various tonics were prescribed by his doctor, but without success.

In desperation, the family procured the services of the famous doctor Zhu Danxi, noted for his special skills and treatments. He came and sat by the gentleman's side, conducted an examination, and listened carefully to the history of the illness. The doctor neither said nor did anything, but finally rose, and, in front of the patient, requested an exorbitant fee from the family for his visit. Taking the money, he bid adieu to the gentleman and left the room. Outside, he wrote a letter, placed it in an envelope, and asked the family to give it to the sick man the following morning. The doctor then departed.

Reading this letter the next morning the patient's blood boiled with rage, for the doctor's words hurled the vilest abuse at him and cursed him roundly. Angered at the thought of how much money had been paid to the doctor for this abuse, he read on. When his eyes came to the words "You should have been in the graveyard a long time ago," he jumped out of the bed, tore the letter to shreds, and cursed the doctor at the top of his voice. All of a sudden he felt a pain in his abdomen, and, without warning, he vomited up all that it contained, including food that had been retained there for some time, and by now had become horribly smelly. His stomach now empty, the gentleman discovered that all his discomfort had miraculously disappeared.

The doctor returned the next day and explained his reasons for doing such a thing. He had concluded correctly that there was no deficiency disorder, but that his patient had been suffering from long-term qi stagnation, and there had been no chance to relieve it. This had developed into a severe constraint disorder, and then retention of food in the Stomach. This type of pattern is called false deficiency and real excess. Thus, if the qi stagnation could be removed, the disorder would be resolved. This is why the doctor deliberately provoked the gentleman—accustomed as he was to suppressing his emotions—to make him angry. This activated the qi to facilitate the removal of the obstruction: the patient vomited up all the retained food in his stomach, after which the qi activity became smooth and the symptoms were relieved. The doctor gave his wealthy patient a few herbs to regulate the body, and soon thereafter the gentlemen had recovered completely.

Psychological disorders correspond to the traditional Chinese medical concept of constraint. Chinese medicine, including both psychological treatment as well as treatment for physical disorders, has helped a great number of people throughout history. As practitioners, it is important that we correctly differentiate among patterns in accordance with the principles of Chinese medical theory.

II. The relationship between emotional disturbances and the Organs

In Chinese medicine the seven emotions (or emotional disturbances) are related to the five yin Organs. Excessive emotion or emotional upset can affect the functioning of a related Organ, and symptoms will therefore ensue.

Excessive joy or excitement can injure the Heart. This is reflected in the saying from chapter 39 of *Basic Questions,* "With excitement the qi becomes lax *(xǐ zé qì huǎn)."* Excessive joy or over-excitement can result in laxness *(huǎn)* of Heart qi, such that the qi becomes difficult to control. In mild cases the patient feels as if energy and strength has been drained from the limbs. In severe cases there will be psychological effects, including very poor concentration. It may also impair the ability of the Heart to house the Heart spirit, causing mania with emotional excitement *(kuáng luàn).*

Anger can injure the Liver. This is reflected in the saying from chapter 39 of *Basic Questions,* "With anger the qi ascends *(nù zé qì shàng)."* This implies that sudden, severe anger can cause a sudden rise of Liver qi. A preponderance of Liver yang or Liver fire can suddenly rise to the upper part of the body. In mild cases there will be dizziness, restlessness, irritability, red complexion, and red eyes. In severe cases there will be sudden fainting or loss of consciousness (syncope).

Obsessive pondering or thinking can injure the Spleen. This is reflected in the saying from chapter 39 of *Basic Questions,* "With pondering the qi clumps *(sī zé qì jié)."* Pondering can lead to obstruction of the qi activity in the middle burner, affecting the upward and downward movement of its qi. The qi will then accumulate in the middle burner. In mild cases there will be poor appetite. In severe cases there can be severe pain in the epigastric and abdominal regions.

Sadness and grief can injure the Lung. This is reflected in the saying from chapter 39 of *Basic Questions,* "With sadness the qi wastes *(bēi zé qì xiāo)."* Excessive grief or sadness can injure and consume the Lung qi, causing shortness of breath, a stifling sensation in the chest, and a very low and weak voice. These are all signs that the qi of the upper burner is being consumed.

Fear and fright can injure the Kidney. This is reflected in the following sayings from chapter 39 of *Basic Questions:* "With fright the qi will be chaotic *(jīng zé qì luàn),"* and "With fear the qi descends *(kǒng zé qì xià)."* Feeling threatened can disturb the qi, and fear can lead to the sapping of qi. Fear and fright can impair the controlling function of the Kidney qi, causing incontinence of urine and stools.

Table 7-1

EMOTION	AFFECTED ORGAN	CHARACTERISTIC SYMPTOMS
Excitement	Heart	Limbs and body weak and drained of energy; mania in severe cases
Anger	Liver	Dizziness, restlessness, and irritability; syncope in severe cases
Obsessive pondering	Spleen	Poor appetite, abdominal and epigastric pain
Grief and sadness	Lung	Stifling sensation in the chest, shortness of breath, weak voice
Fear and fright	Kidney	Kidney incontinence of urine and stools

III. Basic patterns and symptoms

There are various symptoms associated with constraint disorders. Depending on the symptomatology, they can be grouped into two main categories: dysfunctions of the qi, blood, and body fluids, and dysfunctions of the Organs. These two categories of symptoms may occur either individually or together.

Dysfunctions of qi, blood, and body fluids

Emotional upset, or major changes or disruptions in one's environment (including social pressures), can interfere with normal qi activity, impairing the ascending and descending, dispersing, and entering activities of the qi. An impediment to the circulation of qi and blood can lead to various types of accumulation.

QI CONSTRAINT *(qì yù):* When qi activity is obstructed, qi stagnation results. Symptoms may occur locally in one part of the body, or systemically. Typical symptoms are fullness and pain accompanied by a distending sensation.

BLOOD STASIS *(xuè yú):* Qi provides the underlying energy or power to circulate the blood. When the qi stagnates, blood stasis will ensue. Stagnant blood retained in the vessels or internal Organs can cause sharp pain or lumps (masses) locally. The lumps generally remain in a fixed location, and pressure will usually aggravate the pain. In severe cases, there can also be hemorrhaging.

FIRE CONSTRAINT *(huǒ yù):* Qi pertains to yang, which is characteristically warm or hot. Qi constraint can also be described as a type of yang stagnation. When chronic, it can lead to heat from constraint, and if the heat is strong, it can transform into internal fire. The patient will then develop symptoms such as restlessness, irritability, red complexion, red eyes, dry mouth, inclination to drink a lot of liquids, yellow urine, red tongue with a yellow and dry coating, and an overflowing, rapid pulse.

PHLEGM CONSTRAINT and DAMP CONSTRAINT *(tán yù* and *shí yù):* Phlegm and dampness both evolve from disorders of water metabolism. As they accumulate in the body, they become pathogenic. Qi activity provides the underlying energy for the metabolism of water. Qi stagnation will impede the metabolism of water, and eventually lead to retention of water, internal dampness, and phlegm, all of which are excessive in nature and therefore pathogenic. The patient will develop such symptoms as fullness and a stifling sensation in the chest, fullness in the epigastric region, cough, asthma, wheezing, dizziness, sleepiness, poor appetite, nausea, vomiting, diarrhea, or edema.

FOOD CONSTRAINT *(shí yù):* The digestion of food is dependent upon the transportive and transformative functions of the middle burner. Qi stagnation will interfere with the upward and downward movements of the Spleen and Stomach qi. This in turn disrupts the transportation and transformation of food, which is retained in the middle burner. The patient will exhibit such symptoms as poor appetite, distention and fullness in the abdomen, belching, and regurgitation.

In clinical practice, qi constraint *(qì yù)* is the most common pattern, in part because it frequently leads to other constraint disorders *(Fig 7-17).*

Dysfunctions of the Organs

The human body is an organic whole. The normal physiological functioning of the organism relies on the coordination of all the internal Organs. This in turn depends on the control of the qi activity, which, if obstructed, can lead to a disorder in one or more of the Organs. The resulting symptoms, which vary depending on which of the Organs is affected, are summarized below.

LUNG: When the qi activity of the Lung has been disrupted, the qi can stagnate in the upper burner. In mild cases the patient may present with a stifling sensation in the chest and shortness of breath. In severe cases there may be a sudden onset of

Fig. 7-17

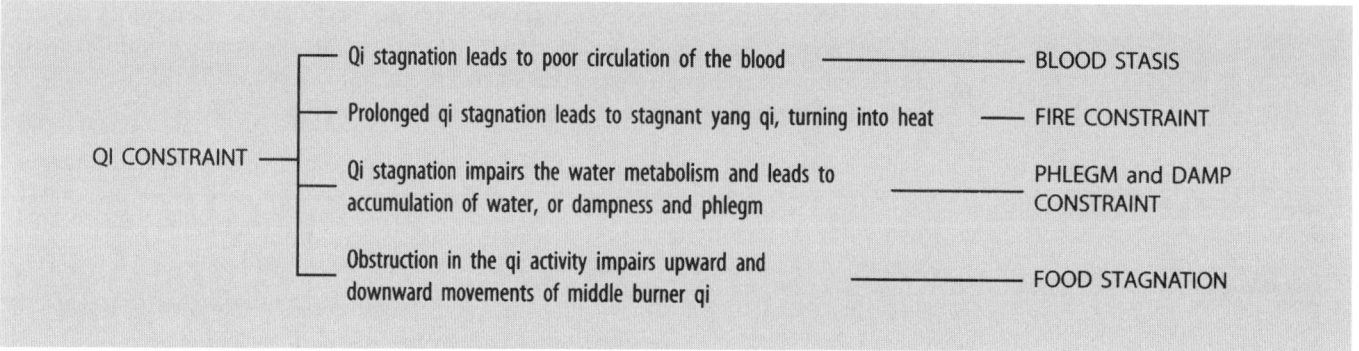

wheezing and a stifling sensation in the chest, or a very bad attack of asthma. There may also be a correlation between the onset or relief of the asthma and the patient's emotional condition.

HEART: The main manifestation of Heart qi stagnation is poor blood circulation caused by obstruction of the qi. The symptoms include palpitations, a slow-irregular or consistently irregular pulse, and pain in the area of the pericardium and chest.

SPLEEN: Disruption in the upward and downward movement of the middle burner qi will present as abnormal appetite: either excessive appetite (overeating), which results in obesity, or depressed appetite or anorexia, vomiting, and nausea.

LIVER: Disruption in the Liver's regulation of the free-flow of qi will affect the body in general, as well as the qi activity in the Organs. Local symptoms may include distention and fullness in the intercostal and hypochondrial regions, irritability, moodiness or depression, bitter taste in the mouth, and a wiry pulse.

KIDNEY: One of the main physiological functions of Kidney qi is controlling defecation and urination. When this function is impaired, the manifestations are usually urinary frequency with a small quantity of urine each time, or urinary difficulty, which leads to retention of urine. With respect to bowel movements, there can be loose stools or diarrhea.

In the early stage of an internal Organ disorder, there is no actual organic damage, just dysfunction. As mentioned above, the onset or relief of symptoms often corresponds with the patient's emotional condition. The sudden appearance, relief, improvement, or worsening of symptoms is an indication that there has been no injury to the Organs themselves, just a disruption in qi activity. Of course, long-term dysfunction of an internal Organ will eventually lead to organic damage. When that is the case, the diagnosis and treatment should focus on the same principles as Organ differentiation and treatment.

Key points for diagnosis

Although constraint disorders may display a variety of symptoms, in general the key points for diagnosis are as follows:

• In most cases, the cause of disease and precipitating factors are very obvious.

• Most of the symptoms are limited to disorders of the qi, such as a dysfunction of qi activity in the channel and collateral system, or a dysfunction of qi activity in one or more of the Organs. Sometimes the blood system can be affected, as in blood stasis for example, but there are seldom any symptoms of blood deficiency or yin deficiency in the early stage of the disorder.

• Constraint disorders are quite often unstable, in that they can change very rapidly. During the intervals between attacks, the patient may appear to be very healthy and symptom-free. The attacks may involve varying degrees of severity, but there are usually no sequelae once the symptoms have been resolved.

Fire and constraint

Two types of pathological change are commonly seen in patients with constraint disorders. These are fire from constraint *(qì yù huà huǒ)* and vigorous fire consuming the qi *(zhuāng huǒ shí qì)*. The latter is often a more advanced variety of the former. The pathogenesis of these two disorders is described below.

FIRE FROM CONSTRAINT: Qi pertains to yang, which is characteristically warm and active. The qi must constantly circulate in order to provide the energy needed to meet the demands of the various physiological functions and activities of the body. The prerequisite of qi activity is that its pathway be free of obstruction. Also, the body temperature must be maintained at a level that is warm enough to keep the qi moving; if it is too cold, it will slow down or constrict the flow of qi. If, as previously noted, an emotional disruption interferes with the Liver's regulation of the free-flow of qi, this will obstruct the circulation of qi, and thereby impair physiological functions. The obstruction of qi will also cause the yang, which pertains to heat, to accumulate in certain parts of the body, producing internal heat and eventually fire, that is, fire from constraint.

VIGOROUS FIRE CONSUMING THE QI: Fire and heat are both yang in nature, and both characteristically rise and disperse. Pathogenic fire and heat can cause the body fluids to evaporate through the pores of the skin, which explains why sweating is a common symptom in patterns of heat. In addition, as they disperse outward from inside the body, pathogenic heat and fire injure (consume) the antipathogenic factors. And while a certain level of body warmth is required for the qi to circulate, pathogenic heat and fire can overheat the body, causing the qi to become overactive. The qi is then said to follow the pathogenic heat out of the body.

As the qi is thus consumed by the pathogenic heat, the patient will begin to exhibit signs of qi deficiency. The most typical manifestations of this can be seen on a hot summer day. If a person is attacked by pathogenic summerheat, besides symptoms involving excessive heat—such as fever, thirst, and a preference for cold beverages—they will also experience dizziness, shortness of breath, general lassitude, and fatigue, which are symptoms of qi deficiency arising from vigorous fire consuming the qi.

Vigorous fire consuming the qi can also be found in patterns of excessive internal heat caused by other factors. The pathogenesis of these patterns is very similar to that of summerheat.

Both the transformation into fire and the consumption of qi can occur in constraint disorders, especially in fire constraint disorder. Stagnant qi can generate pathogenic fire, while pathogenic fire can consume the body's qi. On the surface, it would seem that the two pathological changes are contradictory. How can both conditions occur in the same patient? In fact, however, the stagnant qi that transforms into fire *is* the obstructed qi in the body. This qi has already lost its normal physiological function, and has been transformed into excessive pathogenic qi; it no longer circulates, but accumulates locally. When this stagnant qi transforms into fire, it becomes very strong and consumes the antipathogenic factors. Although the patient develops manifestations of qi deficiency, this does not resolve the stagnation of qi.

Diagnostic procedure for constraint disorders

Constraint disorders are very changeable, and there is a wide range of manifestations. Because of the involvement of different Organs, there are a number of different patterns, the most common of which are listed below *(Fig. 7-18)*.

Fig. 7-18

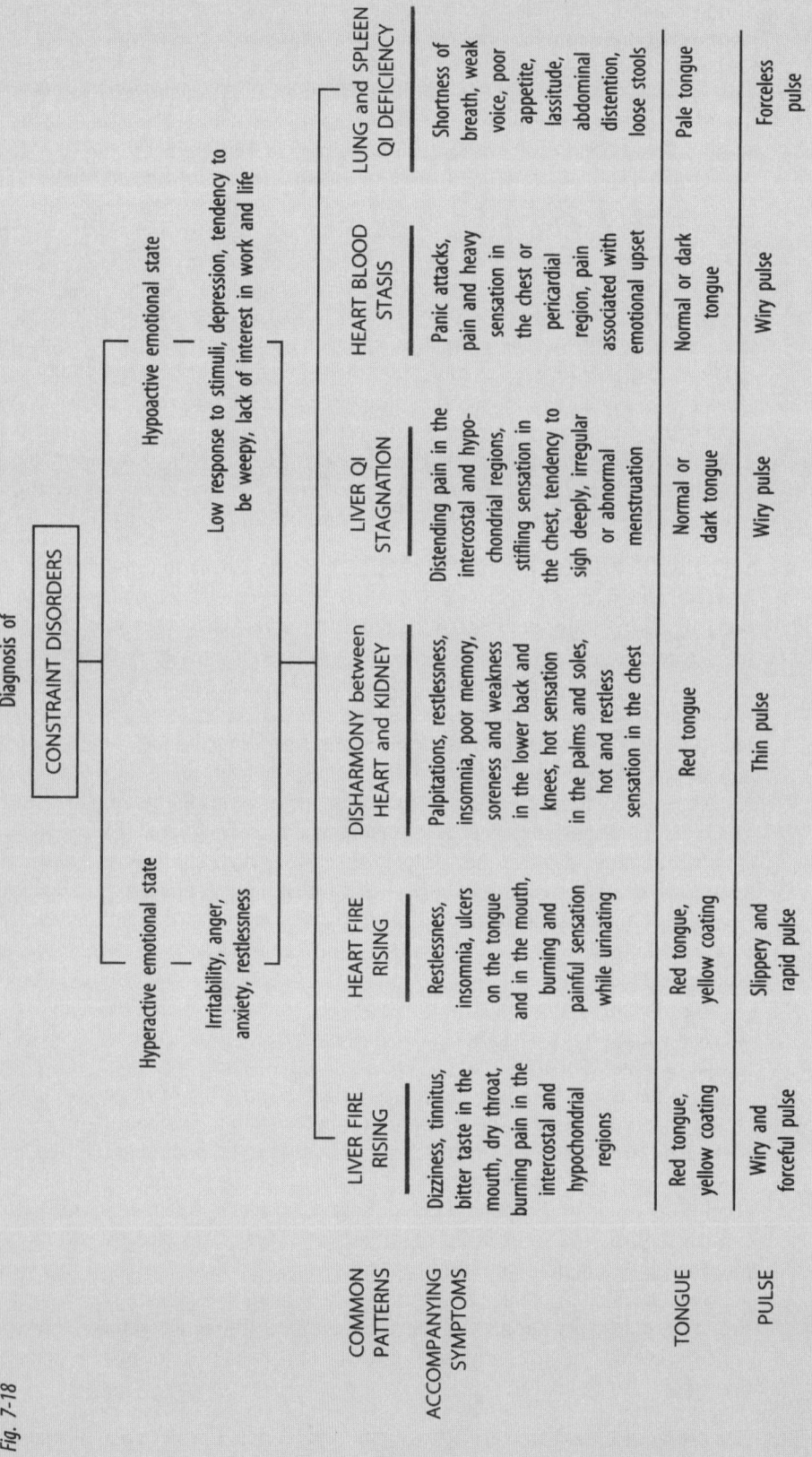

Diagnosis of

CONSTRAINT DISORDERS

Hyperactive emotional state

Irritability, anger, anxiety, restlessness

Hypoactive emotional state

Low response to stimuli, depression, tendency to be weepy, lack of interest in work and life

	LIVER FIRE RISING	HEART FIRE RISING	DISHARMONY between HEART and KIDNEY	LIVER QI STAGNATION	HEART BLOOD STASIS	LUNG and SPLEEN QI DEFICIENCY
COMMON PATTERNS						
ACCOMPANYING SYMPTOMS	Dizziness, tinnitus, bitter taste in the mouth, dry throat, burning pain in the intercostal and hypochondrial regions	Restlessness, insomnia, ulcers on the tongue and in the mouth, burning and painful sensation while urinating	Palpitations, restlessness, insomnia, poor memory, soreness and weakness in the lower back and knees, hot sensation in the palms and soles, hot and restless sensation in the chest	Distending pain in the intercostal and hypo-chondrial regions, stifling sensation in the chest, tendency to sigh deeply, irregular or abnormal menstruation	Panic attacks, pain and heavy sensation in the chest or pericardial region, pain associated with emotional upset	Shortness of breath, weak voice, poor appetite, lassitude, abdominal distention, loose stools
TONGUE	Red tongue, yellow coating	Red tongue, yellow coating	Red tongue	Normal or dark tongue	Normal or dark tongue	Pale tongue
PULSE	Wiry and forceful pulse	Slippery and rapid pulse	Thin pulse	Wiry pulse	Wiry pulse	Forceless pulse

Hypochondrial and Intercostal Pain

CASE 37: **Male, age 70**

Main complaint

Severe pain in the right hypochondrial and intercostal regions

History

Two weeks ago the patient caught a bad cold with a fever and a cough. Although these symptoms had more or less disappeared, yesterday he suddenly developed a severe pain in the right hypochondrial and intercostal regions, accompanied by a hot, burning sensation. The pain has been continuous and without relief. Because the patient has a history of coronary artery disease, he assumed that the pain was related to that condition and therefore took the heart medication that had been given to him, but without result.

This morning he was sent to the emergency department of the hospital. The pain and burning sensation is the same as it was yesterday evening, and he also feels restless, irritable, and hot over his entire body. He does not feel cold, has no shortness of breath, and there are no palpitations. He has little energy at the moment and suffers from intense lassitude. His mouth feels dry and he is drinking a lot of liquids. He has no appetite. His urine is yellow and reduced in quantity, and his stools are dry.

The checkup revealed groups of small red papules in a band around the fifth intercostal space on the right side of the chest. The skin between the groups of papules is normal and there are no blisters. The disorder has been clearly diagnosed as herpes zoster (shingles).

Tongue

Red, with a yellow, thick, and greasy coating

Pulse

Rapid and slightly floating

Analysis of symptoms

1. Severe pain around the intercostal and hypochondrial regions—pathogenic factor in the Liver channel.

2. Hot, burning sensation in a local area with groups of papules—pathogenic fire and toxin from the inside of the body accumulating on the skin.

3. No shortness of breath or palpitations—no injury to the Heart qi.

4. Generalized hot sensation with no feeling of being cold or aversion to cold; restlessness and irritability—internal heat.

263

5. Dry mouth and drinking lots of liquids, reduced quantity of yellow urine, and dry stools—injury to body fluids by heat.

6. Red tongue, yellow and thick coating, and rapid pulse—pattern of heat.

7. Forceful pulse—pattern of excess.

Basic theory of case

Each of the channels has its own pathway. In clinical practice we can determine which channels, collaterals, and Organs have been affected by a pathogenic factor by examining the location of the disease or symptoms.

The leg terminal yin channel, which is associated with the Liver, begins at the big toe, travels up the medial aspect of the leg to the external genital region, and then continues to the lower abdomen. After passing through the abdomen, it connects with the Liver and then with the Gallbladder. It then ascends, passing through the hypochondrial and intercostal regions before reaching the head. It travels up the back of the throat on its way to the nose, after which it connects with the eye and finally reaches the top of the head, where it connects with the governing vessel. The Liver channel also has two branches, one of which goes from below the eye to the cheek, and then around the inside of the mouth and lips; the other rises from the Liver to the Lung, where is connects with the arm greater yin Lung channel.

From this description we can say that, as the Liver channel runs along the surface of the body on the medial aspect of the lower limbs, around the external genitalia, and through the hypochondrial and intercostal regions, symptoms and disorders that occur in these areas are mainly associated with the Liver channel. In addition, the Liver and Gallbladder have an interior/exterior relationship: the Gallbladder channel passes along the lateral side of the body, and disorders of the Liver and Gallbladder often interact.

Shingles (herpes zoster) largely corresponds to the disorder in traditional Chinese medicine variously known as snake cluster sores *(shé chuàn chuāng)*, fire rash around the waist *(chán yāo hǔo dān)*, and dragon [rash] around the waist *(chán yāo lóng)*. This disorder is frequently marked by sudden attacks. The most tell-tale characteristic is violent pain accompanied or followed by reddish papules that rapidly turn into blisters, and that gather together like a belt on one side of the body. In mild cases there will only be slightly red papules without blisters. Shingles frequently occur around the chest and hypochondrial region, and thus the disorder is associated with the Liver channel. Shingles can also appear on the face, chest, lower back, or legs. According to Chinese medicine, the pathogenesis is internal pathogenic heat or fire, or heat and toxins disturbing the channels and collaterals, and thereby obstructing the circulation of qi and blood. This explains such manifestations as the localized burning and hot sensation, violent pain, and severe red rash.

Cause of disease

Pathogenic fire

The diagnosis of pathogenic fire is based on the sudden onset, the hot, burning, and painful sensation locally, red papules, dry mouth, yellow urine, red tongue with a yellow coating, and rapid pulse.

Site of disease

Liver channel

The pain is unilateral in the hypochondrial and intercostal regions, and the papules are located in the same area. This is the domain of the Liver channel.

Pathological change

The distinction between pathogenic heat and fire is based on the degree of severity: pathogenic fire is an extreme form of pathogenic heat. In this case, the hot, burning sensation locally indicates that pathogenic fire is the main cause of the disorder. The Liver channel passes through the hypochondrial region. The pathogenic fire follows the Liver channel and creates a disturbance, causing very severe pain in the hypochondrial and intercostal regions. Because heat characteristically rises and disperses outward, the pathogenic heat and fire in the channels seek to exit the body through the skin. Meanwhile, they disturb the circulation of blood, and accumulate in the small vessels and collaterals of the subcutaneous regions, manifesting as red papules.

The pathogenic fire and toxin affect the general qi and blood of the body via the channel system, which is reflected in the generalized sensation of heat, and the absence of such symptoms as aversion to cold. Because heat and fire consume the body fluids, the patient's mouth is dry, and he tends to drink a lot of liquids. The reduced quantity of yellow urine and the dry stools are further evidence of this injury to the body fluids.

The pathogenic fire and toxin are very strong, disturbing circulation of both the blood and qi. The antipathogenic factors try to dissipate and vent the heat and fire from the body, yet the yang qi is consumed by the pathogenic factors. This accounts for the patient's conspicuous lassitude. The disturbance of the Liver channel's qi activity also affects the upward and downward movements of the Spleen and Stomach qi, and thus their transportive and transformative functions. This is the reason for the loss of appetite, which is not due to an independent disorder of the Spleen and Stomach.

When the Liver's governance of the free-flow of qi is disturbed, it can affect its related function of regulating the emotions. The pathogenic heat and fire can also disturb the Heart spirit. This explains the patient's restlessness and irritability.

The red tongue with the thick, yellow coating and rapid pulse reflect a pattern of excessive heat.

Fig. 8-1

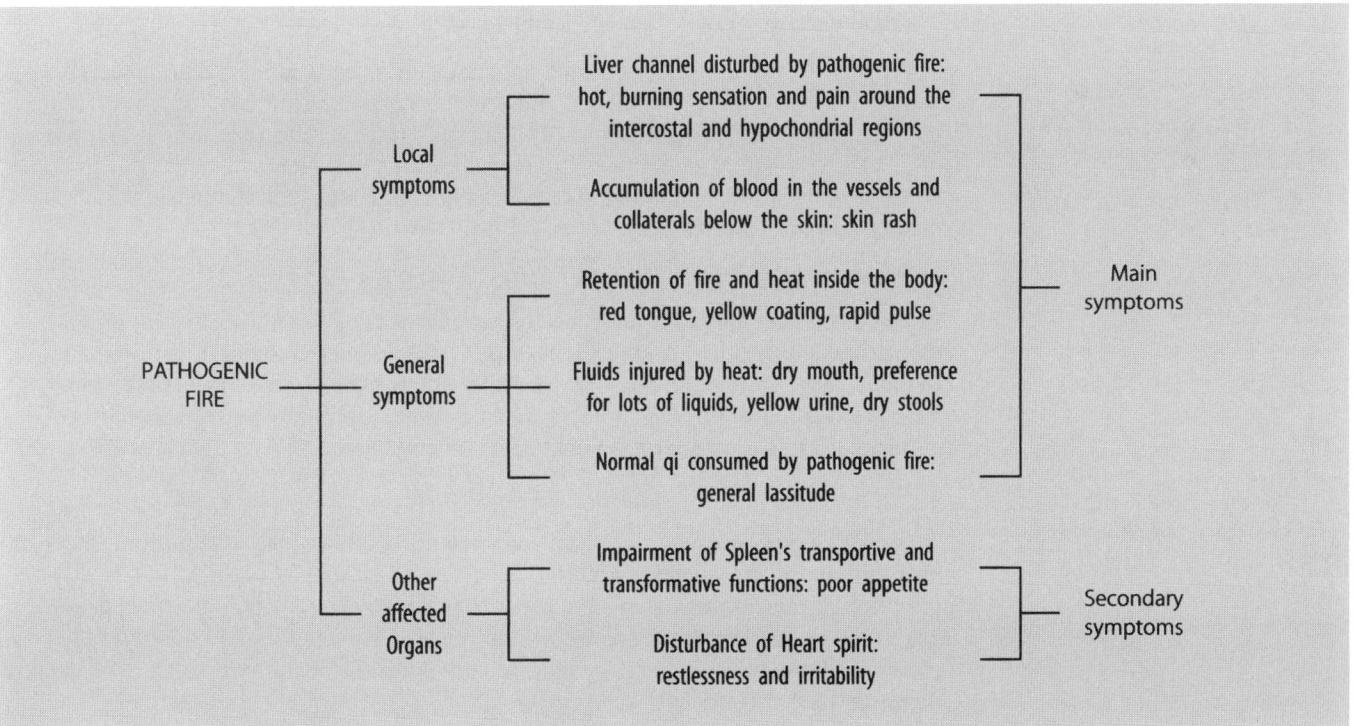

<table>
<tr><td rowspan="7">PATHOGENIC FIRE</td><td rowspan="2">Local symptoms</td><td>Liver channel disturbed by pathogenic fire: hot, burning sensation and pain around the intercostal and hypochondrial regions</td><td rowspan="5">Main symptoms</td></tr>
<tr><td>Accumulation of blood in the vessels and collaterals below the skin: skin rash</td></tr>
<tr><td rowspan="3">General symptoms</td><td>Retention of fire and heat inside the body: red tongue, yellow coating, rapid pulse</td></tr>
<tr><td>Fluids injured by heat: dry mouth, preference for lots of liquids, yellow urine, dry stools</td></tr>
<tr><td>Normal qi consumed by pathogenic fire: general lassitude</td></tr>
<tr><td rowspan="2">Other affected Organs</td><td>Impairment of Spleen's transportive and transformative functions: poor appetite</td><td rowspan="2">Secondary symptoms</td></tr>
<tr><td>Disturbance of Heart spirit: restlessness and irritability</td></tr>
</table>

Pattern of disease   The main symptoms, as well as the localized skin symptoms, are mostly located on one side of the intercostal and hypochondrial regions. This is evidence that the disorder involves the channel and collateral system. The symptoms of internal excessive fire and consumption of the body fluids by heat indicate that the disorder is also in the interior.

The pattern of heat is reflected in the hot, burning sensation and localized red papules, thirst, yellow urine, red tongue with a yellow coating, and rapid pulse.

The excessive nature of the pattern is reflected in the severe and continuous pain that had only begun one day before, together with the tongue and pulse signs.

Additional notes

1. What is the cause and source of the pathogenic fire?

Pathogenic fire can be of either external or internal origin. In clinical practice, an internal cause is the most common. In this case, however, the patient caught a cold two weeks before the present onset, which means that an external factor is the most probable cause. The exterior symptoms are now gone, but the pathogenic factor, which was not alleviated, has penetrated deeply into the channel system. There, it has obstructed the qi in the channels and collaterals, which has transformed into fire. In view of the sudden onset and the channel-disturbing symptoms, we may conclude that the source of the disturbance was external.

Fig. 8-2

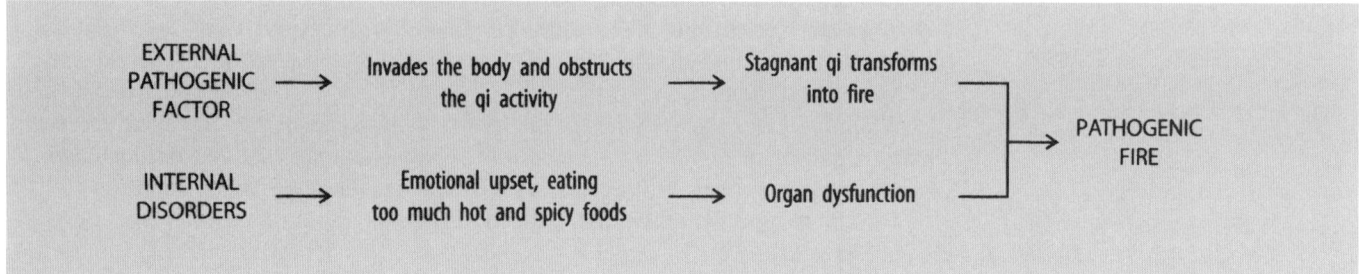

2. Is there a pattern of deficiency in this case?

The patient's general lassitude and poor appetite were caused by the excessive pathogenic fire consuming the qi, and the subsequent disturbance of the Liver's governance of the free-flow of qi. Although the symptoms are very similar to those of qi deficiency, they do not constitute a pattern of qi deficiency. This is confirmed by the nature of the pain, which is severe and continuous, and the pulse, which is neither thin nor forceless.

3. What does the slightly floating quality of the pulse signify?

In general, a floating pulse indicates an exterior pattern. We know that in this case the pathogenic factor was external in origin, that it entered the body and remains in the channel system, having only partially entered the Organs. The pulse, therefore, is still slightly floating; here, it does not indicate a purely exterior pattern, but corresponds to a disorder of the channels and collaterals.

4. What is the cause of the greasy tongue coating?

A greasy tongue coating usually indicates retention of dampness. At present, however, the symptoms suggest heat from excess, with no indication of dampness. The other tongue and pulse signs—and especially the shingles, which have not pustulated—do not reflect the presence of dampness. Thus the tongue coating neither corresponds with the general symptoms, nor with the local symptoms, and can therefore be disregarded.

Conclusion

1. According to the eight principles:
   Heat, excess, and combination of interior and channel-collateral patterns.

2. According to etiology:
   Pathogenic fire.

3. According to theory of channels and collaterals:
   Pathogenic fire in the Liver channel.

Treatment principles

1. Clear and drain the pathogenic heat from the Liver channel.
2. Alleviate the pain.

Explanation of treatment principle

The basic principle for treating pathogenic fire is to clear the heat and drain the fire. In this case, the heat and fire are retained in the Liver channel; thus, clearing the heat and fire from the Liver channel is the basic principle.

Because the pathogenic fire here is associated with stagnant qi, which is a very important pathological change, the removal of the obstruction to the qi activity, as well as from the Liver channel (because of the dry stools), is necessary in order to treat the root of the disorder.

Selection of points

GV-14 *(da zhu)*
LI-11 *(qu chi)*
LI-4 *(he gu)*
hua tuo jia ji (M-BW-35) [thoracic vertebrae 4, 5, 6, 9 & 10]
Ashi points [in the area of the shingles]
GV-34 *(yang ling quan)*
SP-10 *(xue hai)* [left side]
LR-2 *(xing jian)*

Explanation of points

GV-14 *(da zhui)* is the meeting point of all six primary yang channels and the governing vessel. It expels pathogenic wind, disperses exterior patterns, clears heat, and removes obstruction from the channels and collaterals. This is one of the most important points for clearing generalized body heat. In the treatment of excessive heat, the reducing method is used. As this point is connected with all the yang channels, it can remove heat and obstruction from all the yang channels. It also connects the internal and external functions of the body, and drains internal heat out through the surface of the body. Thus, it is very effective for releasing pathogenic heat from the Organs and removing obstruction from the channels.

This point should be punctured to a depth of between 15 and 25mm, and the tip of the needle angled slightly obliquely and upward, following the posterior processes of the vertebrae. A combination of rotating, lifting, and thrusting is used. When punctured properly, the patient feels as if the needle has been extended deep into the body, and experiences numbness in the area. If the needle has not been inserted to the right depth, or the needle sensation is not as it should be, good results will not be obtained.

LI-11 *(qu chi)* is the sea point of the arm yang brightness channel. It expels pathogenic wind, clears heat, and harmonizes the nutritive and protective qi. It is an important point in the treatment of heat, and is excellent for dealing with general heat (wind-heat, damp-heat, toxic heat, etc.) Modern research has shown that this point is useful in treating infections (including staphylococci and beta-streptococci). In this case, where there is a pattern of excessive heat, this point serves as one of the main assistants in clearing the heat, removing the obstruction, and regulating the qi.

LI-4 *(he gu)* is the source point of the arm yang brightness channel. It clears heat, alleviates pain, removes obstruction, and relieves exterior patterns. Although it is located on the arm yang brightness channel, it can be used in treating generalized symptoms. In this case it is used to remove the pathogenic factors from the surface of the body, clear the heat, and alleviate the pain.

Hua tuo jia ji (M-BW-35) properly speaking refers to a series of 17 pairs of points, but in this instance only the points on the fourth, fifth, sixth, ninth and tenth thoracic vertebrae are chosen, bilaterally. In the treatment of shingles (herpes zoster), the *hua tuo jia ji* (M-BW-35) points are selected according to the related level of the vertebrae corresponding to the neural segments affected by the shingles. It is usually very easy to pinpoint the tender areas around the affected levels of the vertebrae. In most cases, tenderness is located around one or two vertebrae, but in others, three or four may be affected. The main *hua tuo jia ji* (M-BW-35) point can be ascertained by determining where the tenderness is most severe in conjunction with the area in which the blisters have appeared.

In this case, the affected region is in the fifth intercostal space, but points above and below are also used on the fourth and sixth spaces.

In general, if the points are to be used unilaterally, those on the side corresponding to the diseased skin should be chosen, so that emphasis is given to the affected side. In practice, however, both sides are often needled; the healthy side is used to draw on the assistance of the antipathogenic factors in expelling the pathogenic factors from the diseased side.

The function of these points is to regulate the qi, remove local obstruction, and alleviate the pain. They also balance the relevant Organ functions. Thus, besides choosing points according to the area affected by the shingles, points can also be chosen according to the level of the associated points corresponding to that of the affected Organs. This is why, in this case, points on the ninth and tenth thoracic vertebrae have been chosen, as these points are on the same level as the associated points of the Liver and Gallbladder.

Ashi points. When certain points of tenderness are pressed by the practitioner, English-speaking patients will often cry "ouch!" while Chinese patients will react with "ah!" Theoretically, these points of tenderness are regarded as acupuncture points because tenderness in an indication of stagnant qi or blood. Thus, use of ashi points can directly regulate the qi and blood by removing obstruction.

The points are needled here using the surrounding puncturing method. A 3-edged needle is used to puncture the area around the rash. The distance between each punctured point should be 1 to 1.5 units. The skin is punctured superficially, and the bleeding method is then used, allowing two to three specks of blood to stain a cotton ball. This method—which can be used when the shingles are newly-developed and the stagnant fire is very severe—is a type of rapid reducing method, used to drain and expel pathogenic fire. It produces very good results. Because of the bleeding associated with this method, the practitioner must consider the patient's constitution: if it is weak, the distance between the punctured points can be increased. The skin must be sterilized properly in order to prevent infection.

GV-34 *(yang ling quan)* is the sea point of the leg lesser yang Gallbladder channel, and is the influential point for the sinews. It clears Liver heat, promotes Gallbladder function, strengthens the sinews, removes obstruction from the channels and collaterals, and treats pain in the chest, intercostal and hypochondrial regions (the domain of the Liver and Gallbladder and their respective channels). It is an important point for treating disorders of the Liver and Gallbladder, and is a very effective distant point. In this case, it is used to clear the pathogenic fire from the Liver and Gallbladder.

SP-10 *(xue hai)* is an excellent choice for regulating and cooling the blood, removing obstruction from the channels, and resolving dampness. Because herpes zoster frequently involves retention of dampness, this point can remove (or assist in the removal) of dampness in a damp-heat pattern. In this case it serves as an assistant point and is used to regulate and cool the blood in order to reduce the heat.

LR-2 *(xing jian)* is the spring point of the leg terminal yin channel. It is very effective for clearing and draining heat, soothing spasms, regulating Liver qi, and promoting the Liver function of governing the free-flow of qi. It is also a very effective distant point and is used in treating many disorders associated with the areas through which the Liver channel passes: headache, dizziness, convulsions, deviation of the mouth and eyes, pain in the hypochondrial region, abdominal distention, pain in the urethra, hernia, leukorrhea, and painful menstruation. In this case, the point is used for its potent ability to drain heat, clear pathogenic fire, and soothe the spirit. Because shingles is one of the most painful disorders, the patient's sleep is often affected. There may also be a disturbance of an emotional and psychological nature, which explains why patients may be very restless, irritable, and anxious. This point is useful in controlling these types of symptoms. The point is helpful in overcoming the stage of most severe pain.

Combination of points

GV-14 *(da zhui)*, LI-11 *(qu chi)*, LI-4 *(he gu)*. These three points are grouped as a prescription for treating generalized heat patterns. The combination is very commonly used in clinical practice. LI-11 *(qu chi)* and LI-4 *(he gu)* are both located on the arm yang brightness Large Intestine channel, which is thought to contain much qi and blood. The former is the sea point of this channel, whereas the latter is the source point. The reducing method is used at both points to remove heat. GV-14 *(da zhui)* is the meeting point of the six yang channels and the governing vessel. Thus, this point is also used to reduce generalized heat. The three points together act to clear heat, relieve toxicity, alleviate pain, calm the spirit, and, according to modern research, can be used in treating infections.

Hua tuo jia ji (M-BW-35) and the Ashi points around the rash. This is a commonly used combination for the treatment of shingles. The points and treatment method are described above.

GV-34 *(yang ling quan)* and LR-2 *(xing jian)*. The former is the sea point of the leg lesser yang channel, and the latter is the spring point of the leg terminal yin Liver channel. This is therefore a combination of points on a pair of channels that share an interior/exterior relationship. It is a potent combination for draining heat. Heat in the Liver and Gallbladder can interact with each other through the channel system; the use of this method reduces the number of needles required, and achieves good results.

Follow-up

The patient was treated once daily for a period of six days. After two treatments there was a dramatic reduction in the pain, and the generalized heat was largely alleviated. No new skin rash appeared, and the old rash became dry and smaller. After six days the rash had turned to scabs, the patient was able to sleep more soundly, his urine and appetite had returned to normal, and his general energy was much improved. Because of the patient's age, the use of the surrounding puncturing method was stopped.

Observation was continued for about ten days, during which he was treated three times with acupuncture. By then the patient had completely recovered and there was no need for a further checkup, as there was no pain or rash.

CASE 38: **Female, age 52**

Main complaint

Pain in the right intercostal and hypochondrial regions

History

The patient was busy and working very hard before the onset of the disorder, due to the renovation of her house. She suffered much from anxiety and slept very little. Three weeks ago she began to experience a burning and painful sensation in the right side of the intercostal and hypochondrial regions. She did not pay too much attention to this, attributing it to fatigue. After a few days she noticed that there were red papules and blisters in the areas of pain. The pain became very severe and radiated to her right breast. She went to her doctor, who prescribed antiviral medication, pain killers, and tranquilizers. She completed the course of antiviral medication in one week, but the result was far from satisfactory, as she is still suffering from the severe pain, and the blisters are still there.

The clinical checkup has revealed that the papules and blisters are bunched together in patches. They are red, and some are dry, in appearance. The patient has a dry, burning, and very uncomfortable sensation down the right side of her body. She uses oil on her skin in an effort to counteract this, but the pain is still severe. She does not sleep well on account of the pain. She suffers from extreme restlessness and feels slightly depressed. She is thirsty and drinks a large quantity of liquids, but her appetite has remained basically unchanged. Urination feels hot and the urine is yellow. Her stools are very dry. Her complexion is red.

Tongue	Red, with a yellow, greasy coating
Pulse	Sunken, thin, and wiry; forceless in the right distal position

Analysis of symptoms

1. Lack of rest, anxiety, and being too busy prior to onset—stagnant qi transforming into fire.

2. Severe, violent pain in the right intercostal and hypochondrial regions, radiating to the breast—obstruction in the Liver channel due to pathogenic factor.

3. Localized burning sensation, red and dry papules—pathogenic fire and toxin emerging through the skin.

4. Thirst, drinking large quantity of liquids, yellow urine, and dry stools—consumption of body fluids by pathogenic fire.

5. Red complexion, red tongue—heat pattern.

6. Sunken, wiry pulse—dysfunction of Liver qi in governing the free-flow of qi.

Basic theory of case

Skin rash *(bān zhěn)* is commonly seen in clinical practice, and accompanies a wide variety of illnesses. In Chinese medicine there are two major types. The first is simply termed rash or papules *(zhěn)* and consists of small pimples that occur individually or together in large numbers, in a big patch. They are generally bright red in color. They rise up above the surface of the skin and are therefore palpable to the fingers. When pressed, the redness disappears.

The second type is called spots or macules *(bān)*. This type of rash occurs as either a small or large patch. The color is red or purplish, and there are no pimples. When touched by the fingers, nothing is felt; nor does the color change under the fingers' pressure.

Rashes and spots are generally caused by pathogenic heat, fire, or toxin forcing the blood circulation, and causing the blood to accumulate in the subcutaneous regions of the body. Rashes are usually caused by the blood congesting in the very small vessels, and not going out. When the affected area is pressed, the blood will change position and the color will decrease; the congestion is thus changed. Spots are caused by pathogenic heat injuring the vessels and forcing the blood out, resulting in a certain amount of subcutaneous hemorrhaging. When the skin is pressed over spots, the color does not change since the blood, which has been forced out of the vessels, cannot move elsewhere. The first of these types of rashes is relatively mild, while the second is severe. The early stage of shingles (herpes zoster) pertains to a rash *(zhěn)*.

Another kind of skin problem is blisters. The cause of blisters is associated with pathogenic dampness, which accumulates in the subcutaneous layer. Blisters are also very commonly encountered in shingles *(Fig. 8-3)*.

Cause of disease

Emotional disturbance and pathogenic damp-heat

Before this problem began, the patient was very busy and anxious, which directly affected the Organs, interfering with the qi activity, qi, and blood. It is this combination of factors which underlies this disorder. That is to say, the emotional disturbance was the initial cause of her condition.

Fig. 8-3

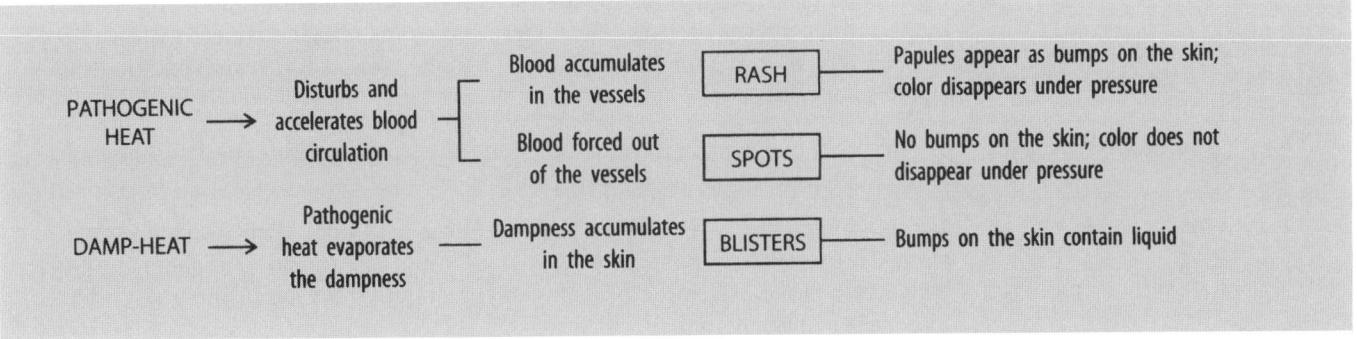

The patient experienced localized pain and a hot sensation, and a large number of blisters appeared on the skin. She also felt thirsty, her urine was yellow and her stools dry, and the tongue coating was greasy. All of these symptoms reflect the presence of damp-heat.

Site of disease

Liver and Liver channel

The onset of the disorder is directly associated with an emotional disturbance, and the localized symptoms (severe pain, skin rash, blisters) are situated in the domain of the Liver channel. This suggests that the site of disease is the Liver.

Pathological change

In Chinese medicine the Liver is responsible for the emotions and the free-flow of qi. A Liver disorder can thus give rise to abnormal emotions, and conversely, a strong emotional disturbance can lead to symptoms or a disorder that involves the Liver. In this case, the patient's overwork and anxiety disturbed the qi and blood activity. Unable to properly circulate, the qi was obstructed, and the stagnant Liver qi has transformed into fire. As the fire emerged from the interior of the body, it followed the channels and eventually disturbed the circulation of blood, which accumulated in the collaterals and small vessels close to the skin. This has led to the burning, hot, and red skin eruptions in the intercostal and hypochondrial regions and breast, through which the Liver channel passes.

The pathogenic fire consumed the body fluids as it emerged from the body and dispersed through the skin. This can be seen in the dryness of the skin, apart from the rash and red papules. The patient's skin therefore feels dry, uncomfortable, and taut. Because the pathogenic heat has also consumed the body fluids, this has caused a deficiency of body fluids. The patient therefore feels thirsty and likes to drink a lot of liquids, her urine is yellow, and stools are dry. The pain, as well as the pathogenic heat and fire which disturb the Heart spirit, affect the patient's sleep. As the pathogenic heat and fire affect the body almost everywhere, the Bladder too is affected, and the patient's urine is hot and burning.

The red complexion, red tongue, and yellow coating are all indicative of interior heat. The sunken, wiry pulse indicates a disorder of Liver qi, here Liver qi stagnation.

The local skin blisters indicate that there is not only heat, but also damp-heat, the existence of which is also shown by the yellow and greasy tongue coating. The damp-heat may be due to dampness and retention of pathogenic water in the body at some previous time; or it may indicate that, after the onset of the disorder, the normal water metabolism was impaired.

Pattern of disease

As the patient's stress is one of the important reasons for the disorder in the internal Organs, there is an interior pattern. Internal heat has affected the Liver channel, causing the severe local symptoms. Thus, there is a combination of an interior and a channel-collateral disorder.

The patient suffers from a dry, hot, and burning sensation in the intercostal and hypochondrial regions, feels thirsty, has yellow urine and dry stools, and a red tongue with a yellow coating. All of these symptoms reflect a pattern of heat.

The very short duration of the illness, and the continuous, severe pain indicate a pattern of excess.

Additional notes

1. How does one explain the contradiction between the pressure of damp-heat and the symptoms of dryness in this case?

We know that fire is a yang pathogenic factor, and that when it becomes very strong, it can cause symptoms of dryness. On the other hand, dampness is a yin pathogenic factor. Retention of dampness can injure the yang of the body, which leads to a pattern of cold.

In this case, there are two types of pathogenic factors: those associated with dryness, which involves fire and heat, and those associated with dampness. The reason for these contradictory symptoms is that, although the body fluids and dampness are essentially composed of water, their effects are completely different: the body fluids nourish the body, whereas dampness, a pathogenic factor, can only cause disease. Pathogenic fire is very active by nature; it does not remain in a fixed location, and tries to exit the body; that is, it disperses from the inside to the outside of the body. This can consume the body fluids on the surface (skin), which becomes very dry and taut. In addition, the pathogenic fire also evaporates the dampness within the body, so that it surfaces and causes blisters. Because dampness cannot nourish the skin, it is unable to compensate for the consumption of the body fluids on the body surface, or to relieve the dryness and tautness of the skin, *Fig. 8-4* that is caused by the fire.

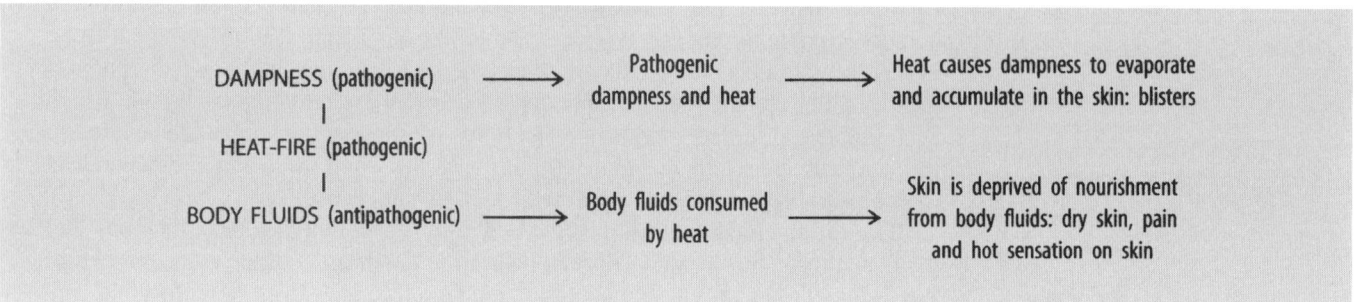

2. The pulse is sunken, thin, and wiry, but is forceless in the right distal position. Why?

The presence of Liver qi stagnation, explained above, accounts for the sunken, wiry pulse, but how can we explain why the pulse is thin and forceless in the right distal position?

The distal position on the right side is the domain of the Lung. The forcelessness in this position is indicative of Lung qi deficiency, which is related to the pathogenic fire consuming the qi *(zhuàng huǒ shí qì)*. The thin pulse reflects that the vessels are not being properly filled, and is associated with the injury to the body fluids caused by pathogenic fire. However, because the deficiency is very mild at this time, it can safely be regarded as insignificant.

3. What is the difference between this case and case 37?

In both cases the patients are suffering from the same disorder, but there are differences with respect to the cause of disease, pathological change, and the site of disease.

With respect to etiology, there is pure pathogenic fire in case 37, while here there are fire and dampness, that is, retention of damp-heat.

With respect to pathological change, in case 37 an external pathogenic factor invaded the body and caused the qi to stagnate in the channel system, which eventually produced fire. Here, it is an emotional disturbance that induced an internal disorder, resulting in an obstruction to the qi activity of the internal Organs, which has produced fire.

With respect to the cause of disease, in case 37 the Liver channel affected the circulation of qi and blood inside the body, but here a disorder of the Liver itself has affected the channels on the body surface.

Conclusion

1. According to the eight principles:
   Combination of heat and excess, and interior and channel-collateral patterns.
2. According to etiology:
   Emotional disturbance (stress and anxiety), damp-heat.
3. According to Organ theory:
   Damp-heat in the Liver and Gallbladder (heat is predominant).

Treatment principle

1. Clear the heat, drain the fire, and alleviate the pain.
2. Remove the dampness.

Explanation of treatment principle

This case, like case 37, is associated with fire in the Liver. Both cases require that the heat be cleared and the fire be drained. The difference is that in case 37 there is only stagnant qi resulting in fire in the Liver channel, where the focus is on removing the obstruction from the channels; in this case, by contrast, the heat is in the Liver itself and so the emphasis is on clearing the heat from the Liver and draining the fire while removing the dampness.

Selection of points

GB-13 *(ben shen)*
hua tuo jia ji (M-BW-35) [thoracic vertebrae 4, 5 & 6 on right side]
Ashi points [around area of shingles]
GB-36 *(wai qiu)* [right side]
SP-9 *(yin ling quan)*
SP-6 *(san yin jiao)* [left side]
LR-2 *(xing jian)*

Explanation of points

GB-13 *(ben shen)* is located 3 units lateral to GV-24 *(shen ting)*, very close to the brain. This point clears heat, relieves pain, expels wind, and soothes spasms. Because of its proximity to the brain, it can settle the emotions, calm the spirit, and relieve convulsions. It can therefore be used in treating a variety of symptoms such as headache, dizziness, vertigo, childhood convulsions, hemiplegia, and epilepsy. In this case it is used to clear the heat, calm the spirit, and relieve both the anxiety and the heat.

Hua tuo jia ji (M-BW-35). See description of points in case 37. Points on the right side of the fourth, fifth, and sixth thoracic vertebrae, which are chosen in this case, regulate the qi, remove obstruction, and alleviate pain.

Ashi points are selected around the area of the skin rash (blisters). The needles are inserted horizontally. These points are used to remove the dampness and heat, alleviate the pain, and facilitate the disappearance of the rash from the skin. Because the damp-heat here has only accumulated in the skin, interstices, and pores, there is no need to puncture too deeply. Deep puncturing can cause the pathogenic factor to penetrate further into the body; hus, only superficial puncturing is necessary.

GB-36 *(wai qiu)* is the accumulating point of the leg lesser yang channel. It clears heat from the Liver and Gallbladder, removes obstruction from the channels and collaterals, relieves toxicity, and is a good point for treating discomfort around the intercostal and hypochondrial regions, as well as skin rash with pain and itchiness. Accumulating points can be used in treating acute heat patterns and hemorrhage. In this case the point has been chosen to release the heat from the Liver and Gallbladder, and to alleviate the pain. It is one of the primary points in the prescription.

SP-9 *(yin ling quan)* is the sea point of the leg greater yin channel. It promotes the functions of the Triple Burner, strengthens Spleen function, and resolves dampness. Because there is damp-heat in this case, in which heat is predominant, and dampness has already appeared on the body surface where it is obstructing the channels and collaterals, this point is used as an assistant to treat the retention of dampness.

Liver and Gallbladder disorders readily affect the Spleen and Stomach. Because this point also promotes the transportive and transformative functions of the Spleen, its use here will prevent the disorder of the Liver and Gallbladder from affecting the middle burner functions.

SP-6 *(san yin jiao)* serves as an assistant point to relieve the dampness in order to assist the other points in removing the heat. The point regulates both the qi and blood, and calms the spirit.

LR-2 *(xing jian)* is the spring point of the Liver channel. It drains heat and calms the spirit. It is an important point for clearing heat from the Liver and Gallbladder, and can also settle the emotions in the treatment of anxiety.

Combination of points

GB-13 *(ben shen)*, SP-6 *(san yin jiao)*, LR-2 *(xing jian)*. This group of points is used in treating Liver and Gallbladder heat, or Liver and Gallbladder damp-heat, with such manifestations as irritability, hot sensations, insomnia, and restlessness. GB-13 *(ben shen)* is very effective in clearing heat and calming the spirit; SP-6 *(san yin jiao)* removes dampness, and LR-2 *(xing jian)* clears heat, especially from the Liver. Together, these three points can regulate the functions of the Liver, Gallbladder, and Spleen, and also calm the spirit.

SP-9 *(yin ling quan)*, LR-2 *(xing jian)*. This two-point combination is useful in treating damp-heat. It is used for damp-heat in the Liver and Gallbladder or for Liver and Gallbladder damp-heat with retention of dampness in the Spleen. SP-9 *(yin ling quan)* strengthens the Spleen and removes dampness, and LR-2 *(xing jian)* releases heat from the Gallbladder and Liver. The former is the sea point of the Spleen channel, and the latter is the spring point of the Liver channel; this combination is therefore comprised of a sea and spring point on two yin channels. In case 37, GB-34 *(yang ling quan)* was combined with LR-2 *(xing jian)*—a combination of a sea and spring point on exterior/interior related channels. As can be seen, the combination in this case is different.

Basic herbal formula

In this case a small prepared herbal pill called Gentiana Longdancao Pill to Drain the Liver *(long dan xie gan wan)* was used for a short period of time. The information given with the pills states that it is comprised of Radix Gentianae Longdancao *(long dan cao)*, Radix Bupleuri *(chai hu)*, Radix Scutellariae Baicalensis *(huang qin)*, Radix Angelicae Sinensis *(dang gui)*, and Rhizome Alismatis Orientalis *(ze xie)*. The composition of these pills is related to, but not exactly the same as, the traditional formula Gentiana Longdancao Decoction to Drain the Liver *(long dan xie gan wan)*.

Follow-up

The fact that this patient's condition had already lasted for three weeks, and that the skin rash was still there, indicated that the damp-heat was very severe. There was also Liver and Gallbladder dysfunction, and stagnant fire caused by the qi obstruction. Both acupuncture and the prepared herbal pills were therefore used to maximize the effect.

Acupuncture was administered every other day, and 6g of Gentiana Long-dancao Pill to Drain the Liver *(long dan xie gan wan)* was taken twice daily (12g per day) to remove the heat, dry the dampness, and settle the spirit. After taking the herbal pills for three days, and receiving acupuncture treatment twice, the blisters began to turn dry, but there was no apparent change in the local dryness and burning sensation. However, the patient's stools were slightly loose, and she had bowel movements two or three times a day. This was caused by the herbal pills. Although the duration of the violent pain was reduced, she still frequently experienced very sharp and severe pain, which affected her daily life and sleep. It was therefore decided to continue taking the herbal pills; even though her stools were still loose, she had only one or two bowel movements a day.

After two weeks of treatment during which acupuncture was administered three times per week, the skin rash gradually disappeared. The local surrounding puncturing was reduced: only the areas around those parts of the rash that had not fully recovered were punctured. There was also some mildly scarred tissue around the right side of the spinous process of the fifth thoracic vertebrae. The patient still experienced obvious pain and tenderness; even when the area was touched very gently, the pain could be very severe. She stated that during the two weeks the pain would sometimes disappear completely, but would then return again. She often experienced the pain during the evenings or when she felt tired, and it was usually alleviated with rest. However, there was no congestion or redness on the skin any more, and no feelings of heat or dryness around the body. The herbal pills were therefore discontinued at this point, and her bowel movements returned to normal.

Acupuncture was continued for another three weeks, two or three times per week. By the end of this time the intervals between bouts of pain had lengthened, but the patient still experienced sudden darts of pain, which lasted for a few seconds. By this stage she was back working half days.

During the following two months the patient only came three times to the clinic for treatment, when the pain was obvious. Thereafter, as the pain largely disappeared and the skin recovered properly, there was no further need to continue treatment.

Generally speaking, shingles (herpes zoster) will often last for three weeks, but if the patient has a weak constitution, or if the pathogenic factor penetrates more deeply into the body, the pain can last up to a few months or even a year. In a very small percentage of patients, the disorder will last for more than a year. Although it is not possible to generalize, it can be said that many patients need both acupuncture and herbal therapy as this can hasten recovery, and more effectively remove the pathogenic factors from the Organs and the obstruction from the channels and collaterals.

CASE 39: **Female, age 42**

Main complaint | Dull pain in both hypochondrial regions

History | About six months ago the patient developed a feeling of discomfort and dull pain in both hypochondrial regions. Because the pain was not very severe, it has not affected her work or daily life too much. She frequently experiences a stifling sensation in the chest, which can be relieved by deeply sighing. Her appetite is normal, but over the last two months she has developed epigastric distention which occurs in the afternoon and becomes worse after lunch and dinner. Sometimes the distention can affect the lower abdominal region. The patient has not experienced any emotional disturbance, such as becoming hot tempered, irritable, or depressed. She has noticed, however, that her hair has become very dry and falls out easily. Both palms also feel very dry, although there are no cracks in the skin, nor does the dry skin flake off. She does not feel thirsty, and she drinks a normal amount of liquids. Her sleep is dream-disturbed. Her bowel movements and urination are both normal, but she has had prolonged menstrual cycles for some time.

Tongue	Pale with a thin, white coating
Pulse	Sunken and thin

Analysis of symptoms

1. Discomfort and pain in both hypochondrial regions—impairment of qi circulation in the Liver channel.
2. Dull pain, not severe, which does not affect the patient's daily life or work—no obstruction by an excessive pathogenic factor.
3. Stifling sensation in the chest, partially relieved by sighing—qi stagnation in the chest.
4. Epigastric distention in the afternoon, worsens after meals—disruption of transportive and transformative functions of middle burner.
5. Dream-disturbed sleep—disturbance of the Heart spirit.
6. Dry hair and loss of hair—malnourishment of the hair.
7. Prolonged menstrual cycle—Liver blood deficiency.
8. Pale tongue and thin pulse—blood deficiency.

Basic theory of case

The Liver channel traverses the hypochondrial region. Thus, when the Liver's function of governing the free-flow of qi is disrupted, pain in the hypochondrial regions results, one of several common symptoms. The pain is most frequently encountered in cases of Liver qi stagnation. However, Liver blood deficiency can also disrupt the Liver's governance of the free-flow of qi.

There is an adage about the Liver which says that while its body is yin, its function is yang *(tǐ yīn yòng yáng).* This means that the Liver stores a large amount of blood, one of the yin substances of the body, and relies on many different types of nutrition. Thus, viewed as an Organ, the Liver itself is categorized as yin. However, functionally it governs the free-flow of qi and regulates the qi activity of the entire body. Because qi is yang, the Liver's functions are therefore categorized as yang. And, because the Liver is thus closely associated with both qi and blood, it has strong aspects of both yin and yang. In its normal state, the Organ relies on the harmony between the qi and blood.

Qi is the commander of blood. When the Liver qi functions normally, the qi activity of the entire body will be properly regulated, and the blood will circulate smoothly through the vessels. Blood, on the other hand, is known as the mother of qi. If there is sufficient Liver blood, there will be an adequate supply of qi, and the Liver's governance of the free-flow of qi will function normally.

In clinical practice, qi stagnation impedes the circulation of blood, which can lead to blood stasis. Conversely, when there is a deficiency of blood, the Liver will be deprived of nourishment, and the Liver qi will lose its power to circulate. It then becomes stagnant and obstructs the general qi activity of the body *(Fig. 8-5).*

Cause of disease

Blood deficiency

In this case the onset has developed fairly slowly. There is no history of an invasion by a pathogenic factor, nor of an emotional disturbance, but the symptoms suggest blood deficiency.

Site of disease

Liver

The patient experiences a dull pain in the hypochondrial regions and a stifling sensation in the chest, relief from which is afforded by deeply sighing. She also has a prolonged menstrual cycle. All of these symptoms are associated with Liver disease.

Fig. 8-5

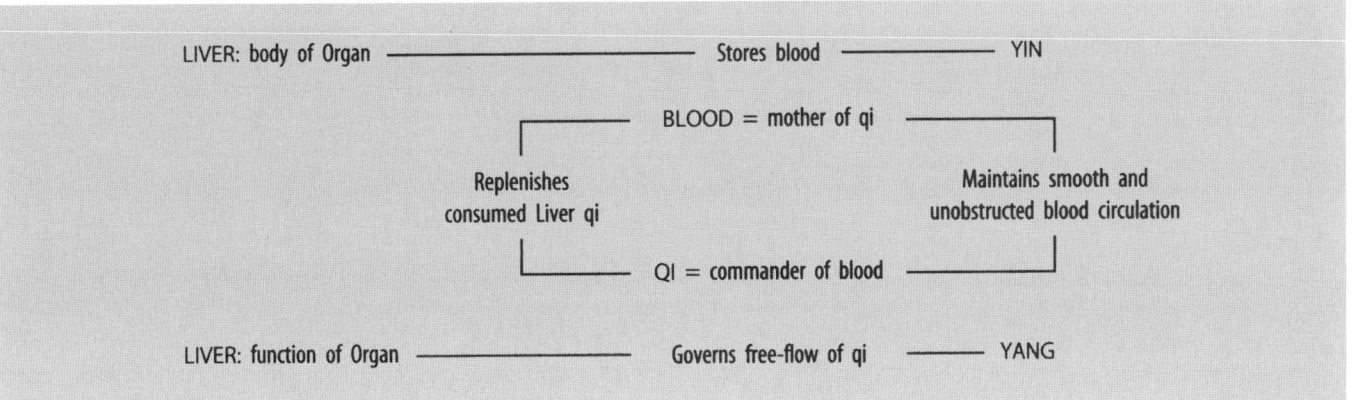

| Pathological change | In this case the patient suffers from disorders of both the Liver qi and Liver blood. |

The stifling sensation in the chest results from the dysfunction in the Liver's governance of the free-flow of qi, which impedes the qi activity in the chest. The patient has developed the habit of deeply sighing, which relieves the qi stagnation in the chest to some degree, and affords her some comfort. The epigastric distention is also related to the Liver's failure in governing the free-flow of qi. This has disrupted the normal qi activity in the middle burner, and caused the qi to stagnate in the epigastric region. Because eating can aggravate the stagnation of qi, the patient notices that the symptoms worsen after meals. The distention in the lower abdomen indicates that the qi activity in this area is also poor, but because the patient's bowel movements and urination are both normal, the impairment of qi activity in the lower burner is very mild.

In Chinese medicine the Liver is regarded as the "sea of blood," and the hair as the "surplus of blood." Blood deficiency thus leads to malnourishment of the hair, which becomes dry and falls out easily. As the blood nourishes the tissues and Organs of the body, blood deficiency can deprive the skin of its nourishment. In this case the patient suffers from dryness and discomfort in the palms. The reason for her prolonged menstrual cycles is that the Liver blood is insufficient, which can lead to deficiency in the conception vessel. The Heart houses the spirit, and Heart spirit relies on nourishment from the blood. Blood deficiency can deprive the Heart spirit of nourishment, and thus the patient's sleep is dream-disturbed.

The dull pain in both hypochondrial regions suggests a dysfunction of the Liver channel. Possible causes of this dull pain—which is typical of this pattern—are impaired qi activity or malnourishment caused by blood deficiency. In this case it can be attributed to both causes *(Fig. 8-6)*.

The pale tongue, that is, the loss of nourishment and luster in the tongue body, indicates blood deficiency. This is also reflected in the thin quality of the pulse, since the blood does not adequately fill the vessels. The sunken pulse suggests an interior pattern.

Pattern of disease This is an interior pattern, as the patient has blood deficiency and qi stagnation, and the site of disease is in the Liver.

The patient does not feel either hot or cold, her bowel movements and urination are normal, and she drinks a normal quantity of liquids: there is a tendency toward neither heat nor cold in this pattern.

The deficiency of Liver blood and loss of nourishment in the body indicates deficiency. The impairment to the free-flow of Liver qi, and the qi stagnation, are forms of excess. Thus, there is a combination of deficiency and excess in this case.

Additional notes 1. What is the relationship between the two Liver disorders, that is, the Liver blood deficiency and Liver qi stagnation?

Fig. 8-6

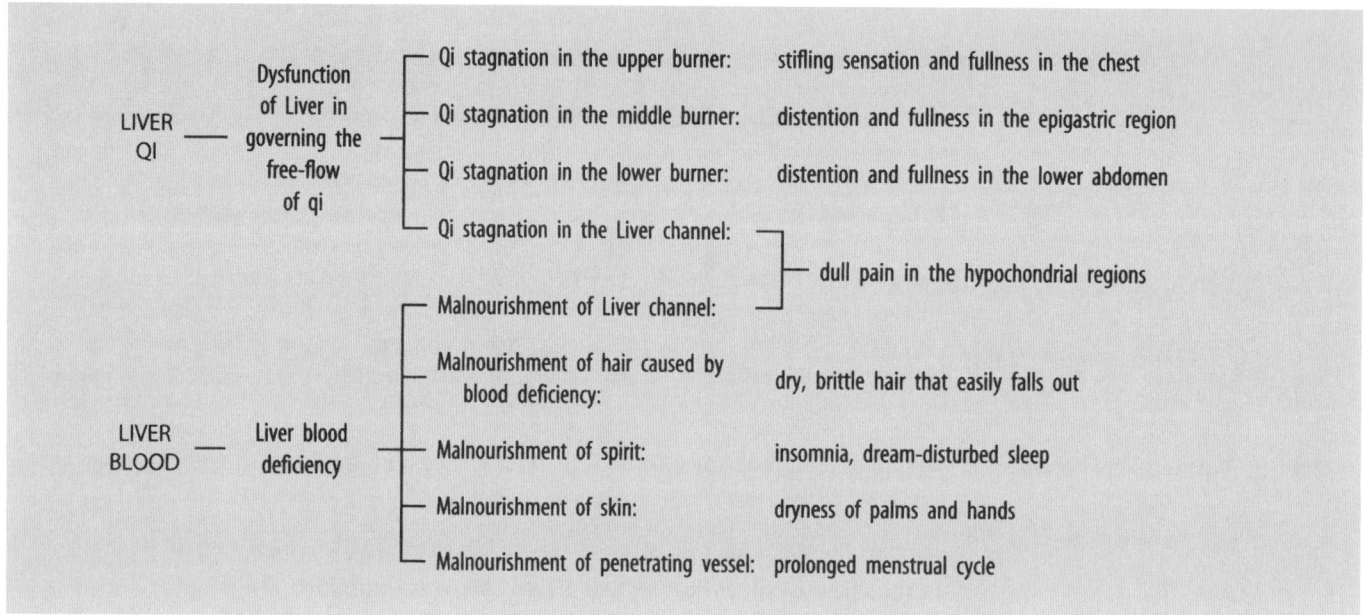

The main symptoms at present are the discomfort in both hypochondrial regions and the stifling sensation in the chest, but the patient has also had a prolonged menstrual cycle for some time. This would indicate that she was previously suffering from Liver blood deficiency which was not properly treated during its early stages. This resulted in malnourishment of the Liver, affecting the Liver's governance of the free-flow of qi, and also led to the disorder of the Liver qi. We can therefore conclude that there is Liver blood deficiency leading to the dysfunction of the Liver in governing the free-flow of qi.

2. What is the relationship between the deficiency and excess in this case?

In this case there is both deficiency (Liver blood deficiency) and excess (Liver qi stagnation). Which pattern predominates?

The patient suffers from a dull pain in the hypochondrial regions, but not a distending pain, and there is no emotional disturbance. This would indicate that the Liver qi stagnation is not very severe.

However, the patient suffers from symptoms involving her periods, hair, and skin, all of which reflect her problem of blood deficiency. These symptoms are much more obvious, and have existed longer, than the Liver qi stagnation. That means that the qi stagnation is secondary in this case, owing to the fact that the blood deficiency occurred earlier than the qi stagnation.

We may therefore conclude that there is a combination of deficiency and excess in this case, but that the pattern of deficiency is predominant.

3. Are there any disorders of the Spleen and Stomach?

This patient suffers from epigastric distention, especially after eating, which indicates a dysfunction in the Spleen and Stomach. As described above, this is due to Liver qi stagnation, or wood overcontrolling earth. The symptom did not originate from a disorder of the middle burner, and the symptom is not particularly severe. Moreover, her appetite is still normal. Therefore, the dysfunction of the Spleen and Stomach, and the disharmony between the Liver and the Organs of the middle burner, need not be regarded as significant in the diagnosis of this case.

Conclusion

1. According to the eight principles:
   Interior, neither heat nor cold, combination of deficiency and excess (deficiency is predominant).

2. According to theory of qi, blood, and body fluids:
   Blood deficiency and qi stagnation.

3. According to Organ theory:
   Liver blood deficiency and Liver dysfunction in governing the free-flow of qi.

Treatment principle

1. Nourish the blood and moisten the body.

2. Soften and nourish the Liver, and regulate the qi.

Explanation of treatment principle

A pattern dryness may be of internal or external origin. Internal dryness can be attributed to either blood deficiency or yin deficiency, or both, which deprives the body of nourishment. In this case, the dryness of both the hair and palms are symptoms of interior dryness, which requires that we nourish the blood. Nourishing and replenishing the blood will have the effect of moistening the hair and skin; it will also treat the menstrual disorder.

The cause of the Liver qi stagnation in this case is that the Liver has been deprived of the blood's nourishment. This creates a disharmony between the yin and yang in the Liver itself: the yin weakens and the yang becomes ascendant. Thus, nourishing the blood is essential to restoring the balance of yin and yang in the Liver, to prevent the Liver qi from becoming overactive, and to restore the Liver to its normal soft and harmonious state. Regulating the qi by nourishing the blood is called softening the liver to regulate the qi *(róu gān lǐ qì)*. This is another example of treating the root of a disease in order to eliminate its superficial manifestations.

Basic herbal formula

Four-Substance Decoction *(si wu tang)* is a basic formula for nourishing the blood, and contains the following ingredients:

Radix Rehmanniae Glutinosae Conquitae *(shu di huang)* 12g
Radix Angelicae Sinensis *(dang gui)* 10g
Radix Paeoniae Lactiflorae *(bai shao)* 12g
Radix Ligustici Chuanxiong *(chuan xiong)* 8g

Explanation of basic herbal formula

This formula was originally used for menstrual disorders, especially reduced menstrual bleeding with pale blood and dysmenorrhea, or severe pain and hard masses in the lower abdominal region. The basic pattern involves blood deficiency leading to a deficiency in the sea of blood, which gives rise to a menstrual disorder that is sometimes accompanied by blood stasis. Thus, the patient will not only have blood deficiency, but also pain or masses in the abdominal region.

In this formula, Radix Rehmanniae Glutinosae Conquitae *(shu di huang)* is sweet and slightly warm. It is associated with the Liver and Kidney channels, and nourishes the blood and yin. Radix Angelicae Sinensis *(dang gui)* is sweet, acrid, and warm, and is associated with the Liver and Heart channels. It nourishes the blood and dispels blood stasis. Both serve as chief herbs in this formula.

The other two herbs serve as deputies. Radix Paeoniae Lactiflorae *(bai shao)* is sour and cold, and is associated with the Liver and Spleen channels. It nourishes the blood. Radix Ligustici Chuanxiong *(chuan xiong)* is acrid and warm, and is associated with the Liver and Gallbladder channels. It dispels blood stasis.

There are only four herbs in this formula, which not only nourishes the blood, but also dispels blood stasis. It is very commonly used in the treatment of blood disorders.

Modified herbal formula

Radix Rehmanniae Glutinosae Conquitae *(shu di huang)* 10g
Fructus Lycii *(gou qi zi)* 15g

Radix Paeoniae Lactiflorae *(bai shao)* 10g

Radix Angelicae Sinensis *(dang gui)* 8g

Fructus Meliae Toosendan *(chuan lian zi)* 8g

Fructus Citri Aurantii *(zhi ke)* 6g

Pericarpium Citri Reticulatae *(chen pi)* 8g

Rhizoma Cyperi Rotundi *(xiang fu)* 6g

Fructus Zizyphi Jujubae *(da zao)* .... 4 pieces

Explanation of modified herbal formula

The basic pathological change in this case is blood deficiency, specifically Liver blood deficiency, which has impaired the Liver's governance of the free-flow of qi. Four-Substance Decoction *(si wu tang)* is used as the basic formula to nourish the blood, with the addition of the following herbs to regulate the qi and remove the qi stagnation.

Fructus Lycii *(gou qi zi)* is mainly associated with the Liver channel; it nourishes and replenishes the yin of the Liver and Kidney. This herb reinforces the basic formula's action in nourishing the Liver. Radix Ligustici Chuanxiong *(chuan xiong)* is omitted from the modifed formula, however, as there is no apparent blood stasis in this case, and we want to avoid injuring the yin and blood, which can occur with warm and acrid herbs.

Fructus Meliae Toosendan *(chuan lian zi)* and Rhizoma Cyperi Rotundi *(xiang fu)* both promote the Liver's governance of the free-flow of qi, and Pericarpium Citri Reticulatae *(chen pi)* regulates the qi of the middle burner. These herbs treat the fullness, distention, and discomfort in the chest, epigastric, hypochondrial, and intercostal regions. Fructus Citri Aurantii *(zhi ke)* removes the qi stagnation and regulates the qi activity in the chest.

Fructus Zizyphi Jujubae *(da zao)* both nourishes the blood and tonifies the qi. It is therefore used to strengthen the antipathogenic factors and also to soothe the Heart spirit, thereby treating the dream-disturbed sleep.

With all these changes, the purpose of the original formula—to nourish the blood and remove the blood stasis—has been modified to nourishing the blood and regulating the qi, which is appropriate to this case.

Follow-up

The patient took one packet of the herbal formula daily, in two doses, for a week, after which the stifling sensation in the chest and the distention in the epigastric region were largely alleviated. In addition, the patient's sleep was improved and no longer dream-disturbed.

Fructus Meliae Toosendan *(chuan lian zi)* and Fructus Citri Aurantii *(zhi ke)* were then removed from the formula. The dosage of Fructus Lycii *(gou qi zi)* was increased to 20g, and Radix Paeoniae Lactiflorae *(bai shao)* to 15g, and 10g of Fructus Ligustri Lucidi *(nu zhen zi)* was added, in order to strengthen the Liver and Kidney. In addition, 12g of Radix Astragali Membranacei *(huang qi)* was added to tonify the qi so as to promote the production of blood.

The patient took the revised formula for a month, during which there was a one-week break. At the end of the month most of the symptoms were alleviated, and the herbal formula was made into pills prepared with honey. The patient took one pill in the morning and one in the evening for a period of three weeks.

Treatment was stopped for one week and then the patient came to the clinic for a checkup. She returned six months later for another. She was very pleased with the result as there was no recurrence in the attacks, and the symptoms had disappeared. The quality of her hair improved: it became more lustrous and less of it fell out. Her periods were also restored to normal.

As can be seen, no particular treatment was given for the dry skin and hair, or for the loss of hair, but as soon as the body's yin and blood were fully replenished, these symptoms cleared up on their own.

CASE 40: **Male, age 49**

Main complaint	Stifling sensation in the chest, sometimes accompanied by pain

History

Over the past year the patient has often experienced a stifling sensation in the chest, occasionally accompanied by sharp, paroxysmal precordial pain. The pain is not very severe; it lasts only a short while, and the location is fixed. It does not radiate to any other area. Occasionally the patient suffers from palpitations. Tiredness, poor sleep, or emotional upset seem to be the precipitating factors. The patient has had several ECG checkups, which show a change in the T wave, which either appears flat or inverted. The diagnosis in conventional medicine is coronary heart disease (angina pectoris). The patient was given conventional medication, but as the drugs gave him a bursting headache and made his face very red, he stopped taking them.

Over the past year the patient has noticed that his physical energy has decreased a little, and that he experiences shortness of breath after physical exertion. However, he does not have any limitation of physical activity and there is no edema. His sleep is not very sound.

Other than these symptoms, he is in good general health and experiences no obvious discomfort. His appetite is good, he drinks a normal amount of liquids, and his bowel movements and urination are both normal.

Tongue

Pale and lusterless with a thin, white coating

Pulse

Sunken and forceless

Analysis of symptoms

1. Chest pain—impairment of qi activity in the chest.

2. Sharp precordial pain—blood stasis in the Heart.

3. Palpitations and unsound sleep—malnourishment of Heart spirit.

4. Shortness of breath after physical exertion—qi deficiency.

5. Pale and lusterless tongue—malnourishment of the tongue due to poor blood circulation.

6. Sunken and forceless pulse—interior deficiency.

Basic theory of case

In Chinese medicine, pectoral qi *(zōng qì)*, also known as ancestral or original qi, is one of the four main types of qi in the human body. One of the sources of pectoral qi is the external environment *(tīan yáng zhī qì*, literally "heavenly yang qi"), which is inhaled by the Lung. The other source is the essence and qi from food *(shuǐ gǔ jīng qì)*, which is transported and transformed in the middle burner by the Spleen and Stomach. When these two elements come together in the chest the result is called pectoral qi. Thus, the functions of the Lung, Spleen, and Stomach directly affect the sufficiency of pectoral qi.

The Heart and Lung are located in the chest, and the physiological functions of pectoral qi are therefore associated with these two Organs. Pectoral qi enters the Lung where it replenishes and supports the Lung qi, and provides energy for the dispersal and downward (descending) movement of Lung qi. Pectoral qi is closely connected with respiration. It also enters the Heart where it replenishes the Heart qi to support its function in governing the circulation of blood and regulating the rhythm of the Heart beat. Thus, pectoral qi is very closely associated with the circulation of blood throughout the body.

Deficiency of pectoral qi can lead to Heart qi deficiency or Lung qi deficiency, which are very common patterns in clinical practice *(Fig. 8-7)*.

Cause of disease

Blood stasis and deficiency of antipathogenic factors

The pain is localized and very sharp, and the tongue is lusterless. This is evidence of blood stasis within the body.

Fig. 8-7

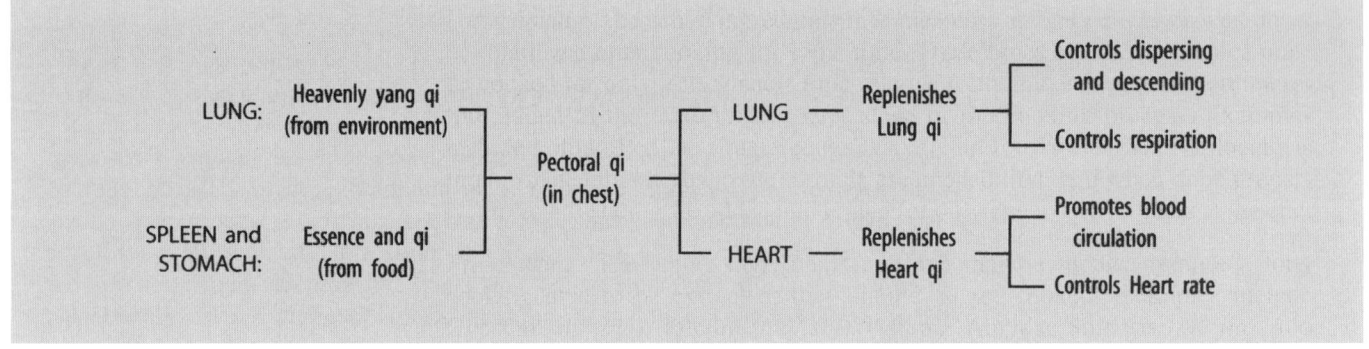

Site of disease	As the cause of the blood stasis is poor blood circulation due to qi deficiency, we can also say that there is a deficiency of antipathogenic factors.

Site of disease

Heart

The patient suffers from a stifling sensation in the chest, palpitations, precordial pain, and unsound sleep, all of which are evidence of a Heart disorder.

Pathological change

In Chinese medicine the Heart governs the movement of blood. The Heart qi provides energy for the circulation of blood throughout the body. Because the Heart qi is replenished by the pectoral qi, deficiency of either Heart qi or pectoral qi can cause poor blood circulation, and even blood stasis.

In this case the patient has suffered from a stifling sensation in the chest for over a year, which indicates that the qi activity in the chest is poor. The reason for this can be either qi stagnation or qi deficiency. Because the patient here has experienced a reduction in his general energy level and suffers shortness of breath after physical exertion, deficiency of qi—or specifically pectoral qi—is indicated. This is why the qi activity in the chest is abnormal and qi stagnation occurs, causing the stifling sensation. The deficiency of pectoral qi also inhibits the Heart qi from circulating the blood, causing sharp precordial pain. This pain reflects the presence of blood stasis, which, in this case, can be attributed to the pattern of qi deficiency.

The Heart governs the spirit, the tranquility of which depends upon nourishment from Heart blood. In this case, because the stasis of Heart blood has impeded the circulation of blood, the Heart spirit is deprived of its nourishment, and is unable to remain tranquil. This accounts for the palpitations and unsound sleep.

The pale tongue indicates that the blood is unable to reach the tongue with its nourishment; this is because the qi lacks the power to properly circulate the blood. The lusterless quality of the tongue is likewise indicative of poor circulation of blood, and is commonly encountered in cases of blood stasis. The thin, white tongue coating reflects the absence of an excessive pathogenic factor in the body. The sunken quality of the pulse indicates an interior pattern, and its forceless quality, qi deficiency.

Fig. 8-8

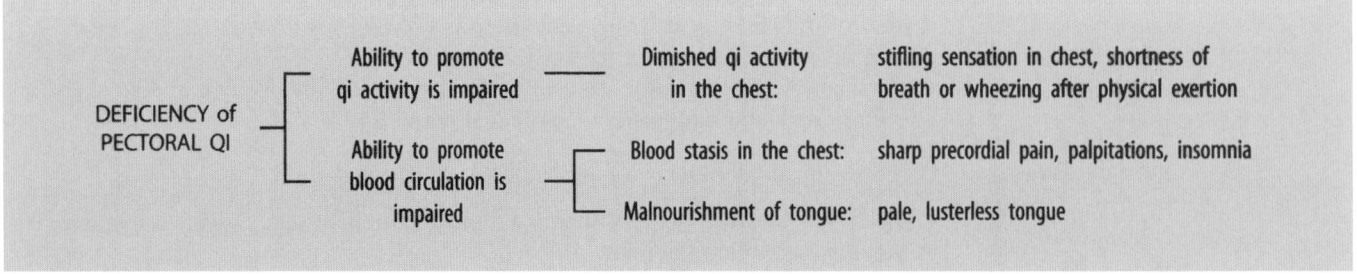

Pattern of disease

As there is no history or evidence of an invasion by an external pathogenic factor, and as the site of disease is the Heart, the pattern is of the interior.

The patient does not suffer from heat or cold, nor is he thirsty; bowel movements and urination are both normal; and the tongue coating is white, not yellow. Thus, there is no tendency toward heat or cold in this case.

Blood stasis obstructing the vessels pertains to excess. The underlying cause of the blood stasis, however, is qi deficiency, which deprives the circulation of its energy; thus, there is also deficiency.

Additional notes

1. Is there a Liver disorder in this case?

The history noted that the patient has been suffering from chest pain, which can be induced by emotional disturbance and a lack of rest. Does this indicate a Liver disorder?

Because the Heart governs the spirit, an emotional disturbance can also directly affect the circulation of Heart qi and blood, and thereby cause an obstruction of the vessels, which causes chest pain. Lack of rest can aggravate the qi deficiency—a common occurrence. There are no other symptoms to suggest Liver involvement. We may therefore conclude that a Liver disorder plays no part in this case, especially since the site of the disease is the Heart.

2. What is the cause of the pectoral qi deficiency?

We have already mentioned that a common cause of pectoral qi deficiency is Lung or Spleen qi deficiency. In this case, besides the general qi deficiency symptoms (stifling sensation in the chest, reduced energy level, shortness of breath after physical exertion), there are no symptoms that are specifically associated with either the Lung or Spleen; we therefore cannot say that there is Lung or Spleen qi deficiency in this case. The cause of the pectoral qi deficiency here is early ageing. The general qi of the body is gradually degenerating, and the qi in the chest has become deficient. Problems associated with ageing can occur when patients are in their fifties. This is an early age, but such cases are common enough in clinical practice.

3. What is the relationship between the problems of deficiency and excess?

This patient's chest pain is a problem of excess, but the shortness of breath after physical exertion, and the reduced energy level, are problems of deficiency. The relationship between the two is that the problems of deficiency lead to the problem of excess. However, based on the symptoms in this case, neither problem is severe, nor is one more severe than the other; they are about evenly matched.

Conclusion

1. According to the eight principles:
   Interior, neither heat nor cold, combination of excess and deficiency of equal severity.
2. According to theory of qi, blood, and body fluids:
   Qi deficiency leading to blood stasis.
3. According to Organ theory: Heart blood stasis.

Treatment principle

1. Tonify the qi.
2. Remove the blood stasis.

Explanation of treatment principle

The basic method for treating blood stasis is to improve the blood circulation and remove the stagnation. Because the causes of blood stasis are varied, there are a number of ways to remove it. The reason for the lack of energy to circulate the blood in this case is the deficiency of qi; tonifying the pectoral qi and restoring the energy for the circulation of blood is therefore essential. This is another example of treating the root of the disease. When normal blood circulation has been restored, the chest pain will be relieved, and the Heart spirit will regain its nourishment. The symptoms associated with the Heart spirit will then spontaneously disappear.

Combining tonification of the qi with dispelling blood stasis will accelerate recovery.

Basic herbal formula

Tonify the Yang to Restore Five-tenths Decoction *(bu yang huan wu tang)* was originally used in treating the sequelae of windstroke, such as hemiplegia. This formula contains the following ingredients:

Radix Astragali Membranacei *(huang qi)* 20g

Radix Angelicae Sinensis *(dang gui)* 6g

Radix Paeoniae Rubrae *(chi shao)* 6g

Lumbricus *(di long)* 3g

Radix Ligustici Chuanxiong *(chuan xiong)* 3g

Flos Carthami Tinctorii *(hong hua)* 3g

Semen Persicae *(tao ren)* 3g

Explanation of basic herbal formula

The indications of this formula are the sequelae of windstroke, such as hemiplegia, deviation of the mouth, difficulty in speaking, loss of strength in the limbs, urinary frequency and incontinence, a white tongue coating, and a moderate pulse. The basic pathological pattern relates to the late stage of windstroke, when the Liver wind has already been extinguished, but the antipathogenic factor has been severely injured, and the blood stasis has not been completely removed. Thus, besides the paralysis, the patient may feel very weak (for example, reduced muscular strength) in the limbs, and suffer from urinary frequency—symptoms involving qi deficiency.

Radix Astragali Membranacei *(huang qi)* is the chief herb in this formula. It is sweet and warm, and is associated with the Spleen and Lung channels. It is very commonly used to tonify qi, the functionfor which it is used in this case to strengthen the circulation of blood.

Radix Angelicae Sinensis *(dang gui)* is sweet, acrid, and warm, and is associated with the Liver and Heart channels. It dispels blood stasis while nourishing the blood. It can remove pathogenic factors, such as blood stasis, from the blood vessels without injuring the blood. This is the deputy herb in this formula.

There are four assistant herbs. Radix Ligustici Chuanxiong *(chuan xiong)* is acrid and warm, Radix Paeoniae Rubrae *(chi shao)* is bitter and slightly cold, Semen Persicae *(tao ren)* is bitter and neutral, and Flos Carthami Tinctorii *(hong hua)* is acrid and warm. These herbs are associated with the Liver, or the Heart and Liver channels, and can assist Radix Angelicae Sinensis *(dang gui)* in regulating the circulation of blood and removing the stasis of blood.

Lumbricus *(di long)* is salty and cold, and is associated with the Liver channel. It can remove obstruction from the channels. This substance serves as the envoy in this formula.

This purpose of this formula is to dispel blood stasis and promote the circulation of blood, but the chief herb, which is administered in a large dose, is very potent for tonifying the qi. The formula is therefore typical of those that tonify qi in order to dispel blood stasis.

Modified herbal formula

Radix Astragali Membranacei *(huang qi)* 10g

Radix Angelicae Sinensis *(dang gui)* 6g

Radix Salviae Miltiorrhizae *(dan shen)* 10g

Radix Ligustici Chuanxiong *(chuan xiong)* 5g

Semen Persicae *(tao ren)* 4g

Flos Carthami Tinctorii *(hong hua)* 4g

Fructus Citri Aurantii *(zhi ke)* 8g

Rhizoma Atractylodis Macrocephalae *(bai zhu)* 8g

Rhizoma Acori Graminei *(shi chang pu)* 5g

Explanation of modified herbal formula

Because it is qi deficiency that led to the stasis of blood in this case, we must tonify the qi in order to remove the blood stasis. Tonify the Yang to Restore Five-tenths Decoction *(bu yang huan wu tang)* serves as the basic formula. However, because neither windstroke nor its sequelae are found in this case, some adjustments are necessary.

Compared with Tonify the Yang to Restore Five-tenths Decoction *(bu yang huan wu tang)*, there are more herbs in the modified formula involving the qi level. Rhizoma Atractylodis Macrocephalae *(bai zhu)* can assist Radix Astragali Membranacei *(huang qi)* in tonifying the qi. Fructus Citri Aurantii *(zhi ke)* is added to regulate the qi and remove the stifling sensation in the chest, thereby assisting the herbs that regulate the blood and remove the blood stasis. Rhizoma Acori Graminei *(shi chang pu)* is acrid and warm, and serves in the original formula to recapture the spirit in order to restore consciousness by opening the orifice of the Heart, which has been blocked by pathogenic wind. Here it is used to remove the obstruction from the qi activity while soothing the spirit.

There are no major changes in the herbs for the blood system. Radix Salviae Miltiorrhizae *(dan shen)* is substituted for Radix Paeoniae Rubrae *(chi shao)* since the former herb is associated with the Heart and is therefore more suitable to this particular case. (The latter herb is associated with the Liver.) Lumbricus *(di long)* is omitted from the modified formula, as the blood stasis exists in the Heart but not in the channels and collaterals.

Follow-up

For two weeks the patient was given one packet of the herbal formula daily, divided into two doses, after which he returned for a checkup. He reported that he experienced no discomfort after taking the herbs, but that there was no change at all in the symptoms. He continued with the same formula for another month and then returned. By then the shortness of breath following physical exertion was gone, and the patient experienced fewer attacks of chest pain. The dosage of Radix Astragali Membranacei *(huang qi)* was increased to 20g, Radix Salviae Miltiorrhizae *(dan shen)* to 20g, and 8g of Tuber Curcumae *(yu jin)* was added in order to strengthen the formula's actions in tonifying the qi, regulating the circulation of qi, and removing blood stasis.

This revised formula was taken for another month, with a one-week break, after which there was no further chest pain. An ECG showed that the T wave still tended to be flat, but it was not inverted. This indicated an improvement of the ischemia. The patient took the herbs for another week and then stopped.

Over the next five years the patient was advised to regularly take a prepared medicine named Salvia Pills *(dan shen pian)*, the main ingredient of which is Radix Salviae Miltiorrhizae *(dan shen)*. During this time the patient experienced only occasional attacks of angina pectoris, which were relieved by taking this prepared medication. ECGs yielded the same result as that folloing the first course of treatment. Only rarely did the patient use conventional medication for the angina pectoris, and there was no continuous or long-term use of this medication.

Although there had been no improvement in the patient's condition after the first two weeks of herbal therapy, this does not mean that the treatment had yielded no results. The problems were still there, but the symptoms had not worsened and there was no discomfort—the patient simply needed to continue taking the herbs. The effect of taking herbs can be slower than that of acupuncture; the practitioner must understand the situation and not abandon treatment or rashly change the prescription.

There are various degrees of severity in coronary heart disease. Mild cases, including those in which conventional medication or herbal treatment is used, may last for many years without any obvious change, whereas severe cases can lead to sudden death. The practitioner must therefore proceed with utmost caution; the patient's symptoms must be monitored, and ECGs should be taken from time to time. Special care should be given to patients with unstable conditions.

If a practitioner is not fully conversant with conventional medication, he or she should avoid interfering with the medication that a patient may be taking for coronary heart disease, especially if the result at the beginning of herbal therapy is not very apparent.

Diagnostic Principles for Pain

Pain is one of the most common symptoms in the clinic. It is a significant, subjective symptom that can undergo various changes, and can occur in a wide range of diseases. In this book and its companion, *Acupuncture Patterns and Practice,* we have discussed many types of disorders that involve pain, including headache, facial pain, pain in the chest and hypochondrial regions, abdominal and epigastric pain, lower back pain, and painful obstruction *(bì)*. Although we have outlined the diagnostic principles for each type of illness at the end of individual chapters, there are two methods that should be followed in diagnosing any type of pain: diagnosis based on the site of the disease, and diagnosis based on the nature of the disease.

Diagnosis based on site of disease

The first step in diagnosis based on the site of a disease is to examine the patient's main complaint, such as headache, lower back pain, or chest pain. From this, one can determine which channel or internal Organ has been affected, or whether the qi, blood, or body fluids have been injured.

I. Disorders of the channels and collaterals

The pain will occur along the pathways of the channels and collaterals, and is generally in a very superficial part of the body. In most cases this type of pain will reflect an invasion by an external pathogenic factor; the disorder often does not last very long. Changes in the patient's environment often affect the symptoms, for better or worse. Pain occurring in the head, face, hypochondrial region, lower back, or in the limbs indicates that the disorder may be in the channels. By determining exactly which area of the body is painful, one can establish which of the channels have been affected. Acupuncture or herbs can then be used to expel the external pathogenic factors, remove the obstruction from the channels, and alleviate the pain.

II. Disorders of the qi and blood

The pain associated with qi and blood disorders usually does not indicate involvement with the pathways of the channels and collaterals; it is generally deeper. Most patients will have no history of an invasion by an external pathogenic factor, but the aggravation or relief of symptoms can frequently be associated with an emotional or psychological disturbance. The symptoms are characterized by obstruction of qi activity or poor blood circulation. If the disorder involves deficiency, these characteristics are usually not very obvious, but there will be a greater vulnerability toward invasion by pathogenic factors. Some cases featuring headache, chest pain, pain in the hypochondrial and epigastric regions, and lower back pain, can be associated with disorders of the qi or blood. Distinguishing whether the disorder is in the qi or blood system, and whether it is deficient or excessive in nature, is important in determining how deep the disease has penetrated, and what treatment method is appropriate.

III. Disorders of the internal Organs

The pain is generally deeper than that of other disorders, and there is a wider range of symptoms, although they are all associated with one or two of the internal Organs. Normally, there will be no recent history of invasion by an external pathogenic factor, and the illness can last quite a long time. The pain usually occurs in the proximity of the affected Organ, or is in a part of the body that corresponds with a related Organ. Both the pain and other symptoms are directly associated with the affected Organ or Organs.

Organ theory is used to differentiate among the Organs in this type of case, and the treatment principle is likewise based on the theory of the treatment of the Organs. However, in patterns of excess, it is very important to remove the obstruction to the qi activity in order to alleviate the pain.

Diagnosis based on nature of disease

By diagnosing the nature of the disease, one can determine the cause of the pain. In general, the particular symptoms, which are affected by the cold or hot nature of the pathogenic factors, or the sufficiency or insufficiency of the antipathogenic factors, will have different characteristics that permit us to diagnose the nature of the disease.

Fig. 8-9   Summary of eight-parameter diagnosis of pain

Pain in cold pattern	Pain is accompanied by a cold sensation and reduced local temperature. Skin may be pale or normal in color. Pain may be aggravated by low temperature or cold weather, and alleviated by warmth.
Pain in heat pattern	Pain is accompanied by a hot or burning sensation. There may be local redness, or redness accompanied by swelling. Heat can be felt by palpation. Pain is aggravated by warmth or very hot weather, while coldness always brings relief.
Pain in pattern of excess	History is usually short, and the pain, which can be colicky or sharp, is severe. Pressure usually aggravates the pain considerably, and patients are therefore advised to avoid it.
Pain in pattern of deficiency	Duration is very long, and the pain is frequently dull. Local massage and pressure can bring relief.

Diagnostic procedure

Having studied the patient's symptoms and the results of the examination, the practitioner should not only be able to find the site of the disease, but also determine the nature of the disease. To assist the practitioner with his or her diagnosis, a summary of the most commonly seen patterns of pain is provided in *Fig. 8-10*. This is followed by individual charts for diagnosing pain in each region of the body: head and face *(Fig. 8-11)*, chest and hypochondia *(Fig. 8-12)*, epigastrium and abdomen *(Fig. 8-13)*, lower back *(Fig. 8-14)*, and limbs *(Fig. 8-15)*.

Fig. 8-10   Differentiating pain

Nature of pain	Related factor	Pattern
WANDERING and RADIATING	Wind	Moving painful obstruction due to invasion of pathogenic wind
COLD	Cold	Severely painful painful obstruction; epigastric and abdominal pain due to invasion of pathogenic cold
BURNING	Heat	Hot painful obstruction; burning pain in the epigastric region due to heat in the Stomach
HEAVY	Dampness	Fixed painful obstruction with heavy and sore joints; heaviness and soreness in the limbs and body due to dampness in the Spleen
DISTENDING	Qi stagnation	Liver qi stagnation affecting the intercostal and hypochondriac regions; stagnation in the middle burner with pain and distention in the epigastrium and abdomen
SHARP	Blood stasis	Chest blood stasis with sharp pain in the chest; blood stasis in the Stomach affecting the epigastrium
DULL	Deficiency	Internal cold in Stomach; Stomach yang deficiency; Kidney yang deficiency
EMPTY	Deficiency	Pain with empty sensation in the head due to deficiency of Kidney essence
CHOLIC	Obstruction	Severe cholic pain caused by Kidney or Gallbladder stones
PULLING	Malnourishment of sinews	Liver blood deficiency leading to spasm and pulling pain in hands and feet, caused by Liver blood or yin deficiency

Fig. 8-11

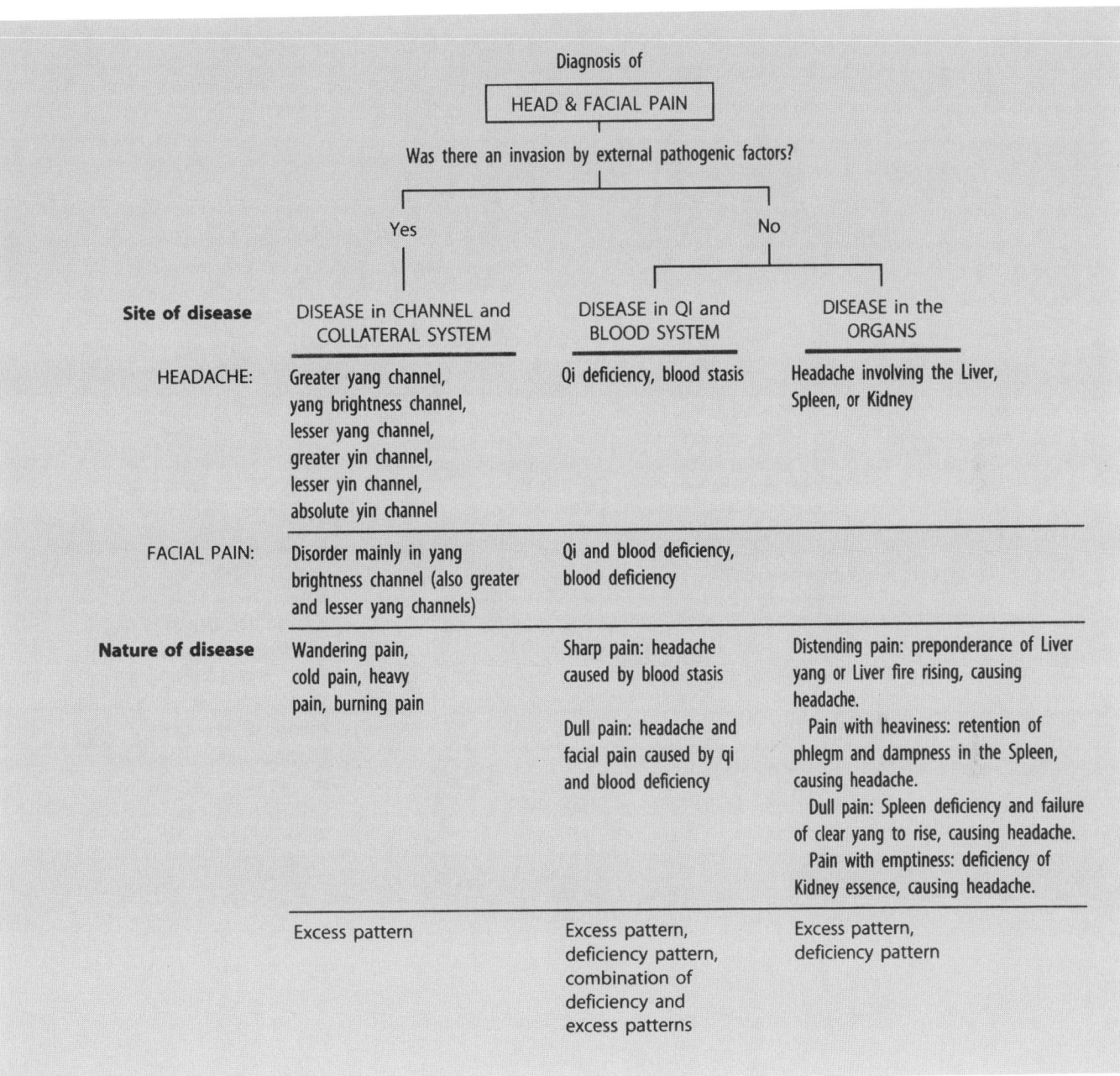

Diagnosis of

| HEAD & FACIAL PAIN |

Was there an invasion by external pathogenic factors?

	Yes	**No**	
Site of disease	DISEASE in CHANNEL and COLLATERAL SYSTEM	DISEASE in QI and BLOOD SYSTEM	DISEASE in the ORGANS
HEADACHE:	Greater yang channel, yang brightness channel, lesser yang channel, greater yin channel, lesser yin channel, absolute yin channel	Qi deficiency, blood stasis	Headache involving the Liver, Spleen, or Kidney
FACIAL PAIN:	Disorder mainly in yang brightness channel (also greater and lesser yang channels)	Qi and blood deficiency, blood deficiency	

Nature of disease	Wandering pain, cold pain, heavy pain, burning pain	Sharp pain: headache caused by blood stasis
		
		Dull pain: headache and facial pain caused by qi and blood deficiency
			Distending pain: preponderance of Liver yang or Liver fire rising, causing headache.
			   Pain with heaviness: retention of phlegm and dampness in the Spleen, causing headache.
			   Dull pain: Spleen deficiency and failure of clear yang to rise, causing headache.
			   Pain with emptiness: deficiency of Kidney essence, causing headache.

	Excess pattern	Excess pattern, deficiency pattern, combination of deficiency and excess patterns	Excess pattern, deficiency pattern

Fig. 8-12

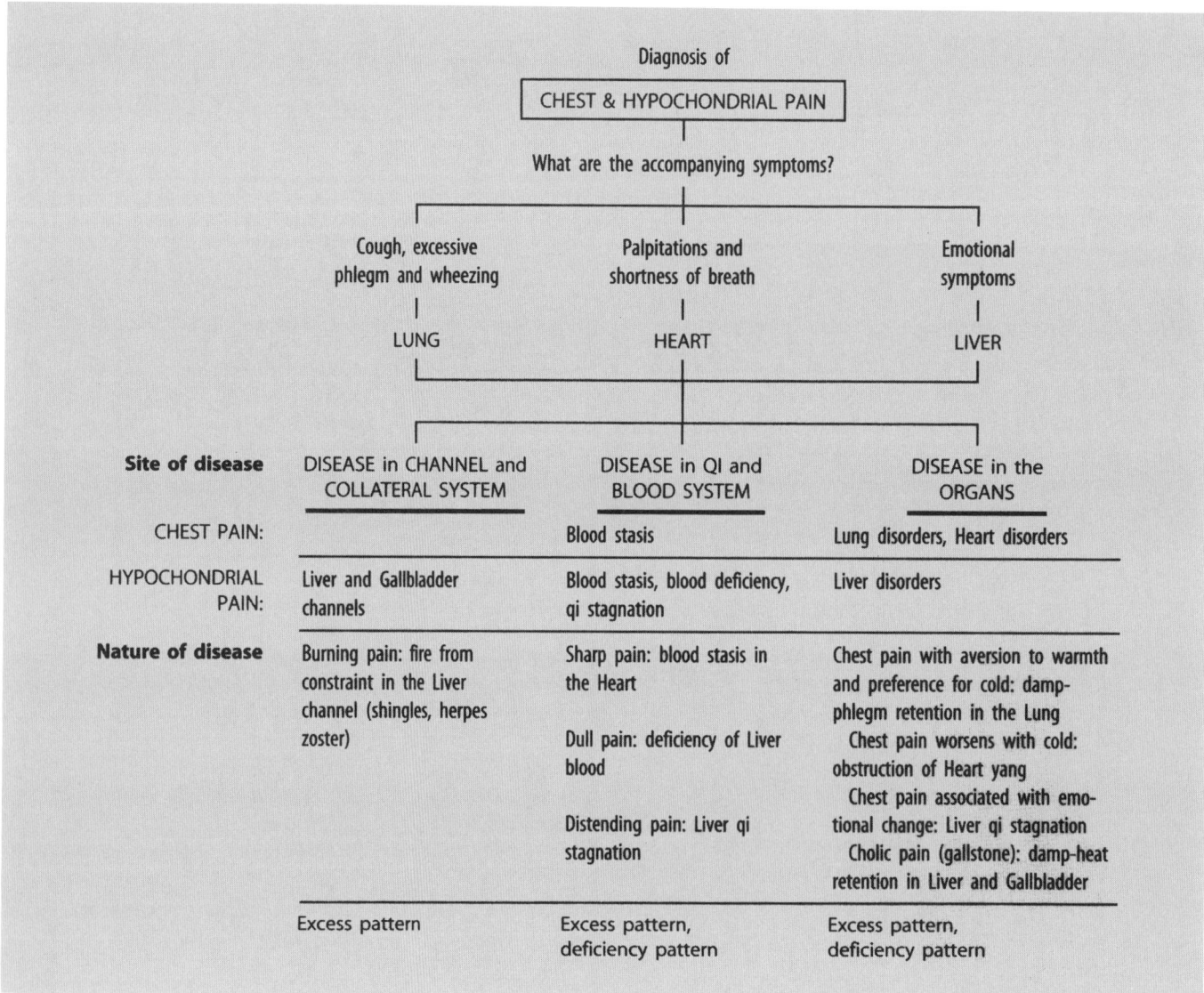

Fig. 8-13

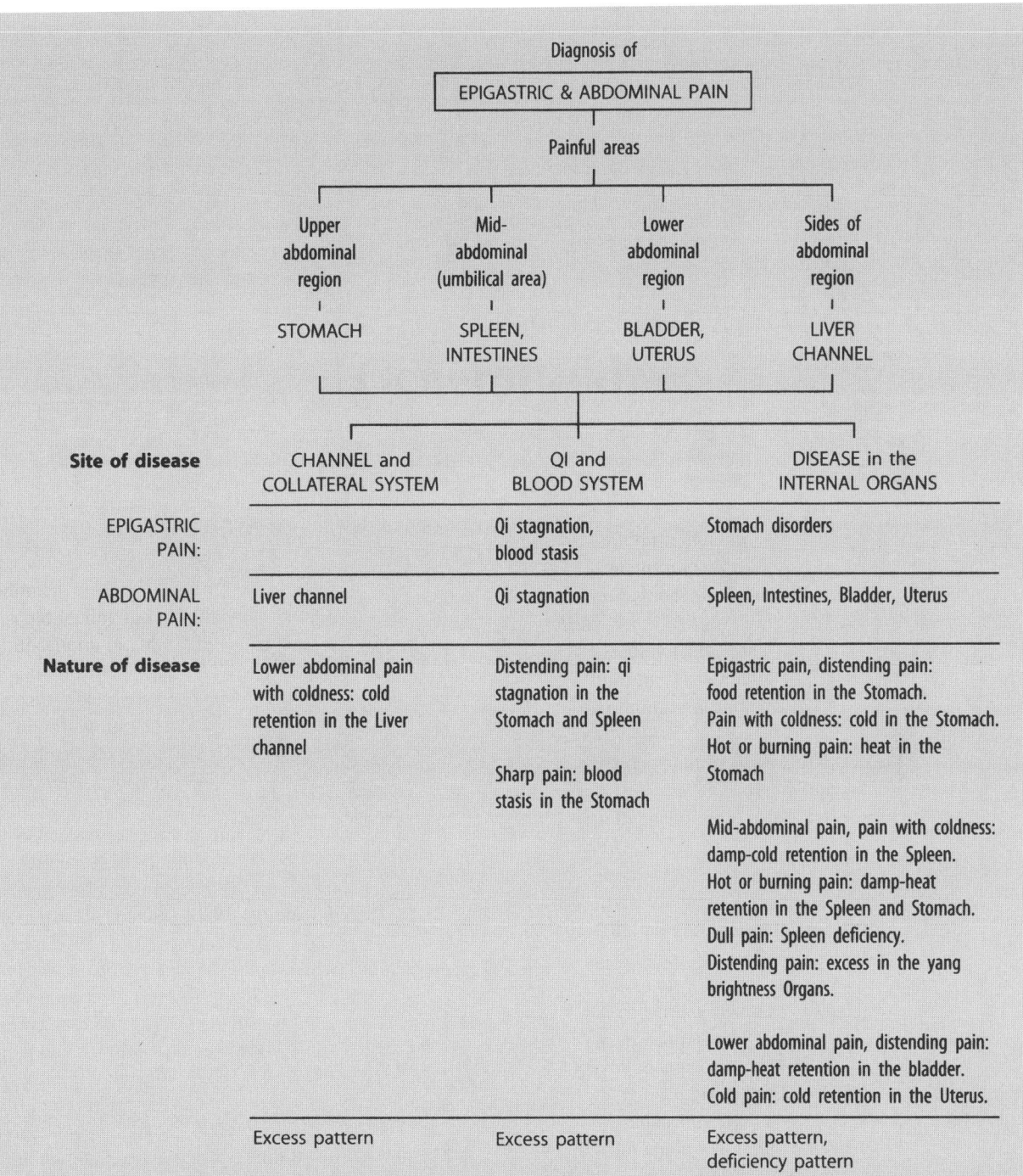

Diagnosis of
EPIGASTRIC & ABDOMINAL PAIN

Painful areas

Upper abdominal region	Mid-abdominal (umbilical area)	Lower abdominal region	Sides of abdominal region
STOMACH	SPLEEN, INTESTINES	BLADDER, UTERUS	LIVER CHANNEL

Site of disease	CHANNEL and COLLATERAL SYSTEM	QI and BLOOD SYSTEM	DISEASE in the INTERNAL ORGANS
EPIGASTRIC PAIN:		Qi stagnation, blood stasis	Stomach disorders
ABDOMINAL PAIN:	Liver channel	Qi stagnation	Spleen, Intestines, Bladder, Uterus
Nature of disease	Lower abdominal pain with coldness: cold retention in the Liver channel	Distending pain: qi stagnation in the Stomach and Spleen Sharp pain: blood stasis in the Stomach	Epigastric pain, distending pain: food retention in the Stomach. Pain with coldness: cold in the Stomach. Hot or burning pain: heat in the Stomach Mid-abdominal pain, pain with coldness: damp-cold retention in the Spleen. Hot or burning pain: damp-heat retention in the Spleen and Stomach. Dull pain: Spleen deficiency. Distending pain: excess in the yang brightness Organs. Lower abdominal pain, distending pain: damp-heat retention in the bladder. Cold pain: cold retention in the Uterus.
	Excess pattern	Excess pattern	Excess pattern, deficiency pattern

Fig. 8-14

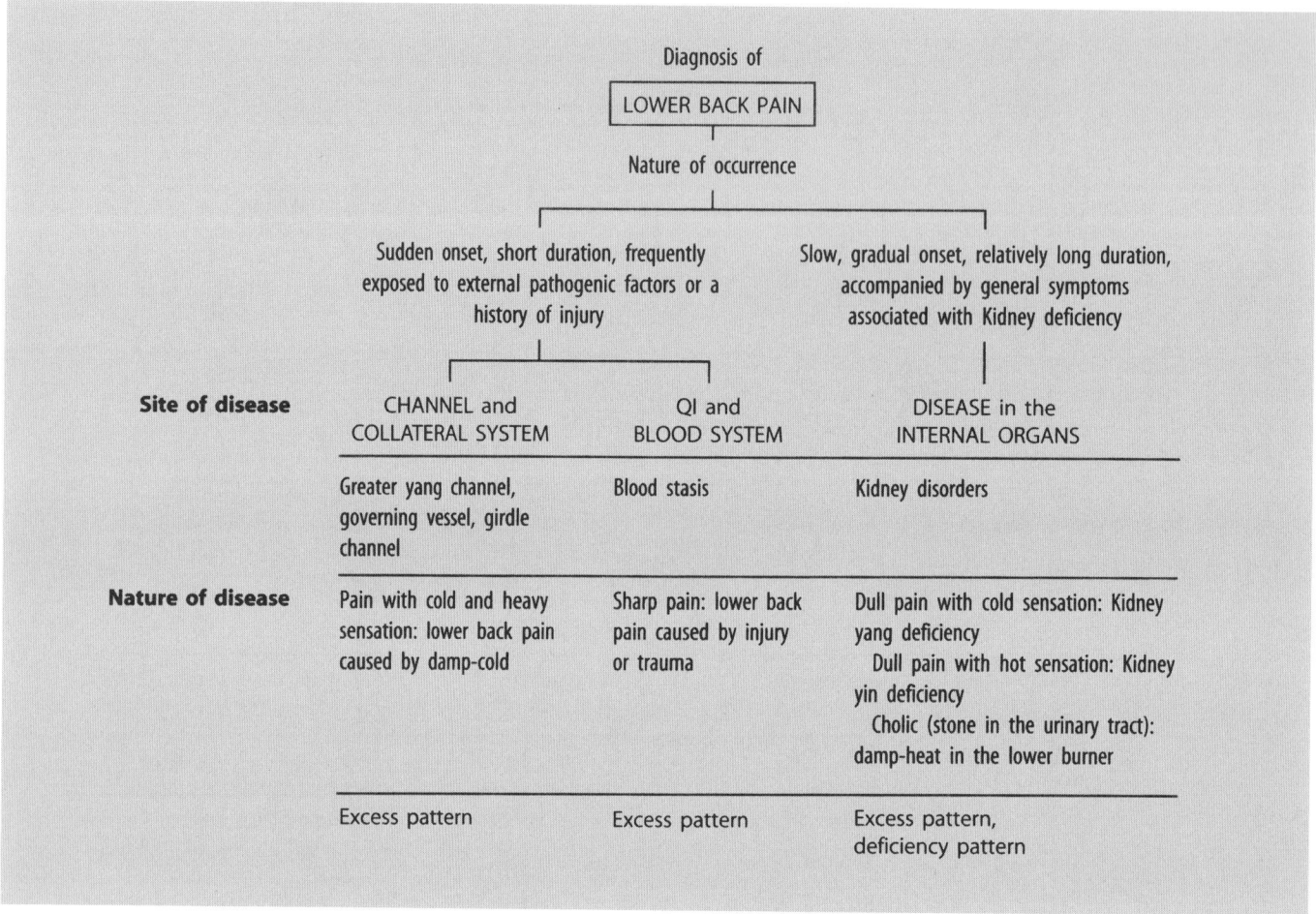

Diagnosis of

LOWER BACK PAIN

Nature of occurrence

Sudden onset, short duration, frequently exposed to external pathogenic factors or a history of injury

Slow, gradual onset, relatively long duration, accompanied by general symptoms associated with Kidney deficiency

	CHANNEL and COLLATERAL SYSTEM	QI and BLOOD SYSTEM	DISEASE in the INTERNAL ORGANS
Site of disease			
	Greater yang channel, governing vessel, girdle channel	Blood stasis	Kidney disorders
Nature of disease	Pain with cold and heavy sensation: lower back pain caused by damp-cold	Sharp pain: lower back pain caused by injury or trauma	Dull pain with cold sensation: Kidney yang deficiency
			Dull pain with hot sensation: Kidney yin deficiency
			Cholic (stone in the urinary tract): damp-heat in the lower burner
	Excess pattern	Excess pattern	Excess pattern, deficiency pattern

Fig. 8-15

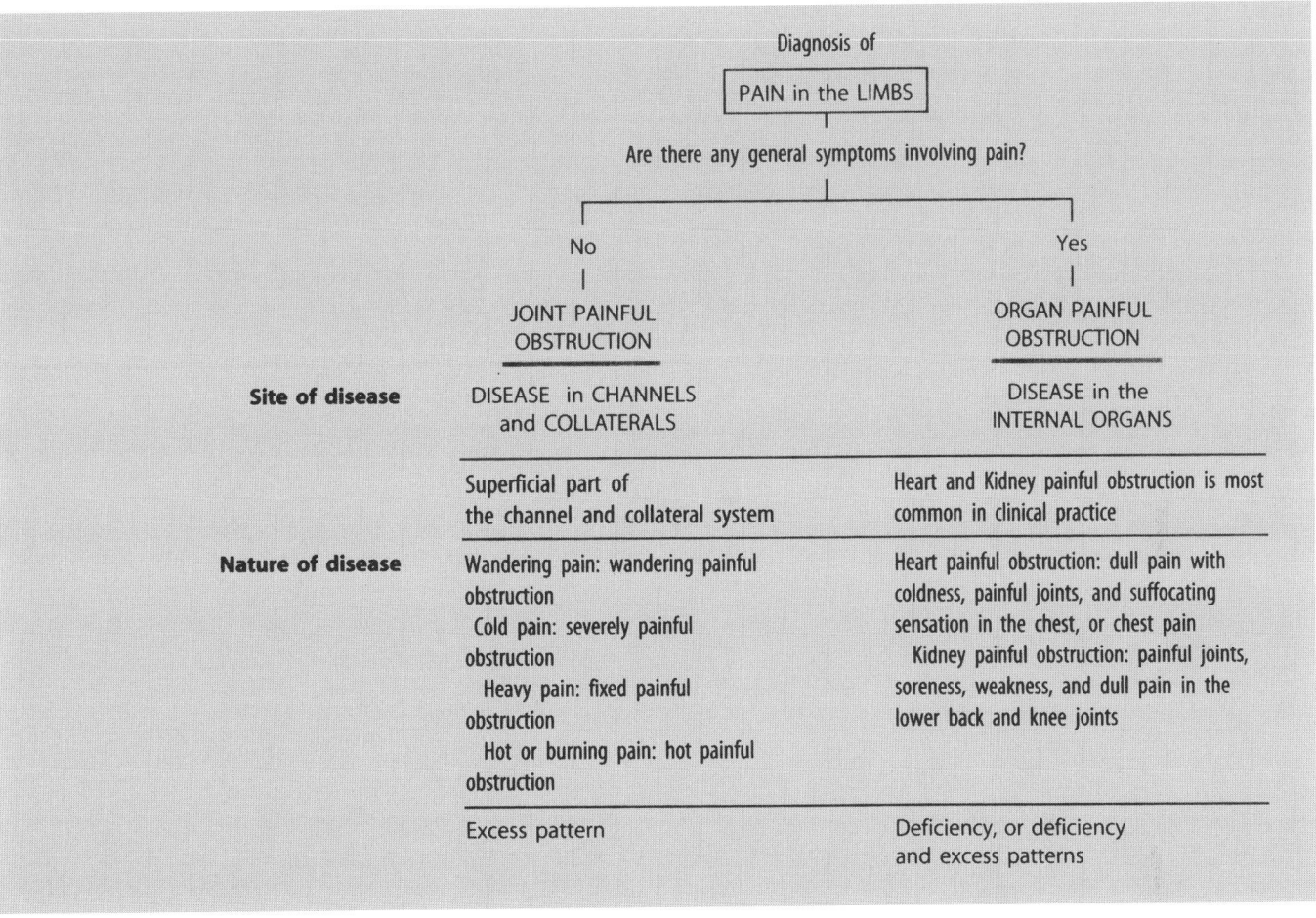

Diagnosis of

PAIN in the LIMBS

Are there any general symptoms involving pain?

	No	Yes
	JOINT PAINFUL OBSTRUCTION	ORGAN PAINFUL OBSTRUCTION
Site of disease	DISEASE in CHANNELS and COLLATERALS	DISEASE in the INTERNAL ORGANS
	Superficial part of the channel and collateral system	Heart and Kidney painful obstruction is most common in clinical practice
Nature of disease	Wandering pain: wandering painful obstruction Cold pain: severely painful obstruction Heavy pain: fixed painful obstruction Hot or burning pain: hot painful obstruction	Heart painful obstruction: dull pain with coldness, painful joints, and suffocating sensation in the chest, or chest pain Kidney painful obstruction: painful joints, soreness, weakness, and dull pain in the lower back and knee joints
	Excess pattern	Deficiency, or deficiency and excess patterns

Appendix

COOKING HERBS

The general principle for cooking Chinese herbal remedies is as follows. One uses a ceramic or pottery pot, but not a metal one, to avoid chemical reactions. The herbs are placed in the pot and cold water is added so that it just covers the herbs. The herbs are soaked in the water for about half an hour before cooking commences. After they have been cooked, the herbs are placed in a sieve, allowing the liquid to drain out. Care should be taken at this point to let the pot and herbs return to room temperature so that the pot does not crack when more cold water is added to the herbs, just covering them, as before. They are then boiled a second time. It should be possible to extract 250-300ml of liquid after each boiling, which means that 500-600ml of herbal soup should be available after both boilings. The two quantities of liquid are mixed together and then divided into two helpings for administration.

If there is excess liquid after boiling, the cooking time should be increased so that the resulting herbal soup is more concentrated. It is better not to throw away any excess soup.

Cooking time depends on the nature of the herbs. Leaves or herbaceous stems require only a very short time—usually just a few minutes, and generally not more than ten minutes. However, stems of xylophyto plants, subterranean stems, and roots of plants require a longer time—about 30 minutes or a little longer. Yet because the constituents of an herbal remedy are often a mixture of different parts of plants, along with minerals and insects, the actual cooking time is somewhat flexible. In such cases, the principal herbs usually dictate the cooking time.

Cooking time can also depend on the purpose of the prescription or formula. Generally speaking, the materia medica used for removing an external disorder, or promoting the dispersing function of the Lung, utilize a lot of leaves, and the cooking time is accordingly short; strong heat is also needed. The herbs should be boiled each time for about three to five minutes, following the procedure outlined above. Formulas used for tonification often utilize roots and stems of xylophyto plants and subterranean stems. The heat is thus turned down so that the mixture can continue to simmer for 30 minutes. As before, the herbs must be boiled twice.

Certain types of materia medica require special cooking methods. Instructions are usually provided with the prescription. The pharmacy will often wrap these materia medica separately and mark them with the relevant instructions for cooking.

The special cooking methods include the following:

1. *Post-cooking.* The active ingredients in some herbs are very easily broken down or volatilized after cooking for some time. These types of materia medica must be cooked for only a very short time relative to the other herbs, and are therefore added to the mixture at a later stage of the cooking process. Examples include Folium Perillae Fructescentis *(su ye)* and Herba Menthae Haplocalycis *(bo he)*. The other herbs in the formula are cooked first, and when done properly, the volatile herbs are added and boiled for only one to two minutes at the end.

2. *Pre-cooking.* The active ingredients in some materia medica require a long cooking time to be extracted; they should be pre-cooked. Examples include Gypsum *(shi gao)*, Talcum *(hua shi)*, Carapax Amydae Sinensis *(bie jia)*, and Concha Ostreae *(mu li)*, all of which should be placed in the pot first and pre-cooked for 20 to 30 minutes (depending on the particular substance) prior to introducing the other herbs.

   In addition, some highly toxic materia medica, like Radix Lateralis Aconiti Carmichaeli Praeparata *(fu zi)*, require a longer cooking time in order to reduce their level of toxicity.

3. *Using a gauze bag.* Some very fine materia medica, including powders, tiny seeds, or plants with a lot of "fur," are difficult to remove from the liquid, and so a sieve cannot be used to separate them. Examples include Semen Plantaginis *(che qian zi)*, Flos Inulae *(xuan fu hua)*, and Talcum *(hua shi)*. These types of herbs should be put into a gauze or loose cotton bag about 5x7cm in size. The bag should be tied at the top and placed in the pot along with the other herbs.

4. *Cooking separately.* Some materia medica, such as Radix Ginseng *(ren shen)*, need to be cooked separately and strained for the resultant liquid.

5. *Dissolving.* Some materia medica, such as powdered Succinum *(hu po fen)*, do not require cooking, as they are already in powdered form. Instead, they are to be mixed with water and drunk. Other materia medica, such as Gelatinum Corii Asini *(e jiao)* and Saccharum Granorum *(yi tang)*, should be added to the herbal soup just before drinking.

Select Bibliography

Anonymous. *Yellow Emperor's Inner Classic: Basic Questions (Huang di nei jing su wen)* 黄帝内经素问. Beijing: People's Health Publishing Company, 1956. [Originally written around 1st century B.C.]

Anonymous. *Yellow Emperor's Inner Classic: Vital Axis (Huang di nei jing ling shu)* 黄帝内经灵枢. Beijing: People's Health Publishing Company, 1956. [Originally written around 1st century B.C.]

Deng Tie-Tao. *Traditional Chinese Medical Diagnostics (Zhong yi zhen duan xue)* 中医诊断学. Shanghai: Shanghai Science & Technology Press, 1984.

Huang-Fu Mi. *Systematic Classic of Acupuncture and Moxibustion (Zhen jiu jia yi jing)* 针灸甲乙经. Beijing: People's Health Publishing Company, 1956. [Originally written in 3rd century A.D.]

Lei Feng. *Discussion of Seasonal Diseases (Shi bing lun)* 时病论. Beijing: People's Health Publishing Company, 1964. [Originally written in the Qing Dynasty.]

Li Ding. *Study of the Channels and Collaterals (Jing luo xue)* 经络学. Shanghai: Shanghai Science & Technology Press, 1984.

Li Shi-Zhen. *Grand Materia Medica (Ben cao gang mu)* 本草纲目. Beijing: People's Health Publishing Company, 1982. [Originally written in the Ming Dynasty.]

Meng Shu-Jiang. *Study of Febrile Diseases (Wen bing xue)* 温病学. Shanghai: Shanghai Science & Technology Press, 1985.

Sun Si-Miao. *Thousand Ducat Prescriptions for Emergencies (Bei ji qian jin yao fang)* 备急千金要方. Beijing: People's Health Publishing Company, 1955. [Originally written in the Tang Dynasty.]

Wang Xue-Tai. *Chinese Complete Collection of Acupuncture and Moxibustion (Zhong guo zhen jiu da quan)* 中国针灸大全. Henan: Henan Science & Technology Press, 1988.

Xi Yong-Jiang. *Study of Acupuncture and Moxibustion Techniques (Zhen fa jiu fa xue)* 针法灸法学. Shanghai: Shanghai Science & Technology Press, 1985.

Xu Ji-Qun, Wang Mian-Zhi. *Formulas for Chinese Materia Medica (Fang ji xue)* 方剂学. Shanghai: Shanghai Science & Technology Press, 1985.

Yan Zheng-Hua. *Chinese Materia Medica (Zhong yao xue)* 中药学. Beijing: People's Health Publishing Company, 1991.

Yang Chang-Sen. *Acupuncture and Moxibustion Therapeutics (Zhen jiu zhi liao xue)* 针灸治疗学. Shanghai: Shanghai Science & Technology Press, 1985.

Yang Ji-Zhou. *Great Compendium of Acupuncture and Moxibustion (Zhen jiu da cheng)* 针灸大成. Beijing: Peoples Health Publishing Company, 1955. [Originally published in 1602.]

Yang Jia-San. *Acupuncture and Moxibustion (Zhen jiu xue)* 针灸学. Beijing: People's Health Publishing Company, 1989.

Yang Jia-San. *Study of the Acupuncture Points (Shu xue xue)* 腧穴学. Shanghai: Shanghai Science & Technology Press, 1984.

Yin Hui-He. *Basic Theory of Traditional Chinese Medicine (Zhong yi ji chu li lun)* 中医基础理论. Shanghai: Shanghai Science & Technology Press, 1984.

Zhang Bo-Yu. *Internal Medicine in Traditional Chinese Medicine (Zhong yi nei ke xue)* 中医内科学. Shanghai: Shanghai Science & Technology Press, 1985.

Zhang Jing-Ze. *Differentiation and Diagnostic Methods for Patterns in Chinese Medicine (Zhong yi zheng hou jian bie zhen duan xue)* 中医证候鉴别诊断学. Beijing: People's Health Publishing Company, 1987.

Zhang Zhong-Jing. *Discussion of Cold-induced Disorders (Shang han lun)* 伤寒论. Edited by Li Pei-Sheng. Beijing: People's Health Publishing Company, 1987. [Originally written in 3rd century A.D.]

Zhang Zhong-Jing. *Essential Formulas from the Golden Cabinet (Jin gui yao lue fang lun)* 金匮要略方论. Beijing: People's Health Publishing Company, 1963. [Originally written in the Han Dynasty.]

Zhang Zong-Jing. *Essentials of the Golden Cabinet with Annotations (Jin gui yao lue quan jie)* 金匮要略诠解. Edited by Liu Du-zhou. Tianjin: Tianjin Science & Technology Press, 1984. [Originally written in 3rd century A.D.]

Journals   Beijing College of Chinese Medicine. *Journal of the Beijing College of Traditional Chinese Medicine (Beijing zhong yi xue yuan xue bao)* 北京中医学院学报.

China Academy of Chinese Medicine. *Chinese Acupuncture and Moxibustion (Zhong guo zhen jiu)* 中国针灸.

China Academy of Chinese Medicine. *Journal of Traditional Chinese Medicine (Zhong yi za zhi)* 中医杂志.

China Academy of Chinese Medicine. *Journal of the Guangzhou College of Traditional Chinese Medicine (Guangzhou zhong yi xue yuan xue bao)* 广州中医学院学报.

Shanghai Academy of Chinese Medicine. *Shanghai Journal of Acupuncture and Moxibustion (Shanghai zhen jiu za zhi)* 上海针灸杂志.

Shanghai College of Chinese Medicine. *Journal of the Shanghai College of Traditional Chinese Medicine (Shanghai zhong yi xue yuan xue bao)* 上海中医学院学报.

Tianjin College of Chinese Medicine. *Journal of the Tianjin College of Traditional Chinese Medicine (Tianjin zhong yi xue yuan xue bao)* 天津中医学院学报.

Points and
Herbal Formula Index

General Index

A Note on the Type

The text of this book is set in a digitized version of Times Roman, usually referred to as Times New Roman. In *The Elements of Typographic Style,* Robert Bringhurst describes this typeface as "an historical pastiche drawn by Victor Lardent for Stanley Morison in London in 1931. It has a humanist axis but Mannerist proportions, Baroque weight, and a sharp, Neoclassical finish."

Subheads are set in Myriad, a two-axis multiple master typeface designed by Robert Slimbach and Carol Twombly for Adobe Systems in 1992. It continues the tradition begun by Eric Gill in the late 1920s of applying the principles of the classic roman letter to sans serif types. Taking full advantage of its digital origin, variations of this humanistic type can be generated in any weight and/or width.

The pages of this book were set in Quark Xpress 3.32 for the Power Macintosh. Charts were imported from Aldus Intellidraw 2.0.